Praise for

OUTSIDE THE BOX

CANCER
THERAPIES

"Dr. Stengler and Dr. Anderson expertly provide clear, practical tools
that can possibly save your life or someone close to you. By harnessing the
healing power of nature, *Outside the Box Cancer Therapies*
gives the answers to beating cancer naturally."

— MICHAEL T. MURRAY, N.D.,
co-author of *The Encyclopedia of Natural Medicine*

"Doctors Stengler and Anderson are trusted names in the field of natural
medicine and integrative oncology. This book is an up-to-date resource
for the patient who is seeking to more studious and integrative in their
approach, utilizing the best of natural medicine, and integrating
those therapies into a whole system."

— TORI HUDSON, N.D.,
author of *Women's Encyclopedia of Natural Medicine*

"Cancer is something that touches everyone's lives, and without a doubt,
Dr. Stengler and Dr. Anderson have provided the best resource for beating it!
Outside the Box Cancer Therapies should be in everyone's health library
before the word 'cancer' stops you in your tracks."

— SUZY COHEN, R.Ph.,
syndicated columnist and best-selling author of *Thyroid Healthy,
Lose Weight, Look Beautiful and Live the Life You Imagine*

"The well-researched and referenced protocols will be a life raft to thousands of
people not yet privy to these out-of-the-box therapies. Thanks to their collective
work, I have had the privilege of applying most of the tools they have taught me
into clinical and consulting practice, and it has truly been a game changer for
the lives of many people otherwise given no hope."

— NASHA WINTERS, N.D.,
best-selling co-author of *The Metabolic Approach to Cancer*

OUTSIDE THE BOX

CANCER THERAPIES

OUTSIDE THE BOX
CANCER
THERAPIES

ALTERNATIVE THERAPIES THAT
TREAT AND PREVENT CANCER

DR. MARK STENGLER
& DR. PAUL ANDERSON

HAY HOUSE LLC
Carlsbad, California • New York City
London • Sydney • New Delhi

Library of Congress has cataloged the earlier edition as follows:

Names: Stengler, Mark, author.
Title: Outside the box cancer therapies : alternative therapies that treat and prevent cancer / Dr. Mark Stengler and Dr. Paul Anderson.
Description: 1st edition. | Carlsbad, California : Hay House, Inc., 2018. |
   Includes bibliographical references and index.
Identifiers: LCCN 2017060610 | ISBN 9781401954581 (hardcover : alk. paper)
Subjects: LCSH: Cancer--Alternative treatment--Popular works. |
   Cancer--Adjuvant treatment--Popular works.
Classification: LCC RC271.A62 S74 2018 | DDC 616.99/406--dc23 LC record available at https://lccn.loc.gov/2017060610

Tradepaper ISBN: 978-1-4019-5460-4
E-book ISBN: 978-1-4019-5459-8

12 11 10 9 8 7 6 5 4 3
1st edition, April 2018
2nd edition, May 2019

Printed in the United States of America

This product uses responsibly sourced papers and/or recycled materials. For more information, see www.hayhouse.com.

To our patients with cancer and their supportive loved ones
that we have had the joy of helping throughout the years.
Also, to all the holistic practitioners and doctors
who have provided integrative and holistic care
for their patients, even when it was considered to be
"outside the box."

CONTENTS

FOREWORD

Following my fellowship as a conventional oncologist at the University of California, San Francisco, in the early '70s, I had the privilege of being a U.S. Army resident trained in Anatomic and Clinical Pathology. After duty in Vietnam, I completed an Internal Medicine residency before entering my oncology fellowship.

From the early '70s until the mid '90s, I practiced only conventional oncology, which today I realize was only an enlightened "guessing game." Many of my patients who had Homeopathic and Naturopathic Therapies were alive longer with higher qualities of life than my conventionally-treated patients. This brought me to the conclusion that I needed to become board certified in Homeopathy in order to practice Integrative Oncology. Thanks to Dr. Paul Anderson and Dr. Mark Stengler's work, I am using combinations of IV vitamin C with artesunate, vitamin C with curcumin, and Poly-MVA with DCA.

As an Integrative Oncologist, board-certified in both Medical Oncology and Homeopathy in Nevada for over 18 years, I have carried out 4 separate outcome-based studies using Poly-MVA, Paw-Paw, and IPT. My latest study began in June 2010 and has continued for over seven and a half years, involving over 1,250 patients who thus far have a survival rate of 70 percent.

I now tell my patients if I am giving them the "wrong" drugs, I am hurting them by damaging their immune system and debilitating numerous other organ systems—everything from Chemo-Brain to Cytopenias to damage to the heart, liver, and kidneys.

In *Outside the Box Cancer Therapies,* Dr. Anderson and Dr. Stengler deliver an "out-of-the-box" epiphany of integrative oncology approaches to treat cancer using the best of both alternative and conventional therapies without succumbing to the one-size-fits-all recipe of surgery, radiation, and chemotherapy, otherwise known as "Cut, Burn, and Poison," from Big Pharma and the conventional establishment.

This well-organized book serves as a complete reference for those who are seeking information about cancer treatment or are treatment providers. I am convinced that if conventional oncology does not adapt Dr. Stengler and Dr. Anderson's protocols and protocols similar to mine, cancer will continue to cause the deaths of over 40 percent of all Americans.

I am honored to write a foreword for this enlightening and lifesaving manuscript.

James W. Forsythe, M.D., H.M.D.
Oncologist and author of *The Forsythe Anti-Cancer Diet*

INTRODUCTION

No matter who you are, the word *cancer* has a way of instantly grabbing your attention. Very few of us escape having it touch our lives in some way. If you haven't done battle with this dreaded disease yourself, you no doubt know someone who has.

The statistics are sobering. Even with the most technologically advanced medical system in the world, consider these statistics about the United States:

- Approximately 40 percent of men and women will be diagnosed with cancer at some point during their lifetime.[1]

- An estimated 1.685 million new cancer cases will have been diagnosed in 2016.[2]

- Cancer will kill 595,690 people in the United States each year or 1,630 people per day.[3]

- Cancer accounts for nearly 25 percent of all deaths.[4]

- Nearly 14.5 million people with a history of cancer were alive on January 1, 2014.[5]

- More than a third of people with cancer reported being "seriously or very seriously" concerned about bankruptcy because of medical bills.[6]

But in the midst of all this bad news, there *is* a bright light! According to the American Cancer Society, "a substantial proportion of cancers could be prevented."[7] In other words, doctors who are trained in nutrition, lifestyle modification, stress management, detoxification, hormone balancing, and immune regulation have a unique opportunity to slash the chances of their patients ever receiving a devastating cancer diagnosis. And if you're already battling cancer, cutting-edge holistic therapies can help you win that fight and then provide you the support you need to keep it from ever coming back.

While conventional cancer therapy has its place, it also has its limits. Those limits, and the fear of severe side effects, send a lot of folks looking for ways to incorporate complementary and alternative care into their cancer treatment programs. In fact, according to the National Health Interview Survey, 65 percent of survey responders who had been diagnosed with cancer had used complementary medicine.[8]

One of the frustrations we hear from a very high percentage of our patients with cancer is that their oncologists and conventional doctors are unfamiliar with nutritional and holistic therapies to prevent, treat, and reduce recurrence of cancer. While some oncologists are frustrated that their training never included complementary and alternative therapies, resulting in learning "outside the box" from nonconventional sources, many conventional doctors seem disinterested in the use of holistic therapies no matter the evidence demonstrating its effectiveness and the patients' demands.

Case in point, a study published in the mainstream *Journal of Clinical Oncology* looked at the use of complementary and alternative medicine (CAM) in Mayo Clinic patients with advanced cancer. They found that 88.2 percent had used at least one modality of CAM. The most commonly used therapy was vitamin and mineral preparations.[9] Other research has shown that "between 54 percent and 77 percent of cancer patients receiving conventional therapy use CAMs,"[10] and "up to 72 percent do not inform their treating physician."[11]

That's where we come in. With our extensive combined experience in the clinical use of natural and integrative medicine and integrative cancer research, we have a lot of experience helping people with cancer reduce all too common side effects from chemotherapy, radiation, and surgery. Research-backed therapies we share in *Outside the Box Cancer Therapies* have been proven to effectively reduce many of the sickening side effects of conventional cancer therapies. In fact, many of the protocols we outline have even been shown to extend life span and quality of life compared to exclusive conventional care.[12]

As naturopathic medical doctors, we have unique training in both conventional and holistic medicine.

We are active in both clinical practice and research. This means we help patients fight and prevent cancer on a regular basis. Between the two of us, we have combined more than 40 years of clinical experience.

Due to the demand for this type of medicine and the results we have been able to produce, our clinics have been overflowing with patients. Dr. Stengler practices in Encinitas, California, and Dr. Anderson's clinic is in Seattle, Washington, and his hospital affiliation is in Rosarito, Mexico. We both take research very seriously, and we constantly review numerous medical resources for cutting-edge ways to help prevent and treat cancer.

Dr. Stengler routinely provides this cutting-edge information to hundreds of thousands of people through his newsletter publications, television shows, and best-selling books, and he was recently rated as one of the top 50 functional and integrative medical doctors in the United States.

Dr. Anderson is a highly regarded lecturer and consultant to the ever-growing field of Integrative Medicine. He is a frequently sought after speaker at medical conventions where he updates physicians on the best therapies and research for integrative oncology. Dr. Anderson has also been actively involved in studies that *prove* the effectiveness of alternative and holistic cancer therapies. Due to his affiliation with hospitals and researchers in other countries, he has been able to collaborate on, learn from, and implement clinical therapies for patients that could not be done in the U.S. This has greatly sped up the learning curve for many integrative oncology therapies he is able to teach and write about, as well as integrate into clinical practice.

We both have a passion for helping people using safe and effective therapies for cancer and other health problems. We regard people as very valuable and strive to treat everyone with dignity. All too often patients complain that the medical system treats them like a "number." We understand that those in the medical system typically have the best of intentions in their work, but we also see that the system has become so standardized that a great deal of personalized care is lost. A large portion of the passion we have is to bring back individualized personal care. This includes meeting each person where they are with their state of health and personal feelings, beliefs, and ideas about their care and working with them in a team effort to bring them the best of all appropriate healing methods.

We consider it critically important to provide you, the reader, with the best that integrative oncology has to offer. Our observation is that only bits and pieces of credible integrative oncology information are available. We have resolved that problem by putting it into one resource.

Outside the Box Cancer Therapies is a comprehensive guidebook designed to help patients and their doctors navigate the most effective nutritional and holistic cancer therapies available today. Conventional medical specialties such as oncology are highly technical and specific in their training and with the therapies that are used. In the modern system, no physician can know everything, but in the world of cancer and integrative care, often the feeling "if I didn't learn it in my residency, it must not be a good therapy" prevails. This can encompass simple things such as nutritional therapies or more complex ones such as the large world of integrative oncology. We aim to provide you and your doctors with the details you need to begin using these lifesaving protocols starting today.

We use the phrase integrative oncology for our approach, which is designed to take into account all available resources—conventional and holistic—to help prevent cancer and treat the disease when it does strike. We recognize people are individuals and every case is different. Sometimes conventional care needs to be prioritized. However, in almost every case, one or more holistic therapies can be used to augment that conventional care in order to reduce your side effects and optimize your chance of survival.

Let's look at the case of a woman with metastatic breast cancer. Her conventional care might include chemotherapy, surgery, radiation, and antiestrogen medication. But during treatment, she could benefit from additional holistic therapy such as dietary changes, nutritional supplements, detoxification support, and intravenous nutrient therapy such as cancer-fighting high-dose vitamin C to help ease some of her worst symptoms and side effects such as nausea, fatigue, anxiety, or insomnia. Once she has finished conventional treatment, integrative oncology and naturopathic approaches could be used to reduce her risk of recurrence. This would include focusing on diet and lifestyle choices and possibly using genetic-specific nutritional recommendations (known as "nutrigenomic therapy"). You'll find several cases throughout the book demonstrating how integrative oncology works in the real world.

The field of holistic medicine is quite vast, which can be intimidating to lay-people and doctors alike. But as licensed naturopathic medical doctors, we already use the holistic therapies that are a part of integrative oncology in our own practices. By combining our extensive research into these methods with our own clinical experiences, we will be your guide to using these techniques and therapies to help you in your own fight against this killer disease.

Integrative oncology always puts you, the person with cancer, and your family and support network first. All-or-none approaches to holistic or conventional treatments harm the patient. When your doctor disregards effective approaches, no matter where they come from, he's not doing what's best for you. Balance between the two systems is the key to beating your cancer. We strive to provide that balance here in *Outside the Box Cancer Therapies.*

HOW TO USE THIS BOOK

Outside the Box Cancer Therapies is designed to be easy to use. That means you don't have to spend a lot of time wading through material to figure out how to use it in your own case. We provide very specific protocols and dosages that you can share with your doctor so that you can begin to use them immediately to help you heal. We believe in good science and have included the references for any studies we cite so doctors can look them up for themselves to see the solid research behind the protocols.

As you read through the book, you will not only gain a better understanding of how integrative oncology works, but also a better understanding of cancer itself. There aren't any one-shot wonder cures here. Instead we champion a rich and varied approach, drawing on the best medicine has to offer for the best outcomes imaginable.

There are many factors involved in the development of cancer, and there are equally as many ways to attack the disease and enable your own body to resist it. We urge you to start using proactive approaches such as diet, exercise, and stress reduction immediately. And we encourage you to read up on the specific cancer you are trying to tackle to help you develop a personalized action plan that will give you the greatest chance of surviving and thriving. Being diagnosed with cancer can be frightening, overwhelming, depressing, or a multitude of other emotions. Our decades of experience working with patients who have cancer will help you demystify the process, become empowered and educated, and bring all that integrative oncology has to offer to your journey with cancer.

CHAPTER 1

REAL HOPE WITH
INTEGRATIVE ONCOLOGY

We congratulate you on stepping outside of your comfort zone and being open to cancer therapies that stray from the small and limited box of conventional medicine. This integrative approach to cancer has become increasingly popular and is now being used by millions around the country.

There is a revolution occurring in medicine with a plethora of studies validating naturopathic and holistic therapies. In this chapter, we take a look at real world cases of people we've treated for cancer.

We have always taken the position that patients should be treated like family members, which is why throughout the book you will find that we use the terms *patient* and *person (people)* interchangeably. The term *person* denotes that we value the human beings we are talking about and do not just see them as people with cancer. On the other hand, the term *patient* signifies that one does have a serious condition—cancer—and requires the utmost in medical care. We avoid just using the term *cancer patients,* because we're focused on treating *people* and not just the disease.

CASE HISTORY: ABDOMINAL CANCER

The first case we're going to look at is that of a lovely 84-year-old woman who was diagnosed with metastatic abdominal cancer. For confidentiality purposes, we will call her Rose.

The cancer had wrapped itself around many of the organs in Rose's abdomen. It was discovered when she went in for what was supposed to be a routine gall bladder surgery. Rose's surgeon delivered the devastating news when she woke up: it wasn't her gall bladder that was the problem but rather a serious case of cancer.

Rose's oncologist soon delivered more bad news: there wasn't any safe chemotherapy for her, and further surgery wasn't likely to be of any help either. Her primary care doctor advised Rose that it would be best to get her affairs in order because she wouldn't likely see her 85th birthday.

But Rose was no pushover. She wasn't at all happy about being told to go home and to wait to die. She had been quite healthy all of her 84 years and was still driving her own car and living independently. Like many folks diagnosed with cancer, she began to search for alternative therapies. This is how she came to meet Dr. Anderson and his team in the Seattle area.

At her first office visit, Dr. Anderson was delighted to learn that Rose was unwilling to simply sit and wait for the cancer to take her life. She clearly had a lot more living to do, and he intended to do his best to help her do just that. He reassured Rose that the advice she was given to avoid chemotherapy or surgery was sound. Dr. Anderson agreed with her oncologist that Rose should avoid more surgery or chemotherapy. With her type of cancer and her advanced age, she wasn't likely to survive them. Instead, he began to prepare a personalized plan of care that took into account Rose's individual needs.

Dr. Anderson began by looking at her complete health history, including any past diseases she had and her overall general health. Besides the cancer and Parkinson's disease, which only gave her a mild tremor, Rose was remarkably healthy. She grew much of her food, ate healthily, got lots of exercise, and didn't smoke or drink alcohol.

Her main complaints since her diagnosis were fatigue and increasing digestive complaints. As Dr. Anderson explained to Rose, active cancer depletes nutrients, leading to fatigue. And the cancer was compressing her digestive organs, creating her digestive upset and inability to eat very much.

Once he had gone through her entire history, performed a physical exam, ordered laboratory testing to assure the safety of future therapies, and ordered images of her tumors, Dr. Anderson moved forward with his plan. His job was to work with Rose's own healing capacity to slow or stop the cancer and provide her with the best possible quality of life.

Rose's individualized treatment plan began with encouraging her to continue her already excellent diet. But Rose's progressive fatigue was a significant issue. So she incorporated movement and gentle exercise to fight fatigue and stimulate her immunities. And she was immediately started on twice-weekly rounds of high-dose intravenous vitamin C therapy (HDIVC) for six weeks before being reassessed.

Dr. Anderson and his staff monitored Rose as she progressed through her treatment and altered any therapies or interventions as required. Her first office visit included a test dose of the HDIVC formula.

After the first week of treatment, Rose felt an increase in her energy levels. By week three she said, "Maybe I'm making this up, but I can eat without pain now and can eat more than before." By the fifth week, Rose reported that her digestion problems had gone away. She could eat as much as she wanted, and her energy had improved enough to garden again. (In fact, she felt so good she overdid the gardening one day and pulled some muscles.) By the sixth week, her energy had skyrocketed, and she was entirely free of any abdominal symptoms.

At that point, Dr. Anderson decreased her HDIVC to once a week for the next eight weeks. At week 10 he ordered an abdominal ultrasound to compare with the original imaging to see if the tumor size had decreased. The imaging revealed that there was still plenty of cancer in her abdomen. But despite its presence, Rose continued to feel full of energy, and her digestion issues stayed away.

At week 14 Dr. Anderson was out of town, and a colleague met with Rose for a follow-up visit. Because Rose was doing so well, Dr. Anderson's colleague had Rose stop treatment for a while. Within three weeks she was back in the office fatigued and barely able to eat.

Dr. Anderson restarted her on two HDIVC treatments a week for three weeks. Her energy bounced back, and once again her digestion problems disappeared. Dr. Anderson tapered the treatment down to once a week for 12 weeks, and Rose remained stable. He then began a "withdrawal trial," slowly decreasing the frequency of her therapy over time. She was placed on a maintenance schedule of one HDIVC treatment every four to six weeks.

During this time, Rose celebrated her 85th birthday by calling up the doctor who had told her she wouldn't see that day and let him know she was still alive. Five years later she celebrated her 90th birthday at Dr. Anderson's clinic!

Rose is still alive and symptom-free as of the writing of this book and has celebrated her 92nd birthday. Dr. Anderson spoke to her recently, and she was healthy, active, happy, and free of all abdominal discomfort.

CASE HISTORY: ESOPHAGEAL CANCER

"Barry," was a 68-year-old man who came to see Dr. Stengler complaining of a hoarse voice that hadn't improved for months. He was an avid traveler who had visited many countries. He had consulted with an ear, nose, and throat specialist (ENT) who had diagnosed him with postnasal drip (mucus dripping from his sinuses down his throat).

Based on the specialist's diagnosis, Dr. Stengler initially prescribed specific nutritional supplements and a special diet that typically resolves postnasal drip. After adjusting the treatment a few times in reaction to changing symptoms, Dr. Stengler began to suspect something else was going on. He referred Barry to a different ENT specialist, where testing revealed Barry had esophageal cancer.

Barry's cancer was caused by the human papilloma virus (HPV). He was given a series of radiation treatments as well as chemotherapy. During his conventional cancer treatment, Dr. Stengler recommended nutritional supplements to support Barry's immune system and aid with detoxification. Barry also started on HDIVC and IV ozone (we'll have more on IV ozone later in the book).

At first Barry was doing well, but after several radiation treatments, his throat became extremely sore, making it very difficult to swallow food and to speak clearly. The skin on his neck became extremely red and ulcerated. When Dr. Stengler asked Barry if the oncologist had explained to him how severe the side effects would be, Barry revealed he hadn't been prepared.

When Barry followed up with his oncologist, he was assured that his response was normal. Over time Barry lost 25 pounds and became extremely weak. Dr. Stengler changed his complementary treatment plan to include daily IV therapy with a host of nutrients, as well as intravenous fats. Barry was switched to eating a meal replacement shake throughout the day instead of solid food since he was having difficulty swallowing. In addition, Dr. Stengler added a drink containing glutamine, aloe vera extract, and licorice extract to help heal the ulcerations in his throat.

The holistic therapies soon helped to stabilize Barry's weight and energy levels and kept him from needing a surgically implanted feeding tube inserted into his abdomen. Barry's oncologist didn't have any solutions to help him deal with the severe side effects of radiation and chemotherapy, so he was grateful Dr. Stengler was able to use integrative oncology to help him recover.

These days Barry is doing well and is back to his old self. He receives a monthly IV treatment of ozone and intravenous vitamin C for cancer prevention. Barry reports he plans on having a steak and seafood dinner with Dr. Stengler in the future to celebrate his recovery.

CASE HISTORY: CHILDHOOD LEUKEMIA

Integrative oncology is also used with children. Dr. Anderson was sought out by the parents of a girl who was only four years old. "Sarah" had a rare type of childhood leukemia, the result of a genetic condition that had been diagnosed when she was 11 weeks old.

Sarah had already gone through a bone marrow transplant donated by her brother, who was a marrow "type match." She was also receiving holistic support with diet, lifestyle, and natural medical therapies. Sarah been in remission for most of her young life, but unfortunately, she had recently fallen out of remission.

Sarah's labs showed that her cancer was advancing. The family was told by her oncologists that Sarah's only hope for achieving remission was to attempt another transplant. The problem was that they had no treatment available to help her get into remission. Dr. Anderson recommended an integrative approach to try to put Sarah back into remission and prepare her for the new transplant. Her treatments would include a special diet, supplements, and IV therapies; and she would be monitored through lab testing.

Initially Dr. Anderson tried pediatric dosages of HDIVC. But unfortunately the HDIVC alone didn't work; Sarah's blood work showed the cancer continued to grow. An herbal extract of the artemisia plant—sometimes called wormwood—known as artesunate was then added to her IV treatment. This plant has been used as a malaria medicine in many parts of the world, and Dr. Anderson helped pioneer its use in treating breast cancer and other cancers. Sadly, the combination of IV artesunate and HDIVC still wasn't working. Sarah's blood work showed her cancer was still progressing.

Desperately wanting to help Sarah, Dr. Anderson spoke with her parents about an early stage experimental metabolic therapy that would combine two potential cancer-fighting agents and target a weak point in the cancer cells' abnormal metabolism. He had safely used the therapy to treat an adult with a cancer of the lymphatic system (lymphoma) before.

Sarah's family had an incredibly difficult decision to make. The combo therapy had never been used in a child before, and it had never been used to treat a leukemia. But with no other options available from the world of conventional oncology and time running out, Sarah's parents decided to move ahead with the innovative therapy.

The stakes were, needless to say, very high. Dr. Anderson had to balance his desire to help this little girl get better with his knowledge that the therapy he was proposing, while scientifically plausible, might not actually work. And if the treatment didn't work, Sarah would likely die.

The first lab tests after the therapy was started contained a ray of hope. The cancer wasn't getting better, but for the first time it hadn't gotten worse. The second set of results showed a drop in the number of "bad" cells. And incredibly, the third set of tests revealed the cells were completely gone!

Dr. Anderson continued the therapy for several more weeks to be on the safe side. Then Sarah's brother once again donated cells, and she underwent the transplant. It was a success, and she was discharged from the hospital.

Sarah continued receiving care from Dr. Anderson, which kept her stable and in remission for quite some time. Although her bone marrow biopsies continued to show some minor remnants of leukemia cells, she was able to enjoy a relatively normal life, spending most of her time at home with her family.

Given the type of cancer, it was a long remission. But tragically, three years later, Sarah's leukemia became active again. Although Dr. Anderson tried several treatments, with varying degrees of success, ultimately Sarah passed away, dying not from the cancer directly but from infections she had acquired.

Sarah's parents were grateful for the extra time they had with their daughter, and thankful that during her remission she had been able to enjoy her life to the fullest. Sarah's quality of life had been every bit as important as the quantity of it.

CASE HISTORY: PROSTATE CANCER

"John," a vibrant 70-year-old farmer, was diagnosed with prostate cancer that had spread to his spine and pelvis. Although John told his oncologists he wasn't interested in chemotherapy, he did have a goal. He was determined to see his grandson, who was only nine years old at the time, graduate from high school.

Although Dr. Stengler couldn't make any promises, and there were limitations to what treatments could be started since John lived more than five hours away, he put the farmer on an aggressive holistic program and anticancer diet right away. Because of John's years of pesticide exposure on the farm, he was given a detoxification program to follow for many months. And he began taking specific research-backed herbal extracts to supercharge his overwhelmed immune system and attack the cancer.

The results were stunning. Scans six months later showed a significant decrease in John's tumors, and he reported that he felt perfectly healthy again. Two years later, Dr. Stengler got a call from John. He wanted Dr. Stengler to know he was still feeling great. He said even his doctors were shocked by how well he continued to do despite still having cancer. John continued to follow Dr. Stengler's recommended protocols, and amazingly he was able to attend his grandson's high school graduation!

CASE HISTORY: CHEMO BRAIN AND FATIGUE

"Dawn" was 66 years old and had been vital and active her whole life until being treated for breast cancer that had spread to her lymph nodes. She came to see Dr. Stengler after she had a mastectomy and had been through a series of chemotherapy treatments that wiped her out physically, mentally, and emotionally.

The chemo was administered as a preventative measure in case any cancer cells were still floating around in her blood stream after her surgery. After the second treatment, Dawn lost her hair and became weak. By the time she finished her fourth treatment, she was barely able to function. Her bones and joints ached, she was nauseated all the time, her memory and focus were greatly impaired, and she had severe fatigue.

By the time she met with Dr. Stengler, she was literally in tears and said she regretted her decision to undergo chemotherapy. It had been a month since her last treatment, and she hadn't begun to recover from the side effects of the treatment. Dr. Stengler comforted Dawn and assured her there were natural approaches they could use that could help reverse her side effects.

Since she had flown to Dr. Stengler's clinic, Dawn only had a week to be treated. Dr. Stengler immediately started daily intravenous treatments of nutrients—including glutathione, B vitamins, vitamin C, minerals, and magnesium—to restore energy production in her cells and detoxify her body from the waste products left behind from the chemotherapy. He also prescribed oral supplements to encourage liver and kidney detoxification, as well as healthy fats to support brain and nervous system health.

Dawn noticed a significant improvement after her second intravenous treatment. By the fifth day of treatment, she was downright astounded by the progress she had made. And by the last day of treatment, she reported an incredible 85 percent improvement in her overall symptoms.

During a phone call two weeks later, she told Dr. Stengler that her family and friends kept telling her what a dramatic difference they could see in her mood and energy levels. She was no longer suffering from severe "chemo brain," and her bones and joints no longer ached. Dawn was able to resume her demanding schedule with energy to spare.

THE TAKEAWAY

These are just a few of the hundreds of successful cases we've been involved in. You will find many more case histories throughout this book that demonstrate the important role integrative oncology can play in anyone's fight against cancer, yours included. *Outside the Box Cancer Therapies* will take an in-depth look at some of the most exciting, cutting edge holistic and alternative cancer therapies available, including step-by-step instructions and the resources you need to start using them in your own life right away.

CHAPTER 2

ROOT CAUSES
OF CANCER

C ancer is a complex disease with many known causes. Cancer harms the body when altered cells divide uncontrollably to form masses of tissue called tumors (except in the case of leukemia, where cancer prohibits normal blood function by abnormal cell division in the bloodstream). Tumors can grow and interfere with the digestive, nervous, and circulatory systems, and they can release hormones that alter body function.

The causes of cancer have been the topic of great discussion, discovery, and debate for a century now. This chapter provides an overview of the updated ideas that have the most scientific validity as well as their relationship to the success of the types of therapies we describe in this book.

Homeostasis is the ability of the body system or cell to return to its normal healthy state after being challenged. Disruption of homeostasis typically occurs at the beginning of cells becoming cancerous. The immune system (and even cells themselves) are supposed to stop abnormal cells from replicating, which is why we do not all develop cancer. If that immune process does not complete that mission, however, an abnormal cell (not experiencing homeostasis) can then replicate and create other cancer cells.

After this rudimentary "birth" of cancer, there are two primary considerations in the beginning of cancer and during its promotion and growth: the factors affecting the ability to return to homeostasis and the triggers that fuel cancer growth and evasion of the immune system.

Before we outline these two crucial areas, let's examine the modern scientific hallmarks of cancer as agreed upon by the oncology community:

> The hallmarks of cancer comprise eight biologic capabilities acquired by incipient cancer cells during the multistep development of human tumors. The hallmarks constitute an organizing principle for rationalizing the complexities of neoplastic disease. They include sustaining proliferative signaling, evading growth suppressors, resisting cell death, enabling replicative immortality, inducing angiogenesis, activating invasion and metastasis, reprogramming energy metabolism, and evading immune destruction. Facilitating the acquisition of these hallmark capabilities are genome instability, which enables mutational alteration of hallmark-enabling genes, and immune inflammation, which fosters the acquisition of multiple hallmark functions. In addition to cancer cells, tumors exhibit another dimension of complexity: They contain a repertoire of recruited, ostensibly normal cells that contribute to the acquisition of hallmark traits by creating the tumor microenvironment.[1]

While potentially missing some subtle hallmarks of cancer, this definition outlines the many ways in which cancer needs to be addressed in its prevention and treatment. For the purposes of this book, we will summarize the main areas of carcinogenesis by dividing them into the main theories of cancer initiation as well as the main triggers and fuel and resistance factors, all of which relate to the hallmarks just discussed.

CANCER INITIATION

Once we have a situation where the immune system and your own cells' internal machinery have failed to stop a cancer cell from existing, there are multiple theories regarding why that cancer cell stays alive and replicates.

The three major theories regarding the initiation of cancer growth involve genetics (the genome), cell design / mechanics (the cytome), and metabolism (the metabolome). In reality they all occur to one degree or another and, if closely studied, can even affect one another. As we describe the three major theories of cancer, we want to point out that when multiple theories exist, it normally means they all have merit and that there is truth in all. They just happen to be looking at the problem (or question) from differing vantage points.

THEORY ONE:
THE GENETIC THEORY

Cancer genes are broadly grouped into "oncogenes" and "tumor suppressor" genes. There are other classes of genes in this area, but these best describe the theory. Think of an oncogene as the gas pedal on your car, where a mutation in an oncogene would be like a continuously pressed accelerator.[2] A non-mutated suppressor gene acts as the brake that inhibits tumor growth. This genomic theory has been the prevailing theory and focus of research for the past five decades. It has shown to be a target of some therapies that are genetically based, but those do not always work. In recent years the understanding of the human genome has not led to as many cancer "cures" as originally thought. It will continue to be an ever-expanding area of research and hopefully treatment development, but the important thing to consider for now is the control of those things that cause or fuel cancer via genomic means (carcinogens) and either avoiding them or mitigating them.

THEORY TWO:
THE CANCER STEM CELL / TROPHOBLASTIC THEORY

The older trophoblastic theory proposed by the British embryologist and histologist Dr. John Beard is in many ways a precursor to the modern "cancer stem cell" theory. The trophoblastic theory of cancer states that trophoblastic cells, which are involved in the formation of the placenta, may receive a signal that causes them to become cancerous.[3] The cancer stem cell theory proposes that "among all cancerous cells, a few act as stem cells that reproduce themselves and sustain the cancer, much like normal stem cells normally renew and sustain our organs and tissues. In this view, cancer cells that are not stem cells can cause problems, but they cannot sustain an attack on our bodies over the long term. . . . The theory, therefore, is that cancer stem cells arise out of normal stem cells or the precursor cells that normal stem cells produce."[4]

Why would one theory differ from the other if they are similar? The reason really is changes in science and technology over time allowing for better explanations and mechanistic descriptions. The trophoblastic theory began in the 1920s, and the cancer stem cell theory many decades later. But if it seems the trophoblastic idea has died out in the scientific literature, one can find publications as recent as 2008[5] and 2015.[6]

A 2008 paper by A. R. Burleigh outlines not only the trophoblastic theory but also the connection it has to the more modern cancer stem cell theory. The Burleigh paper made the connection between these theories, which are really over a half century apart:

> The trophoblastic theory of cancer, proposed in the early 1900s by Dr John Beard, may not initially seem relevant to current cancer models and treatments. However, the underpinnings of this theory are remarkably similar to those of the cancer stem cell (CSC) theory. Beard noticed that a significant fraction of germ cells never reach their final destination as they migrate during embryonic development from the hindgut to the germinal ridge. In certain situations, upon aberrant stimulation, these vagrant germ cells are able to generate tumors. Simplistically, the CSC theory surmises that a small population of tumorigenic cells exists, which initiate and maintain tumors, and these cells have a likely origin in normal stem cells. Both these theories are based on the potential of a single primitive cell to form a tumor. This has a major implication for cancer therapy, in that only a small percentage of cells need to be targeted to ablate a tumor.[7]

Recent publications have validated this theory's mechanisms, science, and potential for therapy.[8]

THEORY THREE:
THE METABOLIC THEORY

For the past 50 years, cancer researchers have focused on targeting the genetic mutations of cancer. In the 1920s, the Nobel Prize winner, Dr. Otto Warburg proposed that cancer was essentially a disease of deranged cell metabolism.[9] This inspired the idea of cancer as a metabolic disease, or the "metabolic theory" of cancer.

As with all things, as science progresses, the technology allows deeper insights into these theories and the mechanisms they are built upon. One of many such revelations is that the energy-producing parts of the cell (the mitochondria) are essentially damaged in cancer, which helps drive a different metabolism in a cancer cell versus a normal healthy cell. And while we can now "see" the changes and differences between healthy and cancerous cells, we can also see that what Warburg described is essentially still true.[10]

Is there a crossover in the genomic theory of cancer and the metabolic theory? To simplify this very deep discussion (which is the topic of many oncology books and some excellent reviews[11]), we will summarize the crossover. First, the fidelity of the nuclear genome (genetic material allowing an organism to develop and grow) is tightly linked to mitochondrial function, so if the mitochondria "go bad," they naturally affect the genome. Cancer activation may be a downstream consequence of changes in energy metabolism (via the damaged mitochondria and genetic changes), creating a cancer "snowball effect," all of which has significant implications for treatment and prevention.[12]

As you can see, there are not really right or wrong ideas but rather multiple ways of examining the existence and persistence of cancer. The only time these ideas get in the way of preventing, treating, or curing cancer is when the approach to treatment relies on only one theory and ignores the others. Our goal is to honor the science and truth in these theories and describe methods of prevention, intervention, and synergy that will help you receive the very best treatment.

TRIGGERS, FUEL, AND RESISTANCE FACTORS

Things that trigger, fuel, or provide resistance to treatment for cancer are critical targets for treatment and prevention. The main triggers, fuel, and resistance factors can be found looking at common cancer risk factors.[13]

In addition to genetics, conventional oncology generally breaks down risk into two categories:

- Toxic influences

- Inflammatory influences

Toxic influences include tobacco smoke, alcohol, other carcinogenic chemicals, mycotoxins, and any other outside (or internally created) toxin.[14]

Inflammatory influences include radiation, obesity and the inflammation it triggers, and infections of all kinds (including dental and oral-pharyngeal infections).[15]

We feel this is an oversimplification that doesn't take into account other important root causes, such as the risk factors for cancer as provided by the mainstream National Cancer Institute (NCI). These include:[16]

- AGE—median age of a cancer diagnosis is 66 years.

- ALCOHOL—increased risk of mouth, throat, esophagus, larynx, liver, and breast cancer. The risk is much higher for those who also use tobacco.

- CANCER-CAUSING SUBSTANCES—commonly recognized ones are tobacco smoke and excessive ultraviolet rays from the sun. The NCI also lists a number of environmental carcinogens:

  - Aflatoxins—family of toxins produced by certain fungi that are found on agricultural crops such as corn, peanuts, cottonseed, and tree nuts.

  - Aristolochic acids—group of acids found in certain types of plants known as *Aristolochia*.

  - Arsenic—naturally occurring substance found in the air, water, and soil. People are exposed to arsenic through smoking tobacco, contaminated drinking water, and food sources.

  - Asbestos—naturally occurring fibrous minerals used in commercial products such as insulation and fireproofing materials, automotive brakes, and wallboard materials. Most exposure today occurs in the construction industry and ship repair.

  - Benzene—substance used primarily as a solvent in the chemical and pharmaceutical industries.

  - Benzidine—used in chemical laboratories in the past for the production of dyes for cloth, paper, and leather.

- Beryllium—metal found in nature. Used in consumer and commercial products such as aerospace components, transistors, nuclear reactors, and golf clubs.

- 1,3-Butadiene—used to produce synthetic rubber products such as tires and plastics.

- Cadmium—a natural element found in the environment. Used to manufacture batteries, pigments, metal coatings, and plastics.

- Coal tar and coal-tar pitch—coal tar is mainly used for the production of refined chemicals and coal tar products. Coal tar pitch is used as a base for coatings and paint, and as a binder in asphalt products.

- Coke-oven emissions—emissions from large ovens used to heat coal to produce coke, which is then used to manufacture iron and steel.

- Crystalline silica (respirable size)—found in stone, soil, and sand. Also found in concrete, brick, mortar, and other construction materials.

- Erionite—naturally occurring fibrous mineral. Most often problematic for road construction and maintenance workers who have been using erionite-containing gravel for road surfacing.

- Ethylene oxide—a substance used to produce other chemicals such as antifreeze.

- Formaldehyde—chemical used in building materials and as an antimicrobial and preservative. It also occurs naturally in the environment.

- Hexavalent chromium compounds—formed with the metallic element chromium found in the earth's crust, air, water, soil, and food. Used as corrosion inhibitors in the manufacture of pigments, metal finishing and chrome plating, stainless steel production, leather tanning, and wood preservatives.

— Indoor emissions from the household combustion of coal—burning coal inside the home for purposes of heating or cooking.

— Mineral oils (untreated and mildly treated)—generally refers to a liquid by-product of the distillation of petroleum to produce gasoline and other petroleum-based products from crude oil.

— Nickel compounds—formed with the metallic element nickel found in the earth's crust. They have many industrial uses, including dental materials.

— Radon—a radioactive gas that is released from the normal decay of the elements uranium, thorium, and radium in rocks and soil.

— Secondhand tobacco smoke (environmental tobacco smoke)

— Soot—by-product of the incomplete burning of carbon-containing materials such as wood, fuel oil, plastics, and household refuse.

— Strong inorganic acid mists containing sulfuric acid—sulfuric acid can be generated from various manufacturing processes.

— Thorium—naturally occurring radioactive metal found in soil, rock, and water.

— Vinyl chloride—colorless gas that is produced synthetically to primarily make polyvinyl chloride (PVC). PVC is used to make plastic products.

— Wood dust

- CHRONIC INFLAMMATION

- DIET

- HORMONES—certain hormones, particularly synthetic hormones, can increase the risk of hormone-dependent cancers, such as breast cancer.

- IMMUNOSUPPRESSION—examples include drugs that suppress the immune system, such as those for transplant recipients. Also includes chronic infections.

- INFECTIOUS AGENTS—infectious agents such as certain viruses are risk factors, for example:

  – Epstein-Barr virus (EBV)

  – Hepatitis B virus and hepatitis C virus (HBV and HCV)

  – Human immunodeficiency virus (HIV)

  – Human papillomaviruses (HPVs)

  – Human T-cell leukemia/lymphoma virus type 1 (HTLV-1)

  – Kaposi sarcoma-associated herpesvirus (KSHV)

  – Merkel cell polyomavirus (MCPyV)

  – Bacteria know to be a risk factor include *Helicobacter pylori* (*H. pylori*). And examples of parasites linked to cancer include *Opisthorchis viverrini* and *Schistosoma haematobium*.

- OBESITY—being overweight or obese is associated with the risk of many types of cancers, including postmenopausal breast, endometrial, esophageal, gallbladder, kidney, pancreatic, and thyroid cancer. It also raises the risk of dying of cancer. Excess body fat increases the levels of estrogen, blood sugar, and insulin, and inflammation, all of which can promote cancer.

- RADIATION—radiation of certain wavelengths, called ionizing radiation, can damage DNA and cause cancer. This includes radiation from nuclear power plants and medical imaging and procedures, including chest X-rays, computed tomography (CT) scans, positron emission tomography (PET) scans, and radiation therapy. Lower energy, non-ionizing radiation from cell phones is now linked to increased risk of certain cancers, such as brain cancer and leukemia. And there is emerging concern about other low frequency electromagnetic fields, such as power lines, electrical wiring, electrical appliances, broadcasting antennas (radio and TV), microwave ovens, cordless telephones, cell-phone base stations, television and computer screens, wireless local area networks (Wi-Fi), and digital electric and gas meters (smart meters).

- SUNLIGHT—UV radiation from the sun is a risk factor, as are suntanning booths.

- TOBACCO—causes many different types of cancer including lung, larynx, mouth, esophagus, throat, bladder, kidney, liver, stomach, pancreas, colon, rectum, and cervix, as well as acute myeloid leukemia.

This list is by no means exhaustive. And as we discuss in Chapter 3, other factors to consider include an unhealthy digestive system, potential environmental carcinogens, and spiritual and psychological stress.

And while a lack of exercise is not generally given as a root cause of cancer, we do know that regular exercise reduces the risk of diabetes, obesity, and being overweight, all of which are known risk factors for cancer.

In Chapter 5, we provide strong evidence that diet is the most important potential cause of cancer.

Other areas of health affect the body's ability to detoxify and maintain optimal immunity, though they have not been shown to cause cancer. One example is body structure and alignment. Posture, vertebral alignment, muscle tone, and other factors influence nerve, circulatory, and lymphatic function. This directly ties into the functioning of all organ systems, including the immune system.

Modalities such as chiropractic, osteopathy, massage, and other forms of body-work are often underestimated components of healthy immune function for preventing and fighting cancer.

The following is a chart of root causes that we assess when patients come to our clinics for primary or integrative cancer care:

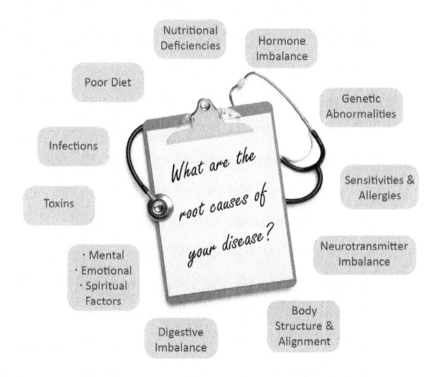

An astounding 30 to 50 percent of cancers can currently be prevented[17] by avoiding risk factors and implementing existing evidence-based prevention strategies. Removing such factors as infections (by appropriate treatment) and toxins (by depuration, or cleansing, and detoxification) can be both treatment and prevention strategies for cancer. The cancer burden can also be reduced through early detection of cancer and management. Many cancers have a high chance of cure if diagnosed early and treated adequately.[18]

Knowing the causes of cancer is important for the prevention and treatment of cancer. Your integrative doctor can help you identify causes from which you may be at risk. Testing techniques have advanced greatly, which allows you to have a much more in-depth risk assessment.

CHAPTER 3

CONTRASTING CONVENTIONAL AND INTEGRATIVE ONCOLOGY

There are similarities and differences when it comes to the medical approaches used by conventional and integrative doctors. By understanding how the two approaches have common ground yet distinct differences in their philosophy, diagnostic methods, and treatments, you will be able to make better choices for yourself or a loved one in the treatment and prevention of cancer.

UNDERSTANDING CURE VS. REMISSION

Both conventional and integrative oncology approaches aim to help people with cancer achieve their goal of a cure. In traditional medical terms, this is defined as "no traces of your cancer after treatment and the cancer will never come back."[1] Obviously, besides never having developed cancer, this would be the best outcome. For some people, this best-case scenario is achieved, and for others, it is not.

The definition of *cure* in oncology is not always that simple, however, because researchers often use five years or more of being cancer-free as the standard for the definition of cure. But even then, since there is always the possibility that a cancer may return, many doctors prefer not to use the term *cure*.

A term that is often preferred by oncologists is *remission*. The National Cancer Institute defines this as "the signs and symptoms of your cancer are reduced. Remission can be partial or complete. In a complete remission, all signs and symptoms of cancer have disappeared."[2]

UNDERSTANDING THE TERM *PROGNOSIS*

A common term that is used in medicine, especially oncology, is *prognosis*. This refers to "the likely outcome or course of a disease; the chance of recovery or recurrence."[3] When you are diagnosed with cancer, it is natural to ask how serious your cancer is and what your chances of surviving it are. This is one of the most difficult issues that doctors and patients speak about when a cancer is diagnosed and during the course of treatment. Patients want to know if their cancer can be successfully treated and/or managed and what the best approach to treatment would be.

The National Cancer Institute lists several factors to consider in evaluating your prognosis:

" •   The type of cancer and where it is in your body

•   The stage of the cancer, which refers to the size of the cancer and if it has spread to other parts of your body

•   The cancer's grade, which refers to how abnormal the cancer cells look under a microscope. Grade provides clues about how quickly the cancer is likely to grow and spread.

•   Certain traits of the cancer cells

•   Your age and how healthy you were before cancer

•   How you respond to treatment"[4]

Prognoses are estimated by using statistics based on large groups of people, but which may not be accurate in predicting your outcome. That being said, they can be helpful in navigating your way through conventional and integrative oncology treatment options. It is good to become familiar with them as you are dialoguing with your cancer care team to assess your best options. As provided by the National Cancer Institute, these are some of the most commonly used statistical terms:

" • CANCER-SPECIFIC SURVIVAL—This is the percentage of patients with a specific type and stage of cancer who have not died from their cancer during a certain period of time after diagnosis." The period of time may be 1 year, 2 years, 5 years, etc., with 5 years being the time period most often used. Cancer-specific survival is also called "disease-specific survival." In most cases, cancer-specific survival is based on causes of death listed in medical records.

• RELATIVE SURVIVAL—This statistic is another method used to estimate cancer-specific survival that does not use information about the cause of death. It is the percentage of cancer patients who have survived for a certain period of time after diagnosis compared to people who do not have cancer.

• OVERALL SURVIVAL—This is the percentage of people with a specific type and stage of cancer who have not died from any cause during a certain period of time after diagnosis.

• DISEASE-FREE SURVIVAL—This statistic is the percentage of patients who have no signs of cancer during a certain period of time after treatment. Other names for this statistic are recurrence-free or progression-free survival."[5]

SURVIVORSHIP

A term that is being used more commonly in the world of oncology is *survivorship.* This can be defined as "the transition from active treatment to recovery."[6] In the case of cancer, it is "the transformation of cancer from a fatal disease to one in which a majority of those diagnosed receive treatments that result in long-term disease-free survivorship."[7]

In terms of cancer survivorship, one oncology nurse and cancer survivor wrote a meaningful insight: "Survivorship is not just about *if* or *how long* patients live, but also about how well they survive and, hopefully, thrive."[8] I think we can all agree with this statement. Survivorship speaks to the concept that instead of treating cancer as a death sentence, it should be treated like a chronic disease. In integrative oncology, when a true "cure" cannot be achieved, the goal is to treat the patient with cancer as if they have any other chronic disease while extending life and improving quality of life.

QUALITY OF LIFE IS KEY

Integrative medicine has always had a primary focus on a patient's quality of life (QoL) for all chronic diseases. In other words, the length of life has much more value if there is a high quality of life. And for most people with cancer, we find their measure of success of treatment is QoL over length of life.

Fortunately, conventional oncology has been increasing its awareness and acceptance of QoL. Long-term cancer survivors have several understandable concerns about their future quality of life, including pain level, side effects from treatment, cognitive function, sexuality/intimacy, energy level, mood, social and emotional support, body image, and spiritual and philosophical views of life.

QoL is also very important for people with advanced cancer who are nearing the end of life. Researchers from Dana-Farber Cancer Institute in Boston found nine key factors that explained the biggest differences in patients' quality of life at their end of life:

- Intensive care stays in the final week of their life

- Dying in the hospital

- Level of patient worry at the start of the study

- Religious prayer or meditation at the start of the study

- Site of cancer care

- Feeding tube use in the final week of life

- Pastoral care inside the clinic or hospital

- Chemotherapy during their last week of life

- Patient-physician therapeutic alliance (relationship) at the start of the study

Your doctor can provide you with a questionnaire that assesses your quality of life score. This type of assessment can help you decide future treatments and understand the short- and long-term consequences. It is critical that you, your family, caregivers, and physicians know your wishes and goals for both end-of-life care as well as any hospitalization or intensive procedures.

DIAGNOSIS AND MONITORING OF CANCER

There is no doubt that conventional diagnostic techniques are recommended for diagnosing cancer. Integrative doctors recommend the same tests to identify what type of cancer one has as well as the staging and grading described earlier. The type of diagnostic tests will depend on one's age, medical condition, suspected type of cancer, types of symptoms, and the results of other lab tests.

The following are common diagnostic tests used to identify cancer:

BARIUM ENEMA: The patient drinks a contrast medium and has an X-ray of the colon and rectum. The contrast solution helps to give clearer images that could identify cancerous growths.

BIOPSY: The collection of tissue from a suspected cancer that is examined under a microscope. The sample is often collected with a needle. It can also be done during surgery or endoscopy with a special tool that removes cells or tissues.

BONE MARROW ASPIRATION AND BIOPSY: The removal of fluid (aspiration) or a small, solid piece (biopsy) from the bone marrow that provides information about blood cells formed in the bone marrow. It can help diagnose blood cancers.

BONE SCAN: A test that looks for cancer that has started in or has spread to the bones. It involves the injection of a small amount of a radioactive substance into a vein, and the entire body is scanned with a scanner that measures radioactivity.

COLONOSCOPY: A thin, flexible tube with a light and camera is inserted in the rectum and moved through the large intestine to look for colorectal cancer and precancerous polyps.

COMPUTED TOMOGRAPHY (CT) SCAN: Also referred to as a CAT scan, an X-ray machine uses multiple X-rays to create a three-dimensional picture of the area being scanned.

DIGITAL RECTAL EXAM (DRE): The doctor inserts a lubricated, gloved finger into the rectum to feel for abnormalities, such as cancerous growths of the lower rectum, pelvis, lower belly, prostate in men, and uterus in women.

EKG AND ECHOCARDIOGRAM: Measures the electrical activity of the heart. This test may be done before, during, and after certain cancer treatments, such as chemotherapy, which can damage the heart.

ENDOSCOPY: The insertion of a thin tube with a light and camera to examine internal areas of body parts, such as the esophagus, stomach, colon, ear, nose, throat, heart, urinary tract, joints, and abdomen.

FECAL OCCULT BLOOD TESTS: A screening test for colorectal cancer which looks for hidden blood in the stool.

LAB TESTS: Blood and urine tests that can help identify substances that can be a sign of cancer. They are tools to help identify cancer but are not relied upon alone to diagnose cancer.

MAGNETIC RESONANCE IMAGING (MRI): It uses magnets create a magnetic field and a computer link creates a 3-D diagnostic image of body tissues to give detailed pictures of areas in the body.

MAMMOGRAPHY: A type of low-dose X-ray that looks for changes in breast tissue, including signs of breast cancer. 3-D mammography, also known as breast tomosynthesis, is a new type of mammogram that puts the images in a three-dimensional picture.

MUGA SCAN: A multigated acquisition scan that uses a radioactive tracer and a special camera to take pictures of the heart as it pumps blood with each heartbeat. It is required during some types of chemotherapy to make sure they are not causing heart damage.

PAP TEST: Also known as a Pap smear, a swab of cells from a woman's cervix. It tests for precancerous and cancerous changes of the cervix.

POSITRON-EMISSION TOMOGRAPHY (PET): The injection of a radioactive tracer that is picked up more by organs and tissues that have cancer and then viewed on a computer image. It allows a doctor to see if cancer is present and if it has spread, and to monitor how a tumor is responding to chemotherapy. It is often combined with a CT scan.

SIGMOIDOSCOPY: The use of a thin, flexible tube with a light and camera that is inserted into the rectum and used to visualize the lower portion of a patient's sigmoid colon and rectum.

STOOL TEST: Stool samples that measure DNA biomarkers can indicate whether there is a low or high likelihood that colorectal cancer or precancer is present.

TUMOR GENOMICS: Genetic typing tests for tumor characteristics specific to certain tumor types and used to guide therapies.

TUMOR MARKERS: Substances measured in blood, urine, or body tissues that are used to monitor how a cancer treatment is working or, at higher levels, may indicate cancer.

ULTRASOUND: An imaging test that uses high-frequency sound waves to create pictures of internal organs and tissues. It does not emit ionizing radiation like an X-ray.

OUTSIDE THE BOX TESTING METHODS

By the time this book is published, there may well be some other method available for the assessment of cancer. While we cannot be encyclopedic in this area, we want to make the reader as aware as possible of the potential assessment abilities available for their cancer care. Certainly not all testing methods are appropriate at all times, which underscores the need for an integrative oncology practitioner to help the patient assess the testing that is best in their own particular case. These are some of the tests used to assess cancer:

8-OHdG (8-OXO-2'-DEOXYGUANOSINE): One of the major products of DNA oxidation. Concentrations of 80HdG within a cell are a measurement of oxidative stress, which is another nonspecific marker of disease regression or progression.[9]

AMAS (ANTI-MALIGNIN ANTIBODY SERUM) TEST: This is an older, nonspecific cancer test aimed at early detection. We include it here for completeness; but in recent times, with the more sensitive testing available, it is rarely used.[10] [11]

CHEMOSENSITIVITY TESTING: A method of using tumor cells in a laboratory to test the sensitivity of those particular cells to specific cancer therapies. There are many labs that perform these tests, and your integrative physician will usually have a preference based on their experience with the lab, location, and long-term outcomes of their testing.[12] [13]

CIRCULATING TUMOR CELL (CTC) AND CIRCULATING TUMOR DNA (CTDNA) TESTING

Circulating tumor cells (CTCs) are cancer cells that have shed from a primary or metastatic tumor and circulate in the bloodstream. The identification and isolation of CTCs in cancer patients can be used with or as an alternative to traditional tissue biopsies in order to evaluate what might be taking place on a real-time basis. This technology may be used to evaluate a patient's prognosis as well as their response to therapy.

CIRCULATING TUMOR DNA (CTDNA): Genetic material that typically mutates and causes cancer (oncogenes) can be found in the bloodstream, and detecting this material in the blood (ctDNA) has become a more common method for profiling cancers. Newer drug therapies are designed to target the specific genetic mutations underlying a patient's disease, and treatment based on this information can enable better treatment outcomes with fewer treatment-related side effects.[14] [15]

HUMAN CHORIONIC GONADOTROPIN (HCG): A hormone normally produced by the human placenta and the basis of pregnancy tests. It is also known to rise in some tumors and to potentially be a trigger for cancer growth. It is used in some cases to follow cancer progress through therapy.[16] [17]

ALPHA-N-ACETYLGALACTOSAMINIDASE (NAGALASE): An enzyme used by cancer cells to develop biochemical strength and can be a laboratory sign of a strengthening cancer process. The two therapies discussed in the Intravenous and Injection chapter (Salicinium and Gc-MAF) interrupt[18] the biochemical pathway for the production of Nagalase and weaken the tumor biology.[19] [20] [21]

IVY GENE TEST: Detects and measures DNA methylation paterns that are consistent with actual cancer presence. The test measures the methylation status of cell-free DNA extracted from blood samples.

TRANSFORMING GROWTH FACTOR-BETA (TGF-BETA): A tissue factor that can be followed to monitor inflammatory and tumor specific progress or treatment. Like many other tissue factors, it is generally nonspecific but can be an important lab test for many cases. It can help predict increased disease activity or decreased disease activity due to either the natural history of the cancer or therapies.[22]

TK-1 TESTING: Thymidine kinase (TK) plays a key role in tissue metabolism in acute or pathological tissue stress. Patients with intermediate and high levels of TK activity in their tumors frequently show a rapid disease progression and generally worse outcomes. This test is often used to monitor cancer progress during active treatment.[23]

OTHER TESTING

IODINE AND SERUM VITAMIN B12: Iodine and vitamin B12 levels are used as very nonspecific markers of tumor spread. This does not mean that these essential nutrients "cause" cancer but rather that during cancer spread, their levels may rise in the blood due to non-nutritional biochemistry (often due to cancer activity).[24] [25] [26] Again, this does not mean they are involved in the cancer but have a "bystander effect" that can be monitored.

OTHER BIOCHEMICAL MEASUREMENTS

Many times, lab tests used for other purposes will change during a cancer process and can be used (mainly as nonspecific markers) for tumor activity. These can include alkaline phosphatase, gamma-glutamyl transpeptidase (GGT), lactate dehydrogenase (LDH), C-reactive protein (CRP), erythrocyte sedimentation rate (ESR), D-dimer, fibrinogen, and others. One colleague regularly monitors the "trifecta" (ESR, CRP, LDH) as a way to catch early cancer activity during treatment. Like many of the previously mentioned tests, they are often nonspecific.

PHILOSOPHY OF MEDICINE

The distinct field known as "philosophy of medicine" explores the unique issues that come with the field of medicine and health care in general. There are professional journals, books, and societies dedicated to discussing and trying to answer the questions that arise from these issues.

Many believe the origin of the philosophy of medicine goes back to Hippocrates, the ancient Greek physician (460–375 B.C.) who has been regarded as the father of medicine. He has been revered for his medical ethics, and the Hippocratic oath is named for him, which has been used as a guide of conduct for the medical profession throughout the ages.

What does philosophy have to do with cancer? The answer is that a physician's view of what cancer is and how it is caused, and the treatments with which they are most familiar and comfortable will greatly influence the way they treat cancer. In other words, their philosophy of the medical treatment of cancer will greatly affect their bias in terms of treatment.

THE WHOLE IS GREATER THAN THE SUM OF ITS PARTS

Conventional oncology often has a reductionist approach, where one looks for fundamental mechanisms or processes that are causing cancer. For example, you test and find a genetic cause. The treatment would then focus on targeting the genetic cause with a pharmaceutical agent.

Another example of this reductionist approach focuses on cancer as the abnormal replication of a region of cells, where surgery is used to remove or conventional treatment (e.g., radiation, chemotherapy, and cryotherapy) is used to destroy the region of abnormal cells or tissue.

The reductionist approach can be effective. For example, if a patient has an early stage melanoma (malignant skin cancer), and it is properly removed surgically, the patient could be cured. However, many common cancers are much more complex, and the reasons for why the cancer comes back can often be poorly understood in traditional medicine.

On the other hand, integrative oncology embraces a more holistic approach. Integrative doctors still recognize there are several causes for cancer and that they should be assessed. If a region or regions is known to have cancerous cells/tissues then conventional therapy would often need to be targeted to this region. Yet cancer, even localized cancer, is often a whole-body problem that can be identified in one or more regions of the body. Localized treatment may be needed, but addressing the whole person (mind, body, and spirit) would result in a higher likelihood of treating the root causes more effectively, as well as summon a variety of anticancer mechanisms and benefits.

For example, if one had breast or prostate cancer that had not metastasized and surgery was warranted, it would still be prudent to address diet, environmental toxins, stress levels, and nutrient deficiencies so that the body would be healthier to both fight the cancer and to reduce the risk of recurrence. The same would be true even if one had metastatic cancer.

HALLMARKS OF CANCER

The understanding of cancer continues to evolve. It used to be believed that cancer was a mass of proliferating cells, but now it is known that cancer involves complex tissues composed of multiple distinct types of cancerous and normal cells that interact with one another.[27]

INTEGRATIVE MEDICINE PHILOSOPHY

Since most people are aware of what conventional medicine practices involve, we are going to introduce integrative medicine philosophy. As naturopathic medical doctors, we believe most comprehensive principles for integrative medicine come from the principles of naturopathic medicine. The American Association of Naturopathic Physicians defines them as follows:

" • THE HEALING POWER OF NATURE (VIS MEDICATRIX NATU-
   RAE): Naturopathic medicine recognizes an inherent
   self-healing process in people that is ordered and intelligent.
   Naturopathic physicians act to identify and remove obstacles
   to healing and recovery, and to facilitate and augment this
   inherent self-healing process.

 • IDENTIFY AND TREAT THE CAUSES (TOLLE CAUSAM): The
   naturopathic physician seeks to identify and remove the
   underlying causes of illness rather than to merely eliminate
   or suppress symptoms.

 • FIRST DO NO HARM (PRIMUM NON NOCERE): Naturopathic physicians follow three guidelines to avoid harming
   the patient:

- Utilize methods and medicinal substances which minimize the risk of harmful side effects, using the least force necessary to diagnose and treat;

- Avoid when possible the harmful suppression of symptoms; and

- Acknowledge, respect, and work with individuals' self-healing process.

- DOCTOR AS TEACHER (DOCERE): Naturopathic physicians educate their patients and encourage self-responsibility for health. They also recognize and employ the therapeutic potential of the doctor-patient relationship.

- TREAT THE WHOLE PERSON: Naturopathic physicians treat each patient by taking into account individual physical, mental, emotional, genetic, environmental, social, and other factors. Since total health also includes spiritual health, naturopathic physicians encourage individuals to pursue their personal spiritual development.

- PREVENTION: Naturopathic physicians emphasize the prevention of disease by assessing risk factors, heredity and susceptibility to disease, and by making appropriate interventions in partnership with their patients to prevent illness."[28]

Integrative doctors seek to treat the root causes of disease. This is very important for cancer in both terms of treatment and prevention. As discussed in Chapter 2, there are several root causes of cancer.

CONVENTIONAL ONCOLOGY

The focus of conventional oncology is to diagnose the type of cancer an individual has and prescribe a treatment that cures or manages the patient.

There are several different options that can be used depending on the type of cancer, how advanced it is, and the health of the patient. Surgery, chemotherapy, and radiation therapy are mainstay therapies. However, as we discuss in Chapter 4, there are several other oncology therapies that are used and many more in development.

THE NEED FOR INTEGRATIVE ONCOLOGY

Research has clearly shown there is a strong desire by the American public for integrative oncology. Why would this be? One reason is the growing acceptance of alternative and holistic medicine. This may be due to the increasing number of studies validating naturopathic and holistic therapies, as well as the influence of European and Asian traditional therapies. Another is that many Americans have either experienced or know someone who has been through the journey of cancer.

The American public has figured out that cancer affects one's life on many different levels. As researchers have documented, ". . . cancer and its treatment have the capacity to affect not simply physical well-being, but also virtually every aspect of an individual's life, including psychological, social, economic and existential health and function."[29]

Since we each have spoken to our patients with cancer for more than two decades of practice, we are very aware of their well-founded fears of the side effects that can impair their quality of life in the short and long term, as well as the risk of death from conventional treatments.

Julia H. Rowland, Ph.D., is director of the National Cancer Institute's Office of Cancer Survivorship. In her career, Dr. Rowland has worked as a clinician, researcher, and teacher in the area of psychosocial aspects of cancer with child and adult cancer survivors and their families.[30] In regard to typical conventional oncology treatment side effects, Dr. Rowland notes:

> ". . . some of these effects (eg, alopecia, nausea, and vomiting) dissipate rapidly once treatment ends, others (eg, fatigue, sexual dysfunction, memory problems) can persist over time, in some cases (eg, lymphedema, pain syndromes), becoming chronic. Still another set of effects may appear months or years after

treatment ends (cardiac dysfunction, osteoporosis, diabetes), the most worrisome of these being recurrent or second cancers."[31]

These concerns of people with cancer can help one understand why they want to incorporate the best of integrative oncology to help them prevent, cope with, and manage these lists of serious side effects.

The official journal of the Multinational Association of Supportive Care in Cancer published a summary of a study of 166 long-term cancer survivors; and the common reasons for complementary health approaches (alternative and holistic therapies) were "to relieve stress (28%), treat or prevent cancer (21%), relieve cancer-related symptoms (18%), and deal with another condition (18%)."[32]

The question is this: Can alternative and holistic therapies accomplish this task? We believe clinical experience and documented research demonstrates that for many people it can!

Integrative oncology generally focuses on four main approaches:

SUPPORT

Most cancer patients that we encounter have started conventional cancer therapy or have already received conventional cancer care. In some cases, they have already been treated and are looking for ways to enhance their recovery and optimize their health, as well as reduce the risk of recurrence.

Using mainly natural, nontoxic therapies, the focus of the provider is to support the patient through their current cancer therapy. For example, this could include multiple types of interventions aimed at many body systems:

- Combating the side effects of fatigue from chemotherapy or radiation

- Helping tissue heal from surgery

- Easing anxiety and depression

- Improving digestive upset, such as nausea, vomiting, diarrhea, and constipation

- Alleviating joint and muscle pain

- Immune support for cancer therapy and preventing/treating infections

- Reducing hot flashes and other hormonal symptoms from hormonal-blocking therapies

- Regimens for protecting against damage to internal organs, such as the liver and heart

- Healing skin burns and rashes

- Maintaining a healthy body weight and fat percentage (too high or too low is problematic)

Specific protocols that we use are provided in Chapter 8.

ENHANCE

An important goal of integrative oncology is to enhance the anticancer treatments that a patient is receiving. The use of natural agents and methods for a direct or indirect cancer effect is a neglected area in conventional oncology. Most traditional oncologists are simply unaware that these types of natural agents or methods exist.

For example, the use of high-dose intravenous vitamin C has been shown in published studies to improve both quality and length of life. (See Chapter 7.) Several supplements, including mushroom extracts, have been shown in human studies to reduce the side effects of chemotherapy and radiation and improve the activity of immune cells that fight cancer.

DETOXIFY/CLEANSE

A tremendous amount of metabolic waste products is produced through therapies such as chemotherapy and radiation. As a result, a person will be more prone to problems such as headaches, fatigue, skin rashes, digestive upset, poor memory and focus, joint and muscle pain, and several other possible symptoms.

Conventional medicine does little to address the need for detoxification during and after these types of therapies. Integrative doctors recognize the critical importance of detoxification and cleansing for the patient to feel better, experience fewer side effects, and have a healthier immune system. Optimally, detoxification should start before a regimen of chemotherapy and radiation and should be maintained to some degree during treatment and especially afterward. (See specific recommendations on detoxification in Chapter 8.)

OPTIMIZE

Once a person has made it through their conventional therapies, there is more work to do from an integrative oncology approach. Now is the time to dig more deeply and try to address the root causes of why one may have developed cancer in the first place.

For example, if one had very poor lifestyle habits such as poor diet and inconsistent exercise, these can be improved. Or if you were exposed to toxins that are known to be carcinogenic, then specific detoxification protocols can be implemented with the help of your integrative doctor. Or perhaps you are overweight, which increases the risk for a variety of cancers. Then now is the time to develop a program for shedding those extra pounds and maintaining a healthier weight.

Your integrative doctor can use modern testing to find out what your body imbalances are. This could include tests for factors that damage the immune system and cell DNA, such as toxic metals (e.g., arsenic, lead, mercury, or nickel) or pesticides. You can also be tested for hormone balance, which is very important for hormone-related cancers such as breast and prostate. In addition, you can be assessed to see if you are deficient in various vitamins and minerals, many of which play a role in a healthy immune system and healthy DNA. Or perhaps you have a sleep problem, such as insomnia or sleep apnea, which is preventing you from having optimal immunity. Another core issue is gut health. The functioning of the digestive system and the important microbiome (gut bacteria) can be assessed and improved. And, of course, how you handle stress is very important for a healthy immune system.

THE GUT CONNECTION

Integrative doctors recognize the vital connection between the digestive tract and the immune system (as well as rest of the body). Seventy percent of your immune system resides in your gastrointestinal system. Highly concentrated in the small intestine, gut-associated lymphoid tissue (GALT) produces white blood cells known as lymphocytes, as well as antibodies. These immune cells fight infection and cancer.

The human digestive tract is also host to trillions of bacteria, many of which play a healthy role in the digestive tract. These good bacteria, also known as flora, have several functions, including immune system enhancement, prevention of infection, manufacturing of several vitamins, and metabolism of hormones.

An important component of the health of the digestive tract and immune system is the health of the small intestine. The human intestinal barrier covers a surface of about 400 square meters,[33] roughly the size of a tennis court! It also requires approximately 40 percent of the body's energy expenditure.[34]

The small intestine provides a barrier to keep harmful microorganisms and toxins from entering the body. At the same time, it allows the absorption of nutrients from the diet into the body and prevents against loss of water and electrolytes. A breakdown in this important barrier can result in severe immune system deficiency and risk of disease.[35]

Thus, the health of one's "intestinal permeability," also referred to as "intestinal barrier," is critical for a healthy functioning immune system and the fight against cancer.

There are many factors that can alter or damage the intestinal barrier, including nonsteroidal anti-inflammatory drugs, alcohol consumption, cow's milk intolerance, a Western-style diet high in carbohydrates and fats, small intestine bacterial overgrowth, pancreatic insufficiency (inability to produce enough digestive enzymes), intestinal infections, stress, intestinal inflammation, changes in the intestinal flora (bacteria), nutrient deficiencies (such as vitamin A and short chain fatty acids), chemotherapy, and radiation therapy (to the pelvis).[36][37]

Conditions related to unhealthy intestinal permeability include gastric ulcers, infectious diarrhea, irritable bowel syndrome, inflammatory bowel disease, celiac disease, allergies, infections, acute and chronic inflammatory states (e.g., arthritis), obesity-associated metabolic diseases, multiple organ failure, inflammatory joint disease, psoriatic arthritis, eczema, psychological conditions, and even cancer (e.g., esophagus and colorectal).[38][39]

Integrative doctors can test for the severity of intestinal permeability and use a variety of natural methods to support and improve digestion and a healthy intestinal barrier. This involves the use of diet, prebiotics (substances that feed the good bacteria in the gut), probiotics (good bacteria), vitamins and minerals, amino acids, herbs, enzymes, and other natural solutions.

Chemotherapy, radiation therapy, and pain medications all contribute to an unhealthy small intestine. To optimize your immune system and health, it is critical that you incorporate a holistic program that supports gut health. We have included very specific digestive support recommendations in Chapters 8 and 9.

THE TOXIN CONNECTION

Americans are exposed to all sorts of environmental chemicals. Some are naturally occurring but most are man-made. Integrative doctors pay special attention to the toxin problem that depletes the immune system and contributes to cancerous changes via DNA damage. The President's Cancer Panel notes: "With nearly 80,000 chemicals on the market in the United States, many of which are used by millions of Americans in their daily lives and are un- or understudied and largely unregulated, exposure to potential environmental carcinogens is widespread."[40]

We are exposed to toxins in our food, such as pesticides in fruits and vegetables, mercury in fish such as tuna, artificial sweeteners, and genetically modified organisms (GMOs). The water supply is contaminated with carcinogenic arsenic, chlorine, and pharmaceutical metabolites. Beauty-care products contain phthalates and parabens, which are known hormone disrupters and suspects in some hormone-related cancers. The air contains a variety of toxins, including benzene, volatile organic compounds, smoke, cadmium, and mercury. Homes may contain mold and a variety of other chemicals. And the list could go on much longer.

The point is that our cells are bombarded with numerous toxins that damage the immune system and our cell DNA. The result can be cancer. And of course, if you are receiving a treatment such as chemotherapy or one of the many other conventional cancer therapies, then you have additional toxins to deal with.

This is why integrative doctors take detoxification so seriously. Cells that have been burdened with toxins are not healthy and provide a more hospitable environment for cancer.

A good integrative program will include natural methods to support detoxification. Three of the key organs of detoxification are the kidneys, liver, and skin. A healthy diet, purified water, and supplements that support detoxification are very important in supporting people undergoing conventional cancer therapy. They are also important in the prevention of cancer.

Techniques that increase the elimination of toxins through sweating, such as exercise or saunas, are time-tested. Another strategy to aid in detoxification is fasting. There are several fasting methods that integrative doctors use but which must be suitable to the health and situation of the patient. Make sure to consult with your integrative doctor for a plan that meets your needs and situation before establishing a treatment strategy.

A great book on the subject of detoxification is *The Toxin Solution* by Dr. Joseph Pizzorno.

THE MANY TOOLS OF INTEGRATIVE DOCTORS

Integrative doctors can help people with cancer through a diverse number of natural and holistic therapies, which are often needed due to the many potential side effects from conventional oncology therapies.

It is helpful to have several holistic healing tools since cancer patients need to be treated individually. These are some of the treatments integrative doctors use:

- Acupuncture

- Bioidentical hormones

- Chiropractic/osteopathic/naturopathic spinal manipulation and body work

- Clinical nutrition

- Counseling

- Herbal therapy

- Homeopathy

- Intravenous and injection therapies

- Massage

- Nutritional supplements

- Physiotherapy

- Therapeutic exercise

STRESS AND THE IMMUNE SYSTEM

When we speak to patients about the time preceding their cancer diagnosis, many state they had intense, prolonged periods of mental or emotional stress. Health experts are certainly in agreement that the effects of uncontrolled stress can be deadly.

According to Lorenzo Cohen, Ph.D., professor of General Oncology and Behavioral Science, and director of the Integrative Medicine Program at MD Anderson, "Stress has a profound impact on how your body's systems function. . . . stress makes your body more hospitable to cancer."[41]

Many studies have demonstrated this connection. The results of at least 165 studies indicate that stress-related psychosocial factors are associated with higher cancer incidence in initially healthy populations. There was poorer survival in patients diagnosed with cancer in at least 330 studies, and higher cancer mortality was seen in at least 53 studies.[42]

In general, our bodies adapt well to short-term stress. However, chronic levels of high stress cause the brain to release hormonal messengers that stimulate our adrenal glands (master stress glands) to release hormones such as cortisol and epinephrine. Long-term exposure of our cells to these stress hormones causes a variety of issues:

- Increased production of free radicals, which leads to DNA damage and impaired immune function

- Increased inflammation through the production of inflammatory proteins known as cytokines, which impair immune function and promote cancer growth

- Direct impairment of immune cell function

- Reduction in the ability of abnormal cells to undergo apoptosis (cell death) and DNA repair, important self-regulating anticancer mechanisms

- Stimulation of the production of IGF-1 (insulin-like growth factor-1), VEGF (vascular endothelial growth factor), and other growth factors that can promote tumor cell growth[43]

In their book *Living with Cancer,* two doctors from Massachusetts General Hospital, Vicki A. Jackson, M.D., M.P.H., and chief of palliative care, and David P. Ryan, M.D. and chief of hematology/oncology, offer several coping strategies in addition to fitness activities and counseling:

DISTRACTION: Take time to be distracted, for example, with TV shows, Internet surfing, or animal watching.

OPTIMISM: Create an event to look forward to. This could be something like attending a child or grandchild's recital, shopping with a friend, or a dream trip.

GRATITUDE: Get in the habit of writing down three things a day that you are grateful for and concentrate on them.

JOY: Take opportunities to stay in the moment and enjoy simple things such as a sunset, a sports event, or connection with a family member or friend.

MEDITATION AND PRAYER: Prayer and spiritual reflection help one stay centered on God and avoid worrying thoughts. Helpful Bible verses include Psalm 94:19 and Philippians 4:6–7.

HUMOR: Humor and laughter are positive coping mechanisms. For example, one can read jokes or watch comedy shows.

FLOW: This refers to any activity that causes one to feel immersed in energized focus, involvement, and enjoyment of the process. For some, this may be painting, for others it could be regular club meetings.

INTELLECTUALIZATION: Focus on treating your cancer like an intellectual puzzle.

PROBLEM SOLVING: This can involve researching options for your cancer, such as alternative therapies.[44]

Here are additional beneficial tips for reducing stress from Cancer.Net:[45]

- Avoid scheduling conflicts

- Be aware of your limits

- Ask for help

- Prioritize your tasks

- Break down tasks into smaller steps

- Concentrate your efforts on things you can control

- Get help with financial problems

Also, a technique of deep breathing with a focus on the lower abdomen can reduce stress hormone levels.

Do not hesitate in seeking counseling or pastoral care. A study with breast cancer patients who received either psychological interventions and advice on minimizing stress or no psychological intervention at all showed that those receiving intervention had a 45 percent reduced risk of breast cancer recurrence and a 59 percent reduced risk of death from breast cancer![46]

GET ACTIVE

Do not underestimate the physical and emotional benefits of regular exercise. A study with female breast cancer survivors who participated in three months of specific exercises, six months of specific exercise, or were sedentary found that those involved in exercise had improvements in cardiovascular endurance, fatigue, and symptoms of depression while those in the sedentary group had no improvement.[47]

A review of the effect of lifestyle factors on breast cancer mortality found that physical activity has the most pronounced effect of all the lifestyle factors on reducing breast cancer recurrence.[48] Physical activity can reduce breast cancer mortality by about 40 percent.[49] Researchers from this study recommended at least 30 minutes of moderate-intensity physical activity at least five days of the week, or 75 minutes of more vigorous exercise, along with two to three weekly strength-training sessions, including exercises for major muscle groups. This recommendation was endorsed by the Canadian Cancer Society and the American Cancer Society.[50]

In a study of 2,705 men with localized prostate cancer, the patients who completed three hours or more of vigorous physical activity had a 49 percent lower risk of death from all causes and a 61 percent reduced risk of dying from prostate cancer, compared with men who completed one hour of vigorous activity per week.[51] Nearly half of the men walked for their activity. Men who walked briskly had a 57 percent lower rate of progression than men who walked at an easy pace.[52]

STRESS HORMONE AND GLAND SUPPORT

Integrative and holistic doctors understand how to support the body's main stress glands, the adrenal glands. These glands respond to the brain's signals for perceived stress (therefore your initial step for stress reduction should be mind-body techniques). Too high adrenaline or cortisol levels lead to immune system suppression and promote inflammation.

Fortunately, there are natural products that help to balance your adrenal stress hormones. One that has been well studied has its origins in India. It is known as ashwagandha and has powerful stress-busting properties.

In a double-blind, randomized, placebo-controlled trial involving 64 volunteers with a history of problems dealing with stress, participants had their blood cortisol levels measured and they filled out a questionnaire that assessed their stress level.

For 60 days one group received a placebo and the other group took one 300 mg capsule of ashwagandha extract twice a day. At the end of the 60 days, those receiving the ashwagandha had a *significant* reduction in perceived stress scores, improving by a full 44 percent. Participants who had received the herb also had an astounding 59 to 89 percent improvement in all categories of their General Health Questionnaire. The ashwagandha-takers walked away with improved sleep quality, productivity, and mental calmness. And perhaps most impressive of all, there was an average 27.9 percent reduction in cortisol levels after the 60 days—quite a remarkable improvement.[53]

Other nutrients that help your adrenal glands to function more healthily include B vitamins, vitamin C, and magnesium. You can also help your nervous system relax gently with nutritional supplements such as L-theanine, GABA, passionflower, chamomile, and others. A number of other natural therapies such as acupuncture, sauna therapy, massage, biofeedback, counseling, and aromatherapy can help you to relax and rejuvenate. Speak with your holistic doctor about the best fit for your situation and symptoms.

MANAGING THE SIDE EFFECTS OF CANCER THERAPY

Integrative medicine has a lot to offer in terms of managing the side effects of conventional cancer care. For most of us who deal with cancer patients, it is one of the most common things we do.

Fatigue, insomnia, depression, anxiety, poor focus and memory (chemo brain), peripheral neuropathy, skin rashes, joint pain, and digestive upset are some of the common issues with which patients with cancer need routine help.

While conventional medicine has pharmaceutical and other therapies to offset these side effects, the use of holistic methods can significantly lessen these side effects and improve the quality of life.

The majority of people who receive chemotherapy and radiation therapy will experience fatigue. This can persist for 5 to 10 years after diagnosis and treatment.

One effective antidote is American ginseng. In a randomized, double-blind trial, published in the *Journal of the National Cancer Institute*, researchers found that 2000 mg of American ginseng (*Panax quinquefolius*) given over an eight-week period was statistically significant in benefit compared to a placebo.[54] (See Chapter 8 for specific protocols for recovery from the side effects of conventional cancer therapies.)

PREVENTION

Let's face it, conventional oncology can be weak in terms of the prevention of cancer. For those of you who have had cancer in the past or those of you who want to incorporate a cancer prevention program, integrative medicine has much more to offer.

A great deal of information is coming out in scientific literature about the role cancer stem cells (CSCs) play in cancer remission and recurrence. Studies published in *The New England Journal of Medicine*[55] and many other established publications underscore the differences in the cancer "parent cells" (CSCs) and the tumor being treated. Much like we see with infections, if treatment is not completed, the original infection will strengthen. Likewise, CSCs can become treatment-resistant after seemingly helpful therapy, which is why the idea of prevention with an "active remission" (actively keeping the CSCs quiet and not reproducing or seeding cancer with integrative therapies) is so critical.

Integrative oncology deals effectively with the root causes of cancer (as described in Chapter 2). This is achieved through improving diet, correcting nutritional deficiencies, identifying and removing toxins, optimizing diges-tion and normalizing intestinal permeability, addressing harmful mental and emotional stress patterns, utilizing nutritional epigenetic approaches (improv-ing genetic expression through diet and other natural agents), and natural immune modulating and anti-inflammatory protocols. All of these integrative strategies have ways of keeping the CSCs under control as well as minimizing their effects over time.

THE TAKEAWAY

You have read in this chapter the many philosophical and treatment differences between conventional and integrative oncology. Conventional oncology plays an important role in the diagnosis and treatment of cancer. But we consider conventional oncology by itself to be incomplete and less humane without the use of the holistic approaches found in integrative oncology. Integrative oncology has a much more encompassing approach to the prevention of cancer, taking into account the individual as a holistic person.

CHAPTER 4

UNDERSTANDING CONVENTIONAL THERAPIES

There are many cancer therapies that are used in conventional oncology. This includes many different mechanisms and strategies for the treatment of cancer. We will review each of these therapies and how they work, and we will describe common side effects so that you can be aware of the risks of these treatments.

SURGERY

There can be many uses for surgery in oncology. One reason is to diagnose cancer. Surgery to diagnose cancer in this case involves removing tissue samples that can then be analyzed in a laboratory. A process called staging is used to assess how much cancer there is in a region and how far it has spread (metastasized). This often includes the lymph nodes and nearby organs.

Another obvious use of surgery is for the removal of cancer, known as curative or primary surgery, with the goal of removing the cancer completely. In certain situations, surgery is used to remove as much of a cancer as possible but cannot remove all of it. While still helpful, additional therapies may be required such as chemotherapy, radiation, or other treatments.

RADIATION THERAPY

The use of radiation for the treatment of cancer was first done with later-stage breast cancer as far back as the late 1800s. Ongoing advances have increased the safety and efficacy of this therapy. Radiation therapy can be used to cure cancer, prevent cancer's return, reduce pain, stop or slow cancer's growth, or shrink the growth of a tumor. It is often used with other oncology therapies such as chemotherapy and surgery.

The use of radiation therapy to fight cancer involves administering energy in the form of photons (X-rays and gamma rays) or particles (neutrons, protons, and electrons). When photons or particles interact with tissues or cells, they generate negatively charged molecules known as free radicals. These free radicals damage the DNA of cancer cells (and often healthy cells), which interferes with the ability of cancer cells to replicate and contributes to cancer cell death. Also, radiation therapy activates the immune response against tumor cells.

Cells treated with radiation can also be stimulated to repair themselves, which is why the correct radiation dose, timing, and frequency of treatments are important.

The major tissue influencer on tumor response to radiation is oxygen.[1] Research has shown that decreased levels of tissue oxygen (known as hypoxia) result in less effective radiation. Or put another way, the more oxygenated tissues are, the more effective radiation therapy can be. In addition, cells that are low in oxygen can repair themselves more easily from the damaging effects of radiation.

When combined with radiation therapy, hyperbaric oxygen therapy (HBOT), which involves breathing pure oxygen in a pressurized tube or tent, has shown improvement for head and neck cancers.[2] This may be one of the reasons why oxidative therapies such as intravenous vitamin C and the use of medical ozone (three atoms of oxygen added to a person's blood) have shown to benefit some types of cancers. (For more information on these holistic therapies, see Chapter 6.)

There are two main types of radiation therapy. The first and most common type of radiation is known as external radiation therapy. It is referred to as external since radiation therapy is generated with a machine and delivered to a specific area of the body with cancer. Diagnostic imaging equipment is used to localize the tumor and tissues that require treatment.

The other main type of radiation therapy is internal radiation therapy, also known as brachytherapy. This involves radiation being placed within tumors or cavities of the body. This therapy may be used temporarily or permanently and allows one to irradiate tumors at close range. One common example is radioactive seed implants used for prostate cancer.

Since healthier cells are damaged during radiation treatments, there can be many side effects. This is known as radiation toxicity. Two of the more common acute side effects of radiation therapy are nausea and fatigue. Chronic side effects may include irreversible problems such as organ damage and even cancer itself. (For information on alternative therapies that may reduce the side effects of radiation therapy, see Chapter 8.)

Potential Side Effects of Radiation Chart

Part of the Body Being Treated	Possible Side Effects	
Brain	• Fatigue • Hair Loss • Nausea/Vomiting	• Skin Changes • Headache • Blurry Vision
Breast	• Fatigue • Hair Loss • Skin Changes	• Swelling • Tenderness
Chest	• Fatigue • Hair Loss • Skin Changes	• Throat changes (i.e. trouble swallowing) • Shortness of Breath • Cough
Head and Neck	• Fatigue • Hair Loss • Mouth Changes	• Skin Changes • Taste Changes • Throat changes (i.e. trouble swallowing)
Pelvis	• Diarrhea • Fatigue • Hair Loss • Nausea/Vomiting	• Sexuality & fertility • Skin Changes • Urinary & Bladder Changes
Rectum	• Diarrhea • Fatigue • Hair Loss • Nausea/Vomiting	• Sexuality & fertility • Skin Changes • Urinary & Bladder Changes
Stomach and Abdomen	• Diarrhea • Fatigue • Hair Loss	• Nausea/Vomiting • Skin Changes • Urinary & Bladder Changes

3

Radiation therapy often results in skin damage known as radiation dermatitis. A study of 40 people with breast cancer who had received radiation therapy for breast cancer were randomized into two groups. In the first group, patients were treated with five grams of supplemental glutamine three times daily. The second group received a placebo. Those receiving glutamine had a significant reduction in radiation dermatitis compared to placebo.[4]

CHEMOTHERAPY

Chemotherapy refers to the use of chemical agents (drugs) to treat cancer. Chemotherapy can be used to cure cancer, prevent cancer's return, reduce pain, stop or slow cancer's growth, or shrink a tumor. It is often used with other conventional therapies, such as radiation and surgery.

The term *chemotherapy* was first coined by German chemist Paul Ehrlich, who focused on developing drugs to treat infectious diseases and cancer. He had some success with infectious disease but not cancer.[5]

The effects of sulfur mustards (mustard gas) as a chemical agent were observed during World War I. Later, during World War II, the effects of an accidental spill of mustard gas and exposure to troops led to the observation of bone marrow damage. This resulted in reduced white blood cell counts and the reduction of swollen lymph nodes. These observations led researchers to theorize this chemical agent might have benefit for cancer with these same signs and symptoms.

Yale researchers then confirmed mustard agents could stop the growth of rapidly dividing cancer cells in mice.[6] The next step of progression occurred in 1943 with the administration of nitrogen mustard to a person with non-Hodgkin's lymphoma, where marked improvement was noted. This research, published in 1946, resulted in a flurry of research of chemotherapy for lymphomas.[7]

A different type of chemotherapy was developed soon after World War II. Drugs that could block folate metabolism were found to be effective for children with leukemia.[8] Today this common anticancer drug is known as methotrexate.

In addition, another program related to World War II involved the evaluation of certain antibiotics for their antitumor effects. An antibiotic known as actinomycin D was developed and shown to have significant antitumor properties and was used for pediatric tumors in the 1950s and 1960s.[9] This drug spurred the development of several antitumor antibiotics.

Like radiation therapy, chemotherapy can kill both cancer cells and healthy cells. Side effects vary depending on the individual and types of chemotherapy. An identical dose of a chemotherapy agent may result in mild toxicity for one person and life-threatening toxicity in another. The most common side effect is fatigue. Other common side effects include nausea, vomiting, decreased blood cell counts, mouth sores, hair loss, and pain.

"Debbie," a 65-year-old new patient of Dr. Stengler's, had recently been diagnosed with metastatic cancer that had spread from her breast to the spine of her neck, ribs, and an area of one of her lungs.

She had already received radiation therapy to her neck (cervical spine), surgery, and had just started chemotherapy. She was started on a regimen of intravenous vitamin C and ozone therapy. Her swollen glands began to shrink, and her energy greatly improved. Today she continues a maintenance regimen of these therapies.

Recent scans by her oncologist had shown tremendous improvement in her cancer lesions.

Many different chemotherapy agents are used by oncologists. These treatments can be administered in several ways, including oral (capsules, tablets, and liquids), intravenous (directly into a vein), by injection into the skin or muscle, intrathecal (injection in the space between the layers of tissue that cover the brain and spinal cord), intraperitoneal (injection into the body cavity that contains organs such as the intestines, stomach, and liver), intra-arterial (directly into an artery), and topical application (often used for skin cancer).[10]

The treatment schedules for chemotherapy vary and depend on several factors. Generally, treatments are given in cycles, such as every day, week, or month. Rest periods give your body a chance to recover and to prevent serious side effects.

In this section, we will describe the common types of chemotherapy, how they work, and potential side effects. For information on alternative therapies that may reduce the side effects of chemotherapy, see Chapter 8.

Alkylating agents that are platinum-based, such as cisplatin, carboplatin, oxaliplatin, pyriplatin, and phenanthriplatin, are given to approximately half of all patients undergoing chemotherapy.[11] These anticancer agents have been shown in multiple studies to cause magnesium deficiency. Symptoms of magnesium deficiency may include muscle cramps, fatigue, anxiety, insomnia, irritability, weakness, seizures, abnormal heart rhythm, migraine headache, loss of appetite, depression, and abnormal nerve sensations.

Research has shown that between 41 percent and 100 percent of patients receiving low-dose cisplatin became deficient in magnesium.[12] Research has also shown that magnesium supplementation during platinum-based chemotherapy significantly reduces the degree of low magnesium levels.[13] It is recommended that everyone on this type of chemotherapy take supplemental magnesium either orally (400 mg daily) or intravenously. Speak with your oncologist and integrative doctor about magnesium supplementation as part of your treatment.

ALKYLATING AGENTS

The first anticancer molecules developed were alkylating agents.[14] They have been used for more than 50 years and continue to be used today. They interfere with a cancer's ability to reproduce itself by damaging its DNA. They are used to treat a variety of cancers including lung, breast, ovary, leukemia, lymphoma, Hodgkin's disease, multiple myeloma, and sarcoma.[15]

Side effects may include toxicity of the bone marrow, intestinal mucosa, and other organ systems, including the testicles and ovaries.[16] The risk of leukemia increases with higher doses of the drug being used.[17] Nausea and vomiting are common side effects that are not well controlled by conventional medications.[18]

There are six major classes of alkylating agents:[19] [20]

- ALKYL SULFONATES

  - Busulfan (Busulfex, Myleran)

- ETHYLENEIMINES/METHYLMELAMINES

  - Altretamine (Hexalen)

  - Thiotepa (Thioplex, Tepadina)

- NITROGEN MUSTARDS

  - Mechlorethamine (Mustargen)

  - Melphalan (Alkeran, Evomela)

  - Chlorambucil (Leukeran)

  - Cyclophosphamide (Cytoxan, Neosar, Cytoxan Lyophilized)

  - Ifosfamide (Ifex)

- NITROSUREAS

  - Carmustine (BiCNU, Gliadel)

  - Streptozotocin (Zanosar)

- TRIAZINES

  - Dacarbazine (DTIC-Dome)
  - Temozolomide (Temodar)

- METAL SALTS

  - Carboplatin (Paraplatin, CARBOplatin Novaplus)
  - Cisplatin (Platinol, Platinol-AQ)
  - Oxaliplatin (Eloxatin)

Research has demonstrated that using fish oil as a supplement improves the effectiveness of chemotherapy without negative side effects.

A one-year study published in the journal *Cancer* looked at the effects of fish oil supplementation in 46 people with a diagnosis of non–small cell lung cancer. All patients received a standard first line of chemotherapy protocol (carboplatin with either vinorelbine or gemcitabine). Keep in mind that the response rate to first-line chemotherapy in patients with non–small cell lung cancer is less than 30 percent. Thirty-one people received chemotherapy while an additional 15 people supplemented fish oil (2.5 grams of EPA and DHA) per day in addition to chemotherapy. Those taking the fish oil had a favorable response rate more than double the chemotherapy only group (60 percent versus 25.8 percent). As well, clinical benefit was significantly improved in the fish oil group (80.0 percent versus 41.9 percent), and the one-year survival tended to be greater in the fish oil group (60.0 percent versus 38.7 percent).[21]

ANTIMETABOLITES

Antimetabolites are drugs that interfere with cancer-cell replication. Their mechanism of action involves the interference of specific phases of cell division. They are used to treat leukemias, as well as cancers of the breast, ovary, intestinal tract, and others.[22]

Several side effects are possible depending on the drug being used. For example, methotrexate may cause bleeding of the digestive tract, elevated liver enzymes, joint pain, diarrhea, sores in the mouth or lips, stomach pain, and swelling of the feet or lower legs.[23]

Antimetabolites are classified according to the substance with which they interfere regarding cancer-cell replication. These include:[24]

- Folic acid antagonist: Methotrexate (Rheumatrex Dose Pack, Trexall)

- Pyrimidine antagonist: 5-Fluorouracil (Adrucil), floxuridine (FUDR), cytarabine (Cytosar-U, Tarabine PFS, Cytosar), capecitabine (Xeloda), and gemcitabine (Gemzar)

- Purine antagonist: 6-Mercaptopurine (Purinethol, Purixan) and 6-Thioguanine (Tabloid)

- Adenosine deaminase inhibitor: Cladribine (Cladribine Novaplus, Leustatin), fludarabine (Fludara), nelarabine (Arranon), and pentostatin (Nipent)

ANTITUMOR ANTIBIOTICS

Antitumor antibiotics are made to fight cancer, and not infection. They interfere with the DNA inside of cancer cells to prevent cell division.

Side effects may include severe nausea and vomiting, hair loss, bone marrow suppression, mucositis, liver disease, skin redness, acne, digestive tract bleeding, cough or hoarseness, fever or chills, lower back or side pain, painful or difficult urination, and bruising.[26][27][28] One of the major concerns with antitumor antibiotics given in high dosages is permanent heart damage.[29]

Different types of antitumor antibiotics include:[30]

- Daunorubicin (Cerubidine)

- Doxorubicin (Adriamycin, Rubex)

- Epirubicin (Ellence, Pharmorubicin PFS, Pharmorubicin RDF)

- Idarubicin (Idamycin)

- Actinomycin-D (dactinomycin, Cosmegen)

- Bleomycin (Bleo 15k, Blenoxane)

- Mitomycin-C (Mutamycin)

- Mitoxantrone (Novantrone)

Curcuminoids (curcumin) are a group of compounds found in the popular spice turmeric. A randomized, double-blind, placebo-controlled trial of 40 men and 40 women aged 25 to 65 years with solid tumors undergoing chemotherapy for eight weeks found that curcuminoid supplementation improved quality-of-life scores and reduced inflammatory blood markers. Participants took 900 mg of a standardized curcumin product daily.[25]

The main types of cancers included colorectal, gastric, and breast cancer. Common chemotherapy agents included docetaxel-cisplatin-5-fluorouracil, topotecan-cyclophosphamide-etoposide, cyclophosphamide-methotrexate-5 fluorouracil, and 5-fluorouracil based regimens.

TOPOISOMERASE INHIBITORS

Topoisomerase inhibitors are chemotherapy drugs that interfere with the action of topoisomerase enzymes. These enzymes are required for the separating of strands of DNA so they can be copied and are essential for preventing and resolving DNA and RNA copying and replication.[31]

These drugs are used to treat certain leukemias, as well as lung, ovarian, gastrointestinal, and other cancers.[32]

Side effects can include diarrhea, constipation, nausea, vomiting, stomach pain, loss of appetite, weakness, fever, pain, abnormal liver-function tests, temporary hair loss, and increased risk of cancer, such as leukemia.[33][34] Some of these medications carry the risk of cardiac toxicity.[35]

These drugs include:[36][37]

- Irinotecan (Camptosar)

- Topotecan (Hycamtin)

- Etoposide (VePesid)

- Teniposide (Vumon)

- Mitoxantrone (Novantrone)

The sleep hormone melatonin, which is available over the counter as a dietary supplement, has been shown in combination with chemotherapy to benefit people with solid tumors. A meta-analysis of eight randomized controlled trials that included chemotherapy in six of the trials concluded that 20 mg of melatonin significantly improved the complete and partial remission as well as one-year survival rate. The effects were consistent across different types of cancer and no severe adverse events were reported.[38]

MITOTIC INHIBITORS

Mitotic inhibitors, also referred to as antimicrotubule agents, contain compounds derived from natural products, such as certain plants. They inhibit mitosis, or cell division, and their mechanism of action is to disrupt structures in cells known as microtubules, which pull the cell apart when it divides. When the activity of microtubules is disrupted, a cell cannot divide properly.

The first class of mitotic inhibitors were the taxanes, which were the result of an investigation of 35,000 plant extracts in 1963, during which an anticancer compound known as paclitaxel (Taxol) was identified in the bark extract of the Pacific yew tree.[39] In 1992, it received approval for the treatment of ovarian cancer and subsequently for several other cancers.[40] Since then other taxanes have been developed, another well-known one being docetaxel (Taxotere).

Side-effect concerns of the taxanes include nerve damage (or neuropathy), low white blood cell count (or neutropenia), bone marrow suppression, nausea and vomiting, and allergic reactions.[41]

Another class of mitotic inhibitors is the vinca alkaloids. Since their introduction 40 years ago, they have been commonly used as chemotherapy agents.[42] They are naturally occurring and extracted from the leaves of the periwinkle plant *Catharanthus roseus* G. Don.[43] They were first used for childhood cancers (blood and solid tumor malignancies) and later for adult blood malignancies,[44] leading the way for semisynthetic vinca alkaloids to be developed, such as vinorelbine, vindesine, and vinflunine.[45]

Two of the major concerns with vinca alkaloids are neutropenia (low white blood cells) and neurotoxicity (nerve toxicity). Other concerns include thrombocytopenia (low platelets), anemia, digestive complaints, hair loss, and vein inflammation.[46]

The next category is known as microtubule antagonists. One of the common chemotherapy drugs in this group is estramustine phosphate, which is used for men with castration-resistant prostate cancer. The most common side effects are nausea and vomiting. Other problems can include gynecomastia, nipple tenderness, fluid retention, and thrombophlebitis.[47]

Next is a class of chemotherapy drugs known as mitotic motor protein inhibitors. They are currently under development and include aurora kinase and polo-like kinase inhibitors as well as kinesin spindle protein inhibitors.

These are common examples of mitotic inhibitors:

- TAXANES
    - Paclitaxel (Onxol, Taxol)
    - Docetaxel (Docefrez, Taxotere)
    - Cabazitaxel (Jevtana)

- EPOTHILONES
    - Ixabepilone (Ixempra)

- VINCA ALKALOIDS
    - Vinblastine (Velban)
    - Vincristine (Oncovin, Vincasar PFS)
    - Vinorelbine (Navelbine)
    - Vinflunine (Javlor)

Chemotherapy-induced peripheral neuropathy (nerve pain and abnormal sensations) is common in patients receiving taxane-derived drugs and other chemotherapy agents, including platinum compounds and vinca alkaloids.

A prospective, randomized, double-blind, placebo-controlled and paralleled clinical study evaluated the effectiveness and safety of the supplement acetyl-L-carnitine (ALC) for the treatment of chemotherapy-induced peripheral neuropathy. Of the 239 participants, 118 people received 3000 mg daily of ALC, while 121 received a placebo. Those taking ALC had significant improvement in peripheral neuropathy symptoms compared to the placebo group. As well, there were no differences in adverse events between the two groups.[48]

TYROSINE-KINASE INHIBITORS (TKI)

Tyrosine-kinase inhibitors (TKI) comprise another class of chemotherapy medication. They were developed from the standpoint of modern genetics and their relation to cancer-cell formation. They inhibit, or block, the family of enzymes known as tyrosine kinase, which plays an important role in the regulation of cell functions, such as cell division (replication), cell metabolism, survival, DNA damage repair, cell motility, and response to the microenvironment.[49] Kinase inhibitors are needed for cell signals and growth factors that are involved in cell division. Genetic mutations of these kinases can lead to oncogenes, which are genes that can turn a healthy cell into a cancerous cell.[50] Over the past 16 years, research has shown that tumors with a kinase mutation are much more likely to respond to treatment with the appropriate TKI.[51]

Several TKI medications, including imatinib and gefitinib, have Food and Drug Administration approval for use in humans. The first TKI, imatinib, was approved in 2001 for the treatment of chronic myeloid leukemia (CML).[52] The very high response rate was a motivating factor for additional research and development in this area.

TKIs have a different mechanism from traditional chemotherapy drugs (although monoclonal antibodies work in a similar way). Since they are more targeted to actual cancer cells and not healthy cells, the potential for toxicity and side effects is greatly reduced compared with traditional chemotherapy. The genetic basis for cancer is now being screened more effectively, and treatment can include TKIs.

Potential side effects vary greatly depending on the TKI being used. Most side effects are mild, but there is the risk of serious side effects, which may cause decreased white blood cell count (increased infection risk), decreased platelets (increased bleeding risk), nausea or vomiting, diarrhea, heartburn, headache, muscle cramps, fluid retention and swelling (especially around the eyes), and rash.[53] TKIs, such as sunitinib, may cause serious liver problems, including liver failure. Also, dasatinib may increase the risk for pulmonary arterial hypertension.[54] In general, TKIs may cause depression.[55]

These are common TKIs:

- Dasatinib (Sprycel)

- Imatinib (Gleevec)

- Nilotinib (Tasigna)

- Sorafenib (Nexavar)

- Sunitinib (Sutent)

HISTONE DEACETYLASE INHIBITORS

Histone deacetylases (HDACs) are enzymes that play an important role in the expression of DNA and act as oncogenes (cancer genes).[56] While one's inherited DNA is fixed, the emerging science of epigenetics has demonstrated that the expression (activity) of DNA can be altered.

Histones are proteins that are contained in cells that provide structural support for tightly packed DNA and regulate the function of DNA. Therefore they play an important role in cell replication and transcribing (passing on information) for the formation of the body's protein building blocks.[57]

HDAC inhibitors have been mainly used in the treatment of hematological (blood) cancers, particularly acute myeloid leukemia (AML). More recently, the condition multiple myeloma has been treated with a specific HDAC inhibitor known as panobinostat.

Many HDAC inhibitors are being investigated for their effectiveness in cancer. Common side effects include nausea, vomiting, loss of appetite, fatigue, fever, anemia, cardiac arrhythmia, diarrhea, neutropenia, and thrombocytopenia.[58]

Here are current HDACs in use:

- Vorinostat (Zolinza)

- Romidepsin (Istodax)

- Belinostat (Beleodaq)

- Panobinostat (Farydak)

DEMETHYLATING AGENTS

Demethylating agents also play a role in altering the expression of DNA, known as epigenetics. The term *methylation* is a term that means the addition of a methyl group (CH3) to a compound, such as a portion of DNA, which influences gene expression and activity. Abnormal DNA methylation is a known factor in some cancers.

These drugs are used for blood cancers, such as chronic myelomonocytic leukemia or bone marrow cancer. They work in part by destroying abnormally dividing cells in the bone marrow.[59][60]

Common side effects include bladder pain, bleeding gums, blood in stool, blood in urine, blue lips and fingernails, blurred vision, body aches or pains, chest pain, chills, coma, congestion, convulsions, cough urination problems, dizziness, drowsiness, fainting, fast or irregular heartbeat, feeling unusually cold, fever, flushed and dry skin, fruit-like breath odor, headache, hives or welts, hoarseness, increased hunger, increased sweating, increased thirst, insomnia, itching, joint pain, light-headedness, loss of appetite, low back or side pain, mood or mental changes, muscle pain or cramps, muscle spasms or twitching, nausea or vomiting, pale skin, pinpoint red spots on skin, runny nose, seizures, shivering, shortness of breath, skin rash, sneezing, sore mouth or tongue, sore throat, sores or white spots on lips or in mouth, stomach pain or bloating, sunken eyes, swelling of various body parts, swollen and painful lymph nodes in neck or armpit or groin, tightness in chest, trembling, trouble swallowing, breathing problems, swelling around anus, urination problems, weight loss, weakness or heaviness of legs, wheezing, wrinkled skin, and yellow eyes or skin.[61][62]

These are common demethylating agents:

- Azacitidine (Vidaza)

- Decitabine (Dacogen)

POLY (ADP-RIBOSE) POLYMERASE INHIBITORS

Poly (ADP-ribose) polymerase inhibitors, also known as PARP inhibitors, are pharmaceuticals used to block the PARP enzyme in cells. Poly (ADP-ribose) Polymerase, or PARP, is an enzyme that helps cancer cells repair their DNA.

Blocking this cell-repair mechanism makes it more difficult for cancer cells to repair their damaged DNA, causing them to die.[63]

PAPR inhibitors are considered a type of chemotherapy known as "targeted therapy," which means they more precisely identify and attack cancer cells. They are most often used along with other cancer treatments.[64]

Several PARP inhibitors are in clinical trials. Currently two main ones have FDA approval. The first is olaparib, which is mainly used for the treatment of advanced ovarian cancer with a specific abnormal inherited gene.[65] The other is niraparib, which is used to prevent the return of cancers, such as those of the ovary, fallopian tube, or peritoneum.[66]

Common side effects may include abnormal kidney function, altered sense of taste, blood in stool, bleeding gums, blood in urine, blurred vision, chills, cold symptoms, cough, dizziness, changes in heartbeat or pulse, digestive upset, headache, muscle or joint pain, nervousness, painful or difficult urination, pale skin, pinpoint red spots on skin, pounding in the ears, rash, troubled breathing with exertion, ulcers, sores or white spots in mouth, unusual bleeding or bruising, and unusual tiredness or weakness.[67][68]

These are common PARP inhibitors:

- Olaparib (Lynparza)

- Niraparib (Zejula)

OTHER CHEMOTHERAPY AGENTS

Several additional chemotherapy agents have different mechanisms of action. We have summarized many them in the following table, along with the types of cancer for which they are used.[69]

DRUG NAME	INDICATED CANCER
Omacetaxine (Synribo)	Chronic Myeolid Leukemi
L-Asparaginase	Pediatric and adult Acute Lymphoblastic Leukemia
Bleomycin	Hodgkin's disease, neoplastic pleural effusion, non-Hodgkin's Lymphoma, squamous cell carcinoma of the following: cervix, nasopharynx, penis, head and neck, vulva, and testicular cancer
Procarbazine (Matulane)	Hodgkin's lymphoma
Vismodegib (Erivedge)	Basal cell carcinoma of the skin
Ado-trastuzumab-emtansine (Kadcyla)	Advanced HER2-positive breast cancer
Temsirolimus (Torisel)	Advanced renal (kidney) cancer
Everolimus (Zortress)	Advanced renal (kidney) cancer, breast cancer, pancreatic neuroendocrine tumor
Thalidomide (Thalomid)	Multiple myeloma, erythema nodosum leprosum
Lenalidomide (Revlimid)	Multiple myeloma, low to intermediate risk myelodysplastic syndrome associated with 5q deletion
Pomalidomide (Pomalyst)	Multiple myeloma

According to the conventional online publication Medscape, several studies from the United States and Europe have found that exposure to chemotherapy treatments can harm nurses and health-care workers.[70]

The article notes that it is well known that medical staff, such as pharmacists, are at risk for exposure and side effects.

The potential for harm also includes the nurses who administer the chemotherapy medications. The article reports oncology nurses in the UK experiencing common chemotherapy side effects, such as significant hair loss, high incidence of miscarriage, and flu-like symptoms.

But there are concerns in the United States, as well. A 2012 study found the overall rate of exposure to the skin or eyes in the past year among oncology nurses who were working in outpatient settings (and not round-the-clock care) of cancer patients as 16.9 percent.[71]

HORMONAL AGENTS

Hormones are chemical substances produced by several glands in the body for a variety of functions. They have different effects in the body, including the proliferation of cells in certain tissues. Hormonal agents are generally used to stop the body's production of hormones or interfere or block cell receptor sites that interact with hormones.[72] Their goal is to stop or reduce the proliferating action of certain hormones on hormone-sensitive tissues, especially the breast, prostate, and uterus (endometrial lining).[73]

Oncologists use hormone receptor tests to determine whether the cancer cells are sensitive to hormones. The hormone receptor test measures the amount of hormone receptors in cancer tissue. Hormones, such as estrogen and progesterone, can attach to these receptors. A positive test means the hormone is likely stimulating the cancer cells to grow, which would indicate treatment by hormonal agents that prevent the receptors from being hormonally stimulated.[74]

Hormonal agents can also be used for paraneoplastic syndromes, or rare disorders where one has symptoms that are triggered by an immune response from substances produced by a cancer. The most common symptom would be fever.[75] They can also be used for symptoms of cancer, such as cancer-related anorexia (loss of appetite).[76]

Hormonal agents are normally given by oral medications or injection, but in some cases, organs, such as ovaries and testicles, are removed surgically to decrease the production of hormones.

Different classes of hormonal agents manipulate the hormonal system in various ways. We will review the major ones.

SELECTIVE ESTROGEN RECEPTOR MODULATORS (SERMS)

Selective estrogen receptor modulators (SERMs) are hormonal agents that work by blocking estrogen receptors in breast tissue and making it more difficult for breast cancers to grow. The term *selective* refers to the fact that SERMs block estrogen receptors in breast tissue but can activate estrogen receptors in other cells, such as bone, liver, and uterine cells.[77]

Tamoxifen is the most commonly used SERM for the prevention and treatment of breast cancer worldwide.[78] It is the only hormonal agent approved by the FDA for the prevention of premenopausal breast cancer, the treatment of ductal carcinoma in situ (DCIS), and the treatment of surgically treated premenopausal breast cancer that is estrogen receptor positive.[79]

The most common side effects of SERMs are fatigue, hot flashes, night sweats, vaginal discharge, and mood swings. They can also cause serious side effects, including blood clots, stroke, and endometrial cancer.[80]

These are common SERMs:

- Tamoxifen (Nolvadex)

- Toremifene (Fareston)

- Raloxifene (Evista)

"Wendy," a 40-year-old mother of two, had recently been treated for breast cancer and was prescribed tamoxifen (Nolvadex) by her oncologist. As a result, she experienced hot flashes and night sweats that woke her up. She also noted that her mood changed often, and she was quite irritable. Dr. Mark was able to help control her symptoms with a homeopathic remedy known as Sepia.

AROMATASE INHIBITORS

Aromatase inhibitors are commonly used hormonal agents for the prevention and treatment of breast cancer. They are preferred over tamoxifen for postmenopausal women with early stage, estrogen-positive breast cancer.[81] They also have fewer serious side effects than tamoxifen.

Aromatase inhibitors work by blocking the enzyme aromatase, which blocks the conversion of sex hormones produced by the adrenal glands into estrogens.[82]

Two drugs in this class, letrozole and anastrazole, have been shown to be superior to tamoxifen in response rates and progression-free survival for metastatic breast cancer.[83]

The most common side effects from aromatase inhibitors are joint stiffness and pain, as well as muscle pain. This can occur in up to 50 percent of users.[84]

These are common aromatase inhibitors:

- Anastrazole (Arimidex)

- Letrozole (Femara)

- Exemestane (Aromasin)

"Patti," a 60-year-old accountant and breast cancer survivor, had been experiencing arthritis in several of her joints. Her oncologist confirmed that this was a side effect of her drug anastrazole (Arimidex). She consulted with Dr. Mark for his recommendations. He recommended supplements that supported cartilage and joint health such as collagen, glucosamine, and MSM. Within two weeks she noticed improvement, and after eight weeks she stated that her arthritis pain and stiffness were 80 percent improved.

SELECTIVE ESTROGEN RECEPTOR DOWN-REGULATOR (SERD)

Selective estrogen receptor down-regulator, also known as SERD, currently refers to one breast cancer drug known as fulvestrant (Faslodex). It competitively binds with estrogen receptors.[85] It is also known as an estrogen receptor antagonist. In other words, it prevents estrogen from activating estrogen receptors in cells. It has an affinity for estrogen receptors approximately 100 times greater than tamoxifen.[86]

Fulvestrant is approved to treat hormone receptor–positive breast cancer in postmenopausal women that has spread to other parts of the body.[87] It is given as an injection.

The most common side effects are hot flashes, nausea, vomiting, diarrhea, constipation, stomach/abdominal pain, sore throat, back pain, and headache.[88]

LUTEINIZING HORMONE RELEASING HORMONE AGONIST (LHRH AGONIST)

Luteinizing hormone is produced by the pituitary gland located at the base of the brain and stimulates the testicles to produce testosterone. LHRH agonists, also known as gonadotropin-releasing hormone blockers or androgen deprivation therapy, stop the production of luteinizing hormone and prevent testosterone production by the testicles.[89] They are given as an injection or placed as small implants under the skin.

LHRH agonists are used for men with prostate cancer in combination with the drug flutamide plus radiation therapy for locally advanced prostate cancer.[90] It is also approved to lessen or relieve symptoms of prostate cancer.[91] Although testosterone replacement has not been shown to cause prostate cancer, once it is already present, testosterone can stimulate further cell division. Thus the focus of this class of medications is suppression of testosterone and its metabolite dihydro-testosterone (DHT).

LHRH agonist therapy is also used for the treatment of breast cancer. By stopping the production of luteinizing hormone, the stimulation of estrogen and progesterone by the ovaries is reduced. This reduces the stimulation of hormone-positive breast cancer receptors.

Side effects for men may include an initial increase in tumor size, hot flashes, breast tenderness or increase in breast tissue, impotence and loss of sex drive, osteoporosis, high blood sugar and diabetes, heart problems, seizures, muscle or back or joint pain and aching, fatigue, and reduction or stoppage of sperm pro-duction.[92 93]

Side effects for women may include an initial increase in tumor size, hot flashes, osteoporosis, muscle or joint pain and aching, fatigue, vaginal dryness, headaches, mood swings, depression, nausea and/or vomiting, high blood sugar and diabetes, heart problems, heart attack and stroke, seizures, and stoppage of the menstrual cycle.[94 95]

These are common LHRH agonists:

- Leuprolide (Lupron, Eligard)

- Goserelin (Zoladex)

- Triptorelin (Trelstar)

- Histrelin (Vantas)

LUTEINIZING HORMONE RELEASING HORMONE ANTAGONIST (LHRH ANTAGONIST)

LHRH is also sometimes referred to as gonadotropin-releasing hormone antagonist (GnRH antagonist). This refers to one current medication known as degarelix (Firmagon). It is a man-made form of a protein that blocks the production of gonadotropin-releasing hormone (GnRH) by the pituitary gland,[96] which prevents GnRH stimulation of testosterone by the testicles and creates what is known as a medical castration.

Like the LHRH agonists, degarelix is used to lower testosterone but does so more quickly. It also has the advantage of not causing initial tumor growth flare-ups like the LHRH agonists.[97]

Side effects may include hot flashes, breast tenderness or increase in breast tissue, osteoporosis, reduction or stoppage of sperm production, elevated liver enzymes, and weight gain.[98]

ANTI-ANDROGENS

Androgen deprivation therapy (ADT), also known as androgen suppression therapy, refers to the reduction or suppression of androgen hormones produced by the testicles and adrenal glands. The use of anti-androgens blocks androgens, such as testosterone, from attaching to the receptors on the surface of prostate cancer cells.[99] These anti-androgens are used to keep cancer cells from growing or to cause them to grow more slowly and are taken daily as pills.[100]

ADT is not typically used as a sole treatment. It can be used in addition to orchiectomy (removal of the testicles) or LHRH agonist or antagonist therapy if these therapies are no longer working. After an LHRH agonist begins, it may be given for a few weeks to prevent a tumor flare-up (increased growth).[101]

Common side effects may include bloating or swelling of the face, arms, hands, lower legs, or feet; blurred vision; congestion; cough or hoarseness; dryness or soreness of the throat; fever; headache; lower back pain; nervousness; pounding in the ears; rapid weight gain; runny nose; slow or fast heartbeat; sweating; tender, swollen glands in the neck; tightness in the chest; tingling of the hands or feet; trouble with swallowing; weight loss; wheezing; pain in the back, pelvis, or stomach; increased nighttime urination; weakness; dizziness; nausea; diarrhea;

constipation; black, tarry stools; bloody or cloudy urine; difficult or burning, painful urination; pale skin; troubled breathing with exertion; unusual bleeding or bruising; chills; insomnia; vomiting; runny nose; muscle aches and pains; and fatigue.[102] [103] The toxicity of nilutamide has limited its use, as it may cause night blindness and pulmonary (lung) toxicity.[104]

These are common anti-androgens:

- Flutamide (Eulexin)

- Bicalutamide (Casodex)

- Nilutamide (Nilandron)

"Don," a 70-year-old real estate agent, had been on aggressive therapy for his prostate cancer. Part of his cancer therapy included the anti-androgen drug bicalutamide (Casodex), which caused several side effects, the most concerning of which was fatigue.

Dr. Mark boosted his energy levels naturally with intravenous nutrient therapy that included B vitamins and magnesium, as well as supplements that supported his adrenal glands. Within four weeks, Don noted the significant improvement of his energy and quality of life.

CYP17 INHIBITOR

Men with advanced prostate cancer are often treated with LHRH agonists and antagonists, or orchiectomy, which can stop the testicles from making androgens such as testosterone. However, prostate cancer cells and other cells in the body can still make small amounts of androgens. The use of a medication known as abiraterone (Zytiga) blocks an enzyme known as CYP17, which works to stop the production of androgens by other cells.[105]

This medication is taken daily as a pill. Since it lowers other hormones in the body, the drug prednisone needs to be taken along with it to prevent certain side effects.[106]

More common side effects may include bladder pain; bloating or swelling of the face, arms, hands, lower legs, or feet; bloody or cloudy urine; blurred vision; bone fracture; chest pain or discomfort; convulsions; decreased urine; difficult, burning, or painful urination; dry mouth; fast, pounding, or irregular heartbeat or pulse; feeling of warmth; frequent urge to urinate; headache; increased thirst; increased urge to urinate during the night; light-headedness, dizziness, or fainting; loss of appetite; lower back or side pain; mood changes; muscle pain or cramps; nausea or vomiting; nervousness; numbness or tingling in the hands, feet, or lips; pain or swelling in the arms or legs without any injury; pounding in the ears; rapid weight gain; redness of the face, neck, arms, and occasionally upper chest; shortness of breath; slow heartbeat; sudden sweating; swelling with pits or depressions on the skin; unusual tiredness or weakness; and unusual weight gain or loss.[107]

OTHER ANTI-ANDROGENS

Enzalutamide (Xtandi) is a newer anti-androgen. It is also an androgen receptor inhibitor that acts on multiple steps of the androgen receptor signaling pathway within the tumor cell.[108] It is used for men with advanced prostate cancer that has not responded to therapy. This medication is taken daily as a pill.

Common side effects may include headache; dizziness; spinning sensation; shortness of breath; weakness or fatigue; increased blood pressure; numbness, burning pain, or prickly feeling under your skin; flushing; back pain; joint or muscle pain; bone pain; swelling in the arms or legs; loss of appetite; weight loss; diarrhea; constipation; and cold symptoms, such as stuffy nose, sneezing, or sore throat.[109]

OTHER SEX STEROID THERAPIES

There are a few other medications that are used to disrupt the hormonal stimulation of cancers, which are described below.

Fluoxymesterone

This drug is an androgen (synthetic testosterone) that has been used in women with metastatic breast cancer who have hormonally responsive cancers but have not responded well to other hormonal therapies such as tamoxifen or megestrol acetate.[110] This medication is taken daily as a pill.

Side effects may include hirsutism (excessive growth of facial or body hair), male-pattern baldness, voice lowering (hoarseness), acne, enhanced libido, erythrocytosis, and elevated liver function tests.

Estrogens

One of the early treatments for prostate cancer was synthetic versions of female hormones known as estrogens. They are not used much anymore due to side effects on the cardiovascular system.[111] Occasionally they are used after typical hormone therapy has failed. Estrogen therapy is usually taken daily as a pill.

Examples of estrogens used with men are Premarin and estradiol.

Megestrol and Medroxyprogesterone

Megestrol and medroxyprogesterone are progesterone derivatives that are different structurally from the progesterone produced in the human body. These medications are given daily as a pill.

In the past, megestrol was used as a hormonal agent for the treatment of advanced breast cancer. Currently megestrol is most often used to treat hormonally responsive metastatic endometrial cancer, and occasionally it is used to treat prostate cancer. It is also used for anorexia and cachexia related to cancer. Also, it is used to control hot flashes in women with breast cancer and in men who have had androgen ablation therapy (androgen deprivation therapy or castration). Although it may cause nausea and vomiting, it has been shown to decrease nausea and vomiting in advanced-stage cancer patients by approximately two-thirds.[112]

Medroxyprogesterone is very similar in its activity as megestrol. It is used more commonly in Europe than the United States for the treatment of breast cancer.[113]

The exact mechanisms of the antitumor effects of these drugs is unclear. Several mechanisms have been reported, including the suppression of adrenal steroid synthesis, suppressed estrogen receptor levels, altered tumor hormone metabolism, enhanced steroid metabolism, and the direct killing of tumor cells.[114]

Common side effects may include nausea, gas, diarrhea, vaginal bleeding, mild skin rash, weakness, and swelling.[115] [116]

Ketoconazole (Nizoral)

Ketoconazole, or Nizoral, is a drug that is mainly known for its antifungal effects. Yet it is used to block the production of hormones, such as androgens, in a manner similar to the drug abiraterone. It may be used to treat advanced prostate cancer in men as it quickly lowers testosterone levels.[117] Since it also blocks the production of the hormone cortisol, men treated with ketoconazole often require a corticosteroid such as hydrocortisone or prednisone. This medication is taken daily as a pill.

Common side effects include nausea, vomiting, stomach pain, itching or skin rash, headache, dizziness, breast swelling, impotence, and loss of interest in sex.[118]

OTHER HORMONAL THERAPIES

Octreotide

Octreotide is a drug and an analog of the natural chemical in the body known as somatostatin. Somatostatin is produced in an area of the brain known as the hypothalamus. It has several functions, including the inhibition of certain chemicals in the body that in part control flushing and diarrhea. Octreotide is a better choice for treatment than somatostatin since it is more stable and longer acting in the body.[119]

Octreotide is used for the treatment of carcinoid syndrome and other hormonal excess syndromes associated with some pancreatic islet cell cancers and acromegaly.[120]

Anti-angiogenesis Agents

The term *angiogenesis* refers to the creation of new blood vessels. This is a normal process for healthy tissues that are damaged and need repair. But in terms of cancer, the process of creating small blood vessels that feed a tumor and allow it to grow is problematic.

Anti-angiogenesis agents, also known as angiogenesis inhibitors, refers to a type of targeted therapy that uses drugs to stop tumors from making new blood vessels.[121] These medications can be taken daily as a pill or intravenously.

Different types of anti-angiogenesis drugs target different mechanisms of stopping blood vessel development so tumor blood supply is cut off. One of the most common drugs is bevacizumab (Avastin), which is a type of monoclonal antibody that recognizes and binds to vascular endothelial growth factor (VEGF). This growth factor protein is involved in the signaling that promotes the growth of new blood vessels. Bevacizumab prevents the activation of VEGF.[122] Other anti-angiogenesis agents, such as sorafenib (Nexavar) and sunitinib (Sutent), have different mechanisms in which they block VEGF activity.[123]

Side effects may include high blood pressure, rash, dry and itchy skin, hand-foot syndrome, diarrhea, fatigue, low blood counts, and problems with wounds healing or cuts reopening. Less common but more serious side effects can include serious bleeding, heart attacks, heart failure, or blood clots.[124]

These are common anti-angiogenesis agents include:

- Axitinib (Inlyta)

- Bevacizumab (Avastin)

- Cabozantinib (Cometriq)

- Everolimus (Afinitor, Zortress)

- Lenalidomide (Revlimid)

- Pazopanib (Votrient)

- Ramucirumab (Cyramza)

- Regorafenib (Stivarga)

- Sorafenib (Nexavar)

- Sunitinib (Sutent)

- Thalidomide (Synovir, Thalomid)

- Vandetanib (Caprelsa)

- Ziv-aflibercept (Zaltrap)

IMMUNOTHERAPY

Immunotherapy is a type of cancer treatment that supports your immune system in fighting cancer as well as infection. It is known as a type of biological therapy, meaning it uses substances made from living organisms to treat cancer.[125]

Different types of immunotherapy include monoclonal antibodies, adoptive cell transfer, cytokines, treatment vaccines, and bacillus Calmette-Guérin (BCG).[126] They are not used as widely as surgery, chemotherapy, and radiation therapy, but the treatment continues to progress with ongoing research.

MONOCLONAL ANTIBODIES

Monoclonal antibodies are laboratory-produced antibodies used to help the immune system target and destroy cancer cells and alter messaging systems to prevent the stimulation of tumor growth.[127]

Monoclonal antibodies are designed to function in several ways to help the immune system fight cancer. More specifically, this includes flagging cancer cells so the immune system can recognize them, triggering cell-membrane destruction, blocking cell growth, preventing blood vessel growth, blocking immune system inhibitors, directly attacking cancer cells, delivering radiation and chemotherapy, and binding cancer and immune cells.[128]

The FDA has approved more than a dozen monoclonal antibodies to treat certain cancers and many more are likely to be developed.[129]

Different classes of monoclonal antibodies have different mechanisms for helping the immune system to fight cancer.[130] The most common type to treat cancer is known as naked monoclonal antibodies. They attach to proteins (antigens) on cancer cells to stimulate an immune response. Another kind is conjugated monoclonal antibodies, which involves the joining of a chemotherapy drug or a radioactive particle that takes these substances directly to the cancer cells. The third class is known as bispecific monoclonal antibodies. These drugs are made up of parts from two different monoclonal antibodies, which allows them to attach to two different proteins at the same time.

Monoclonal antibodies tend to have fewer side effects than chemotherapy drugs.[131] Possible side effects can include fever, chills, weakness, headache, nausea, vomiting, diarrhea, low blood pressure, and rashes.[132]

Following are examples of monoclonal antibodies:

- Abciximab (Reopro)
- Adalimumab (Humira, Amjevita)
- Alefacept (Amevive)
- Alemtuzumab (Campath)
- Basiliximab (Simulect)
- Belimumab (Benlysta)
- Bezlotoxumab (Zinplava)
- Canakinumab (Ilaris)
- Certolizumab pegol (Cimzia)
- Cetuximab (Erbitux)
- Daclizumab (Zenapax, Zinbryta)
- Denosumab (Prolia, Xgeva)
- Efalizumab (Raptiva)
- Golimumab (Simponi, Simponi Aria)
- Inflectra (Remicade)
- Ipilimumab (Yervoy)
- Ixekizumab (Taltz)
- Natalizumab (Tysabri)
- Nivolumab (Opdivo)
- Olaratumab (Lartruvo)
- Omalizumab (Xolair)
- Palivizumab (Synagis)
- Panitumumab (Vectibix)
- Pembrolizumab (Keytruda)
- Rituximab (Rituxan)
- Secukinumab (Cosentyx)
- Tocilizumab (Actemra)
- Trastuzumab (Herceptin)
- Ustekinumab (Stelara)

ADOPTIVE CELL TRANSFER

Adoptive cell transfer is a treatment designed to boost your immune system's T cells (a type of white blood cell) to fight cancer. Researchers take T cells from the tumor, isolate the T cells that are most active against your cancer or genetically modify them to work better against your tumor, and then grow large amounts of these T cells in a lab setting.[133]

You may have treatments to reduce your immunity to prepare you for later treatment with lab-grown T cells.[134] The T cells administered can expand more than a thousandfold after administration.[135] The treatment is given by intravenous therapy.[136]

Potential side effects can vary depending on the tumor target.[137] For example, for melanoma treatment, vitiligo, hearing loss, and uveitis can occur. For colorectal cancer, colitis may occur.

CYTOKINES

Cytokines are signaling proteins made by your body's white blood cells and involved in the immune system's response to cancer.[138] The main types of cytokines to treat cancer include interferons and interleukins.[139] IL-2 and interferon-alfa 2b are two cytokines approved by the FDA for treatment of cancer.[140] These treatments are given intravenously.

Side effects of high-dose IL-2 may include extreme fatigue, low blood pressure, fluid buildup in the lungs, trouble breathing, kidney damage, heart attacks, intestinal bleeding, diarrhea or abdominal pain, high fever and chills, rapid heartbeat, and mental changes.[141] Side effects for interferon-alfa may include flu-like symptoms, such as fever, chills, and muscle aches, as well as fatigue and nausea.[142]

VACCINES

The treatment of cancer with vaccines is progressing. They are designed to treat cancers that have already developed rather than to prevent them.[143] These vaccines contain cancer-associated antigens, which enhance the immune system's response to a patient's tumor cells.[144]

Currently, the one cancer treatment vaccine that has FDA approval is sipuleucel-T.[145] It is used to treat advanced prostate cancer in men.[146] This treatment is given intravenously.[147]

Side effects vary depending on the vaccine. With sipuleucel-T, one may experience back pain, mild nausea, headache, mild body aches, or an allergy reaction to the infusion.[148]

BACILLUS CALMETTE-GUÉRIN (BCG) VACCINE

Bacillus Calmette-Guérin (BCG) is a vaccine that is made from a type of germ known as *Mycobacterium bovis*. A live strain is available as a vaccine for people at high risk for tuberculosis and for the treatment of bladder tumors or bladder cancer.[149] It is the only agent approved by the FDA for primary therapy of bladder cancer known as carcinoma in situ (CIS).[150] BCG therapy has been shown to reduce the risk of recurrence, and ongoing use reduces the risk of progression in patients with high-grade non–muscle invasive bladder cancer.[151]

BCG has been shown to have multiple mechanisms of action, including inducing an immune reaction in the bladder.[152]

The treatment is given directly into the bladder in a liquid solution via a catheter. A typical program starts with treatments every six weeks, and then it is administered monthly to every three or six months. Maintenance therapy is often given for at least one year.[153]

Side effects may include a burning feeling in the bladder and flu-like symptoms, such as fever, chills, and fatigue.[154]

IMIQUIMOD (ALDARA)

Imiquimod, or Aldara, is a drug that is used topically as a cream for early stage skin cancers or precancerous conditions. It is commonly used for superficial basal cell carcinoma or actinic keratoses located on the face[155] and normally applied five times a week for six weeks.[156]

Side effects may include mild skin irritation, itching, dryness, flaking, scabbing, crusting, redness, or hardening of the skin where the medicine was applied.[157]

PHOTODYNAMIC THERAPY (PDT)

Photodynamic therapy, or PDT, refers to the use of specialized drugs known as photosensitizing agents, which are activated with light to kill superficial cancer cells. This type of treatment is also known as photoradiation therapy, phototherapy, or photochemotherapy.[158]

Usually the photosensitizing agent is injected into the bloodstream or put on the skin. Over time the cancer cells absorb the drug, and then light is applied to the area that requires treatment. An interaction occurs where light causes the drug to react with oxygen and form a chemical that kills cancer cells. This therapy may also activate the immune system to kill cancer and destroy blood vessels that feed cancer.[159]

Studies have shown that PDT can be as effective as surgery or radiation therapy for the treatment of certain kinds of cancers and precancers.[160]

PDT is FDA-approved for non–small cell lung cancer, esophageal cancer, and precancerous changes of Barrett's esophagus. It is also used for the treatment of very early, superficial skin cancers known as actinic keratoses.[161]

Advantages of this type of therapy include not having long-term side effects when used properly, being less invasive than surgery, having a short treatment time, being done as an outpatient, targeting the area of cancer precisely, can be repeated many times at the same site (unlike radiation), usually little to no scarring, and often costing less than other cancer treatments.[162]

Limitations of PTD include that it can only treat superficial areas where light can reach, does not treat metastatic cancer, causes light sensitivity of the skin for a period of time, and cannot be used in people with certain blood diseases.[163]

These are FDA-approved photosensitizing agents:[164]

- Porfimer sodium (Photofrin)

- 5-aminolevulinic acid (Levulan)

- Methyl aminolevulinate (Metvix)

Light sources used for this therapy include laser, intense pulsed light, light-emitting diodes (LEDs), blue light, red light, and many other visible lights (including natural sunlight). The best light source depends on the ideal wavelength for the particular drug used and the target tissue.[165]

Side effects may include mild skin irritation, pain, and swelling.[166] [167]

LASER THERAPY

The word *laser* stands for light amplification by stimulated emission of radiation. Laser light has a specific wavelength that can be focused into a very narrow beam. This allows for a powerful and precise therapy that allows for cutting or destroying small areas.[168] [169]

A limited number of doctors offer laser therapy for the treatment of superficial cancers. Examples of cancers treated with laser include basal cell skin cancer, very early states of cervical, penile, vaginal, vulvar, and non–small cell lung cancer.[170] In certain cases they can be used for small cancers of the head and neck.[171] There are clinical trials underway using lasers to treat cancers of the brain and prostate, and others.[172]

Laser is also used to relieve certain symptoms of cancer, such as bleeding or obstruction.[173] An example of where it can be used is a tumor in the throat (trachea) that is restricting air flow. Laser can also be used to remove polyps of the colon or stomach.[174]

Laser treatments are often given through a flexible endoscopy (a thin, lighted tube that allows the doctor to look at tissues inside the body). Using lasers combined with photosensitizing agents, known as photodynamic therapy, is also common. (See the photodynamic therapy section in this chapter for more information.)

There are three main types of lasers used in cancer treatment, and they are named for the liquid, gas, solid, or electronic substance that is used to create the light. The main laser types are carbon dioxide (CO_2), argon, and neodymium: yttrium-aluminum-garnet.[175]

Advantages of laser treatment include more precise and exact cutting than scalpels (blades) and a sterilization effect on the edges of body tissues that reduces the risk of infection. Laser heat seals blood vessels, which results in less bleeding, less swelling, less pain, or less scarring, and laser treatment often requires a shorter operating time and less cutting and damage to healthy tissues. Procedures can be done in outpatient settings, and healing time is often shorter.[176]

Some of the limitations include the fact that fewer doctors and nurses are trained to use lasers, that effects of some laser treatments many not last as long, and that treatments can be expensive.[177] [178]

STEM CELL TRANSPLANT

Stem cell transplant refers to a procedure that restores blood-forming stem cells in people who had their bone marrow destroyed by chemotherapy, disease, or radiation therapy.[179] [180]

Blood-forming stem cells, also known as hematopoietic stem cells, are how all of the blood cells in your body begin.[181] Most stem cells are found in the bone marrow. They grow into different types of blood cells that include white blood cells (immunity), red blood cells (carry oxygen), and platelets (blood clotting).

Stem cells are given to the patient intravenously. They travel through the bloodstream to the bone marrow, where they hopefully take the place of the cells that were destroyed by treatment or disease.

Sources of stem cells include the bone marrow, blood, or umbilical cord.[182] There are three main kinds of transplants:[183]

- *Autologous,* where the stem cells come from the patient (the one receiving the treatment)

- *Allogenic,* where the stem cells come from another person that match the patient's

- *Syngeneic,* where the stem cells come from your identical twin

Stem cells are generally given to help people recover from high doses of radiation and chemotherapy, or both. They are most often used to help people with leukemia and lymphoma, but they may be also used for neuroblastoma and multiple myeloma.[184] However, they can be used to directly treat cancer, such as in multiple myeloma and leukemia.[185]

Stem cell transplants can cause side effects, such as bleeding and an increased risk of infection.[186] Those with an allogenic transplant are at risk of white blood cells from the donor attacking organs in their body.[187] Also, stem cell transplants are very expensive, with cost estimates varying between $350,000 to $800,000.[188]

CHAPTER 5

FOODS THAT PREVENT AND FIGHT CANCER

Few topics conjure up more confusion than what foods are effective in the prevention and treatment of cancer. At one end of the spectrum, health food enthusiasts (often without medical education) advise raw, whole-food diets no matter the type of cancer or state the patient is in. Conversely, there is the typical medical oncologist who is overly casual when it comes to nutritional recommendations for their patients. It is not uncommon that our patients tell us their oncologist has told them, "Eat whatever you want since diet has nothing to do with your cancer treatment!"

Certainly, we are in much more agreement with the whole-food camp. Yet we have several distinctions and greater flexibility based on what research demonstrates and the unique needs of the patient. Experience will tell you that no one size fits all in terms of medical treatment.

Nutrition is critically important in the fight against cancer. It just makes sense that the foods we eat can hinder or enhance our health. Obviously, a disease such as cancer requires the patient to focus on a diet to enhance their health.

Malnutrition is a serious problem for people with cancer. For example, an observational study of almost 2,000 adults with cancer found that "91% had nutritional impairment, 9% were overtly malnourished, 43% were at risk for malnutrition, and 40% of patients were experiencing a loss of appetite.[1] Dr. Patrick

Quillin, author of *Beating Cancer with Nutrition,* has found in his research that "malnutrition kills greater than 40% of cancer patients."[2]

One of the tenets of a holistic approach for preventing and treating cancer is to provide a healthy environment for normal cell division. This is achieved through sound nutrition, detoxification, and the avoidance of environmental carcinogens.

Conventional oncology has focused intensively on the link between genetics and cancer. However, there is emerging evidence supporting epigenetics, where environmental influences such as nutrition can affect genetic expression in a positive manner. As stated in the journal *Nutrition and Cancer,* "The potential reversibility of epigenetic changes suggests that they could be modulated by nutrition and bioactive food compounds. Thus, epigenetic modifications could mediate environmental signals and provide a link between susceptibility genes and environmental factors in the etiology of cancer."[3]

The foods we eat can have an impact on the messages our cell DNA receives for cell division, good or bad. An article in the journal *Cancer Treatment and Research* notes, "Many natural dietary agents which consist of bioactive compounds have been shown to be effective in cancer prevention and treatment and these nutraceuticals often mediate favorable epigenetic changes."[4] It goes on to provide scientific documentation on better-known anticancer food, such as green tea and the phytochemical sulforaphane from cruciferous vegetables, and how they influence cancer prevention and treatment through epigenetics.[5]

The medical community agrees that a healthy diet plays a role in the prevention of cancer, yet its importance is often understated. Unfortunately, oncologists and family physicians often provide little to no information on clinical nutrition specific to cancer prevention and treatment. Many have little to say in regard to a nutritional approach to cancer that is based on research. In our opinion, the common conventional medical approach of informing patients to "eat healthy" is not helpful. Eating healthy means different things to different people. We will help you to sort through the foods and diets that should be considered.

There has been compelling evidence that good nutrition can help fight cancer. For example, well-known diet and lifestyle researcher Dean Ornish, M.D., led a group of researchers who studied the effect of diet (plant-based, very low fat) and lifestyle changes in men with prostate cancer. In this study, 93 men with prostate cancer were randomly assigned to either have usual care or to be in an experimental group given diet and lifestyle changes. After one year researchers found that

PSA (prostate-specific antigen) levels decreased (improved) in the experimental group and worsened (increased) in the control group receiving usual care. None of the experimental group required conventional treatment due to an increase of PSA or progression of the disease based on MRI imaging compared with six men in the control group who did require conventional treatment. Also impressive was the fact that tumor growth in vitro was inhibited 70 percent in the experimental group but only 9 percent in the comparison group.[6]

In another multiyear study, researchers followed approximately 1,500 women who had been treated for early stage breast cancer. They found that the combination of consuming five or more daily servings of vegetables/fruits and exercise (equivalent to walking 30 minutes, six days a week) resulted in a 50 percent reduction of death from breast cancer.[7]

Conventional physicians have increasingly agreed that good nutrition is important in the fight against cancer. In their book *The Essential Cancer Treatment Nutrition Guide & Cookbook*, Jean LaMantia, R.D., and Neil Berinstein, M.D., state, "Certain foods can reduce inflammation and boost your immune system, while other foods are carcinogenic, feeding the cancer by promoting uncontrolled cell division."[8]

In November 2007, "Food, Nutrition, Physical Activity and the Prevention of Cancer: a Global Perspective," the most comprehensive report ever completed on the links between food, nutrition, physical activity, and cancer, was published. It was a collaboration between the American Institute for Cancer Research and the World Cancer Research Fund International and involved over 7,000 scientific studies that were independently reviewed by 21 world-renowned scientists.[9] This research has been ongoing and updated through the Continuous Update Project.[10] Their updated 2017 report included the following conclusions about nutrition and cancer:[11]

Strong Evidence on What Increases the Risk of Cancer

- Foods preserved by salting increase the risk of cancer of the stomach.

- Alcohol increases the risk of cancer of the bowel (colorectum), breast (both pre- and post-menopause), liver, mouth, pharynx and larynx (mouth and throat), esophagus (squamous cell carcinoma), stomach.

- Mate (South American herbal tea) increases the risk of cancer of the esophagus (squamous cell carcinoma). However, the evidence of the risk is only apparent when drunk scalding hot through a metal straw.

- Cantonese-style salted fish increases the risk of cancer of the nasopharynx.

- Processed meat increases the risk of cancer of the bowel (colorectum) and stomach. Examples of processed meat include bacon, salami, and ham.

- Red meat increases the risk of cancer of the bowel (colorectum). Examples of red meat include beef, pork, lamb, and goat.

- A high glycemic load (measure of how much one's blood sugar is raised by foods) increases the risk of cancer of the endometrium (lining of uterus).

- Aflatoxins (toxins produced by certain fungi through the inappropriate storage of food) increase the risk of cancer of the liver. It is generally more of an issue in warmer regions of the world. Foods that may be affected include cereals, spices, peanuts, pistachios, Brazil nuts, chillies, black pepper, dried fruits, and figs.

Strong Evidence on What Decreases the Risk of Cancer

- Non-starchy vegetables decrease the risk of cancer of the mouth, and pharynx and larynx (mouth and throat). Examples of non-starchy vegetables include broccoli, cabbage, spinach, kale, cauliflower, carrots, lettuce, cucumber, tomatoes, leek, swede (rutabaga), and turnip.

- Fruit decreases the risk of cancer of the lung, mouth, and pharynx and larynx (mouth and throat).

- Foods high in fiber decrease the risk of cancer of the bowel (colorectum). Examples of foods high in dietary fiber include vegetables, fruit, nuts, seeds and pulses (dried legumes), and whole-grain varieties of cereals, pasta, rice, and bread.

- Whole grains decrease the risk of cancer of the bowel (colorectum). Examples of whole grains include brown rice, whole-grain bread, oats, and bulgur wheat.

- Coffee decreases the risk of cancer of the liver and endometrium (uterine lining).

- Dairy products and calcium decrease the risk of cancer of the bowel (colorectum).

- Alcohol decreases the risk of cancer of the kidney. The evidence is only apparent when drinking up to 30 grams (about two drinks) a day.

Based on this worldwide research, scientists from the project recommend the following with regard to diet:

- Avoid high-calorie foods and sugary drinks.

- Enjoy more grains, vegetables, fruit, and beans.

- Limit red meat and avoid processed meat. Eat no more than 500 grams (18 ounces; cooked weight) a week of red meat, such as beef, pork, and lamb. Eat little, if any, processed meat, such as ham and bacon.

- For cancer prevention, don't drink alcohol.

- Eat less salt. Limit your salt intake to less than 2,400 mg of sodium a day by adding less salt and eating less food processed with salt.

- Avoid moldy grains and cereals. They may be contaminated by aflatoxins.

This international research reflected that different foods had a different association with the risk of different cancers. Next, we will summarize the strong evidence between common cancers and foods that are more likely to increase or decrease their risk based on the research published by the World Cancer Research Fund International, from 2007 to the present.[12] This type of information can be helpful for you in your dietary planning depending on what type of cancer you have, what cancer you may have had a history of, and what has been common in your family history. We also have other specific recommendations based on additional research in Chapter 9. *These recommendations are based on strong evidence, unless other circumstances are noted.*

Colorectal cancer

- Whole grains decrease the risk of colorectal cancer

- Foods containing dietary fiber decrease the risk of colorectal cancer

- Dairy products decrease the risk of colorectal cancer

- Red meat increases the risk of colorectal cancer

- Processed meat increases the risk of colorectal cancer

- Approximately two or more alcoholic drinks per day increases the risk of colorectal cancer

Breast cancer (both premenopausal and postmenopausal)

- Alcoholic drinks increase risk

Esophageal cancer

- Alcoholic drinks increase the risk of esophageal squamous cell carcinoma.

- Regularly consuming mate, as drunk very hot in the traditional style in South America, increases the risk of esophageal squamous cell carcinoma.

Stomach cancer

- Approximately three or more alcoholic drinks per day increase the risk of stomach cancer.

- Foods preserved by salting increase the risk of stomach cancer. Research mainly relates to high-salt foods and salt-preserved foods, including pickled vegetables and salted or dried fish, as traditionally prepared in east Asia.

- Processed meat increases the risk of stomach non-cardia cancer.

Bladder cancer

- Drinking water containing arsenic increases the risk of bladder cancer.

Kidney cancer

- Alcoholic drinks decrease the risk of kidney cancer, when consuming up to 30 grams (about two drinks) a day. There is insufficient specific evidence for higher levels of drinking—for example, 50 grams (about three drinks) or 70 grams (about five drinks) a day.

Liver cancer

- Approximately three or more alcoholic drinks a day may cause liver cancer.

- Foods contaminated by aflatoxins (toxins produced by fungi) increase the risk of liver cancer. (Aflatoxins are produced by inadequate storage of food, and are generally an issue related to foods from warmer, developing regions of the world.) Foods that may be affected by aflatoxins include cereals, spices, peanuts, pistachios, Brazil nuts, chillies, black pepper, dried fruit, and figs.

- Drinking coffee is linked to a decreased risk of liver cancer.

Prostate cancer

- None given

Breast cancer
Common general recommendations for dietary changes for breast cancer survivors include:

- Eat foods containing fiber

- Eat foods containing soy

- Have a lower intake of total fat and, in particular, saturated fat

Ovarian cancer

- Limited evidence that non-starchy vegetables may decrease risk[13]

Endometrial cancer

- Decreased risk from coffee

- Increased risk from higher glycemic load

Cervical cancer

- Limited evidence that carrots decrease risk

Pancreatic cancer

- Foods containing folate decrease risk

- Limited evidence that fruits decrease risk

- Limited evidence that red meat increases risk

Lung cancer

- Fruit and vegetable intake significantly reduces risk in current smokers

Mouth, pharyngeal, and laryngeal cancer

- Non-starchy vegetables, fruits, and foods containing carotenoids decrease risk

- Alcoholic drinks increase risk

- Mate (South American herbal tea) increases risk (only apparent when drunk scalding hot through a metal straw)

Nasopharynx cancer

- Limited evidence that non-starchy vegetables, fruits decrease risk

- Cantonese-style salted fish increases risk

Gallbladder cancer

- Limited evidence peppers (capsicums), fish, coffee, tea, and alcohol decrease risk

Prostate cancer

- Foods containing lycopene and selenium decrease risk

- Limited evidence that pulses (legumes) and foods containing vitamin E decrease risk

- Diets high in calcium increase risk

- Limited evidence that processed meat, milk, and dairy products increase risk

Skin cancer

- Arsenic in drinking water increases risk

Thyroid cancer

- Vegetables decrease risk

- Fish decreased risk in areas where iodine deficiency was common

Testis Cancer

- Milk and dairy consumption increased incidence of testis cancer

Lymphoid and hemopoietic (blood) cancers

- Increased vegetable and fruit intake were associated with reduced incidence

- Meat or red meat were associated with increased incidence

- Alcohol reduced the incidence of non-Hodgkin's lymphoma, particularly Burkitt's lymphoma

- Increased milk and dairy consumption was associated with increased incidence of non-Hodgkin's lymphoma

FRUITS AND VEGETABLES

Beyond this colossal research by the World Cancer Research Fund International, many epidemiological (population) and case-control studies have proven that diets rich in fruit and vegetables resulted in a significantly reduced risk of several cancers.[14] One of the obvious foundations of a cancer-specific diet is an increased intake of fruits and vegetables.

Plant foods are the source of phytochemicals, the naturally occurring plant chemicals that fight cancer and other diseases. They are another big reason why research has shown an association between plant foods and a decreased risk of several cancers. Laboratory studies have shown that phytochemicals have the potential to do the following:[15]

- Stimulate the immune system

- Block substances we eat, drink, and breathe from becoming carcinogens

- Reduce the kind of inflammation that makes cancer growth more likely

- Prevent DNA damage and help with DNA repair

- Reduce the kind of oxidative damage to cells that can spark cancer

- Slow the growth rate of cancer cells

- Trigger damaged cells to destroy themselves before they can reproduce

- Help to regulate hormones

Thousands of phytochemicals are contained in plant foods. A daily diet that contains a variety of vegetables, fruits, whole grains, and beans will provide these cancer fighters for your body. Researchers have found that phytochemicals from fruits and vegetables have multiple anticancer mechanisms that are complex and likely arise from their multitudinous synergistic combinations.[16]

A study published in the journal *Food Chemistry* found that when a number of fresh vegetables were juiced, they added to a variety of cancer cell lines derived from stomach, kidney, prostate, breast, brain, pancreatic, and lung cancer. Overall the tumor cells derived from prostate and stomach cancer had reduced proliferation from the extracts. The other tumor cells were also inhibited by the vegetable extracts but just not to the same high degree of sensitivity.[17]

In this same study, vegetables with very high activity on cell proliferation included Brussels sprouts, cabbage, curly cabbage, garlic, green onion, kale, leek, and spinach. Vegetables with high activity were asparagus, beet, broccoli, cauliflower, fiddlehead, green bean, radish, red cabbage, rutabaga, and yellow onion. And vegetables with intermediate effect were celery and eggplant.[18]

Keep in mind that this study does not necessarily mean these vegetables will have similar anticancer effects when taken orally; this study only tested cancer cell lines rather than active subjects who ingested the juices. However, it does demonstrate the anticancer properties of these vegetables. There is probably no magic bullet food for cancer, but rather the synergistic effect among many anticancer foods will be most effective.

The following chart from the American Institute for Cancer Research describes the cancer-fighting phytochemicals.[19]

PHYTOCHEMICAL	PLANT SOURCE	POSSIBLE BENEFITS
Carotenoids (such as beta-carotene, lycopene, lutein, zeaxanthin)	Red, orange, and green fruits and vegetables, including broccoli, carrots, cooked tomatoes, leafy greens, sweet potatoes, winter squash, apricots, cantaloupe, oranges, and watermelon	May inhibit cancer cell growth, work as antioxidants, and improve immune response
Flavonoids (such as anthocyanins and quercetin)	Apples, citrus fruits, onions, soybeans, and soy products (tofu, soy milk, edamame, etc.), coffee, and tea	May inhibit inflammation and tumor growth; may aid immunity and boost production of detoxifying enzymes in the body
Indoles and Glucosinolates (sulforaphane)	Cruciferous vegetables (broccoli, cabbage, collard greens, kale, cauliflower, and Brussels sprouts)	May induce detoxification of carcinogens, limit production of cancer-related hormones, block carcinogens, and prevent tumor growth
Inositol (phytic acid)	Bran from corn, oats, rice, rye and wheat, nuts, soybeans, and soy products (tofu, soy milk, edamame, etc.)	May retard cell growth and work as antioxidant
Isoflavones (daidzein and genistein)	Soybeans and soy products (tofu, soy milk, edamame, etc.)	May inhibit tumor growth, limit production of cancer-related hormones, and generally work as antioxidant
Isothiocyanates	Cruciferous vegetables (broccoli, cabbage, collard greens, kale, cauliflower, and Brussels sprouts)	May induce detoxification of carcinogens, block tumor growth, and work as antioxidants
Polyphenols (such as ellagic acid and resveratrol)	Green tea, grapes, wine, berries, citrus fruits, apples, whole grains, and peanuts	May prevent cancer formation, prevent inflammation, and work as antioxidants
Terpenes (such as perillyl alcohol, limonene, carnosol)	Cherries, citrus fruit peel, and rosemary	May protect cells from becoming cancerous, slow cancer cell growth, strengthen immune function, limit production of cancer-related hormones, fight viruses, and work as antioxidants

Besides eating an increased number of fruits and vegetables, juicing is an excellent way to increase your intake of fruits and vegetables and their inherent phytochemicals.

ACID-ALKALINE BALANCE

Many books have been published over the years recommending a diet that promotes "blood alkalinization" and reduces "blood acidity." Many of our patients ask about this approach. As it turns out, there is something to this concept, but not in the way most authors have described.

Your blood has a mildly alkaline pH (different from urine and saliva) and works to maintain a narrow blood plasma level pH of 7.4 (with an average range between 7.35 and 7.45). Your acid-alkaline balance has much to do with how your kidneys respond to food. Your kidneys determine whether the nutritional composition of the food ultimately produces an alkaline or acidic effect in the blood, and they coordinate your body's response.

People often make the mistake of thinking of food as acidic in terms of its taste or reaction in the stomach. While an acidic food like tomatoes may trigger heartburn, this is different from its effects on your blood pH.

Doctors use the term *net endogenous acid production (NEAP)* to describe how food impacts your blood pH. In everyday terms, your body pH is related to the acidic or alkaline metabolic *effect* of food, not whether a specific food happens to be acidic.

Our ancient diet was higher in potassium than sodium and higher in bicarbonate than chloride. Potassium is a natural buffer against an acidic pH. People used to eat a 10:1 ratio of potassium to sodium, and this is what our biology is best suited for. But modern processed foods have flipped this ratio to 3:1 in favor of sodium.

Most fruits and vegetables promote alkaline since their final metabolite is often bicarbonate.[20] Meat, eggs, and dairy increase sulfuric acid, which is acid producing. NaCl, or salt, is also acid forming, whereas potassium salts and magnesium are alkalinizing.[21]

You can see that the standard American diet would push most people toward a tendency to a net acid trend. Blood pH from chronic acid-promoting diets is near the low-normal range (7.36 to 7.38) as compared to the higher alkaline end of the range (7.42 to 7.44). Please note that you cannot measure this pH on your own; it requires special arterial blood testing at a research institution.

There are no studies showing a direct link between a diet-caused acidic blood pH and cancer. However, it has been established that a diet-induced acidosis may influence molecular activities at the cell level, which may promote cancer formation.[22] This may be another reason why diets rich in fruits and vegetables and lower in animal protein are generally cancer protective.

DIET AND INFLAMMATION

Chronic inflammation is a risk factor for the development and progression of cancer. The National Cancer Institute states, "Over time, chronic inflammation can cause DNA damage and lead to cancer."[23] There can be many causes of chronic inflammation, such as infection, gut bacteria imbalance, smoking, obesity, diabetes, toxins, and lack of exercise. One of the main causes that you are most able to control is diet.

Dr. Frank Hu, professor of nutrition and epidemiology in the Department of Nutrition at the Harvard School of Public Health, agrees that a healthy diet is necessary to combat inflammation. He states, "Many experimental studies have shown that components of foods or beverages may have anti-inflammatory effects."[24] And he recommends a diet rich in fruits and vegetables to reduce inflammation.[25]

Research has shown that diets high in saturated fat and trans fat increase inflammation,[26] whereas foods high in omega-3 fatty acids are associated with decreased markers of inflammation.[27] In terms of carbohydrates, high glycemic load diets (amount and quality of carbohydrates on the glycemic index) increase the production of inflammatory chemicals known as cytokines.[28] [29]

In general, plant foods are anti-inflammatory while animal products (with the exception of fish) can be inflammation promoting. The most well-studied diet for reducing markers of inflammation is the Mediterranean diet, which we will discuss shortly.

THE ROLE OF SUGAR AND CANCER

Many patients have reported to us that their oncologist told them it was fine to consume simple sugar products as they had no effect on their cancer. Is this good science? We don't think so.

Research has shown that approximately half of the U.S. adult population has either diabetes or prediabetes.[30] Many people are unaware that they have one of these conditions.[31] Generally, diabetes is defined as a fasting plasma glucose level of 126 mg/dL or higher, or a hemoglobin A1C blood value of 6.5 percent or greater.[32] For prediabetes, the fasting plasma glucose level is 100 mg/dL to 125 mg/dL and an A1C between 5.7 percent and 6.4 percent.[33] Your doctor can test these levels for you or drugstores carry home testing kits.

The underlying mechanism for most people with elevated blood glucose levels (type 2 diabetes, prediabetes) is insulin resistance. The term *insulin resistance* refers to the cells of your muscles, fat, and liver not responding to or accepting insulin properly. Since insulin transports glucose to your cells, the end result is a high blood glucose level. The pancreas then produces more insulin in response to the higher blood glucose levels.

A less common form of diabetes is insulin-dependent diabetes (type 1 diabetes). This occurs when the pancreatic cells do not produce enough insulin. As a result, insulin replacement is required. Some people with uncontrolled type 2 diabetes are also treated with insulin.

Emerging evidence has demonstrated a link between insulin resistance and a variety of precancerous or cancerous conditions.[34] The excessive release of insulin is considered to be carcinogenic. This may be why people with type 2 diabetes who require insulin therapy have a higher risk of colorectal cancer. Other research shows that increasing doses of human insulin increases cancer mortality and risk of malignant cancer.[35]

There are several mechanisms by which insulin resistance promotes cancer growth. This includes the activation of signaling cascades that promote tumor growth, activation of growth factors such as IGF and IGF-binding proteins, activation of inflammatory mediators, and increased levels of free hormone levels, such as estradiol.[36]

People have insulin resistance due to a variety of reasons, including stress, medications, being overweight, environmental toxins, diet, and a lack of exercise. The typical North American diet is loaded with simple carbohydrates, which means lots of sugar. Simple carbohydrates in such foods as breads, pastas, sodas, cookies, pastries, and candies spike blood sugar levels, which results in the release of insulin.

The World Health Organization recommends an ideal amount of daily sugar intake that would be less than 5 percent of an adult's calories from added sugar or from natural sugars in honey, syrups, soft drinks and sugar-sweetened beverages, and fruit juice. For a 2,000-calorie diet, this would be 25 grams.[37]

Many people consume much more than this in just one meal-replacement bar or soda. To put this in perspective, the average American consumes 82 grams (19.5 teaspoons) of sugar daily![38] This, of course, leads to cancer-related insulin resistance and obesity, another risk factor for cancer.

One area of confusion is the topic of grains. Refined grain products are a major contributor of simple sugar and insulin resistance/diabetes in our country. The average American whole-wheat bread product has a higher glycemic index rating (how slowly or quickly a food increases blood glucose levels) than Coca-Cola![39]

The other issue to be aware of when eating carbohydrates, in addition to the glycemic index (available online), is the amount of the carbohydrates you are eating, known as the glycemic load. If your carbohydrate intake is too low, you could feel tired and lose weight, which are symptoms to be monitored if you have cancer.

Below is a table of common carbohydrates and their glycemic index and load ratings:[40] The lower the glycemic index and glycemic load, the less the spiking effect of sugar and insulin on the body.

FOOD	GLYCEMIC INDEX (glucose = 100)	SERVING SIZE (grams)	GLYCEMIC LOAD PER SERVING
BAKERY PRODUCTS AND BREADS			
Banana cake, made with sugar	47	60	14
Banana cake, made without sugar	55	60	12
Sponge cake, plain	46	63	17
Vanilla cake made from packet mix with vanilla frosting (Betty Crocker)	42	111	24
Apple muffin, made with rolled oats and sugar	44	60	13
Apple muffin, made with rolled oats and without sugar	48	60	9
Waffles, Aunt Jemima®	76	35	10
Bagel, white, frozen	72	70	25
Baguette, white, plain	95	30	14
Coarse barley bread, 80% kernels	34	30	7
Hamburger bun	61	30	9
Kaiser roll	73	30	12
Pumpernickel bread	56	30	7
50% cracked wheat kernel bread	58	30	12

FOOD	GLYCEMIC INDEX (glucose = 100)	SERVING SIZE (grams)	GLYCEMIC LOAD PER SERVING
White wheat flour bread, average	75	30	11
Wonder® bread, average	73	30	10
Whole wheat bread, average	69	30	9
100% Whole Grain® bread (Natural Ovens)	51	30	7
Pita bread, white	68	30	10
Corn tortilla	52	50	12
Wheat tortilla	30	50	8
BEVERAGES			
Coca Cola® (U.S. formula)	63	250 mL	16
Fanta®, orange soft drink	68	250 mL	23
Lucozade®, original (sparkling glucose drink)	95	250 mL	40
Apple juice, unsweetened	41	250 mL	12
Cranberry juice cocktail (Ocean Spray®)	68	250 mL	24
Gatorade, orange flavor (U.S. formula)	89	250 mL	13
Orange juice, unsweetened, average	50	250 mL	12
Tomato juice, canned, no sugar added	38	250 mL	4
BREAKFAST CEREALS AND RELATED PRODUCTS			
All-Bran®, average	44	30	9

FOOD	GLYCEMIC INDEX (glucose = 100)	SERVING SIZE (grams)	GLYCEMIC LOAD PER SERVING
Coco Pops®, average	77	30	20
Cornflakes®, average	81	30	20
Cream of Wheat®	66	250	17
Cream of Wheat®, instant	74	250	22
Grape-Nuts®	75	30	16
Muesli, average	56	30	10
Oatmeal, average	55	250	13
Instant oatmeal, average	79	250	21
Puffed wheat cereal	80	30	17
Raisin Bran®	61	30	12
Special K® (U.S. formula)	69	30	14
GRAINS			
Pearled barley, average	25	150	11
Sweet corn on the cob	48	60	14
Couscous	65	150	9
Quinoa	53	150	13
White rice, boiled, type non-specified	72	150	29
Quick cooking white basmati	63	150	26
Brown rice, steamed	50	150	16

FOOD	GLYCEMIC INDEX (glucose = 100)	SERVING SIZE (grams)	GLYCEMIC LOAD PER SERVING
Parboiled Converted white rice (Uncle Ben's®)	38	150	14
Whole wheat kernels, average	45	50	15
Bulgur, average	47	150	12
COOKIES AND CRACKERS			
Graham crackers	74	25	13
Vanilla wafers	77	25	14
Shortbread	64	25	10
Rice cakes, average	82	25	17
Rye crisps, average	64	25	11
Soda crackers	74	25	12
DAIRY PRODUCTS AND ALTERNATIVES			
Ice cream, regular, average	62	50	8
Ice cream, premium (Sara Lee®)	38	50	3
Milk, full-fat, average	31	250 mL	4
Milk, skim, average	31	250 mL	4
Reduced-fat yogurt with fruit, average	33	200	11
FRUITS			
Apple, average	36	120	5

FOOD	GLYCEMIC INDEX (glucose = 100)	SERVING SIZE (grams)	GLYCEMIC LOAD PER SERVING
Banana, raw, average	48	120	11
Dates, dried, average	42	60	18
Grapefruit	25	120	3
Grapes, black	59	120	11
Oranges, raw, average	45	120	5
Peach, average	42	120	5
Peach, canned in light syrup	52	120	9
Pear, raw, average	38	120	4
Pear, canned in pear juice	44	120	5
Prunes, pitted	29	60	10
Raisins	64	60	28
Watermelon	72	120	4
BEANS AND NUTS			
Baked beans	40	150	6
Black-eyed peas	50	150	15
Black beans	30	150	7
Chickpeas	10	150	3
Chickpeas, canned in brine	42	150	9
Navy beans, average	39	150	12

FOOD	GLYCEMIC INDEX (glucose = 100)	SERVING SIZE (grams)	GLYCEMIC LOAD PER SERVING
Kidney beans, average	34	150	9
Lentils	28	150	5
Soy beans, average	15	150	1
Cashews, salted	22	50	3
Peanuts	13	50	1
PASTA AND NOODLES			
Fettucini	32	180	15
Macaroni, average	50	180	24
Macaroni and Cheese (Kraft®)	64	180	33
Spaghetti, white, boiled, average	46	180	22
Spaghetti, white, boiled 20 minutes	58	180	26
Spaghetti, whole-grain, boiled	42	180	17
SNACK FOODS			
Corn chips, plain, salted	42	50	11
Fruit Roll-Ups®	99	30	24
M & M's®, peanut	33	30	6
Microwave popcorn, plain, average	65	20	7
Potato chips, average	56	50	12

FOOD	GLYCEMIC INDEX (glucose = 100)	SERVING SIZE (grams)	GLYCEMIC LOAD PER SERVING
Pretzels, oven-baked	83	30	16
Snickers Bar®, average	51	60	18
VEGETABLES			
Green peas	54	80	4
Carrots, average	39	80	2
Parsnips	52	80	4
Baked russet potato	111	150	33
Boiled white potato, average	82	150	21
Instant mashed potato, average	87	150	17
Sweet potato, average	70	150	22
Yam, average	54	150	20
MISCELLANEOUS			
Hummus (chickpea salad dip)	6	30	0
Chicken nuggets, frozen, reheated in microwave oven 5 minutes	46	100	7
Pizza, plain baked dough, served with parmesan cheese and tomato sauce	80	100	22
Pizza, Super Supreme (Pizza Hut®)	36	100	9
Honey, average	61	25	12

SUGAR ALTERNATIVES

We do not recommend the use of artificial sweeteners as they are associated with health problems. Dr. Susan E. Swithers, a professor of behavioral neuroscience at Purdue University, reviewed published studies on artificial sweeteners and warned, "Frequent consumers of these sugar substitutes may . . . be at increased risk of excessive weight gain, metabolic syndrome, type 2 diabetes, and cardiovascular disease."[41] And one controversial study that followed approximately 125,000 people over 22 years found that in men, greater than one daily serving (12 ounces) of diet soda containing aspartame increased risks of non-Hodgkin's lymphomas and multiple myeloma in men but not women.[42]

If you avoid artificial sweeteners and use natural sweeteners such as Lo Han, xylitol, raw honey, and stevia, you will consume much less sugar. You can also switch from fruit juices and soda or other sweetened beverages to flavored sparkling water and herbal teas, or consume berries, other fruits, and small amounts of dark chocolate to satisfy your sweet tooth.

THE WARBURG EFFECT

Our cells rely primarily upon oxygen to create energy in our cell energy-producing factories known as the mitochondria. Aerobic respiration, or the use of oxygen to create energy, is very efficient. Our cells, however, also generate energy (ATP) from a process known as fermentation, or glycolysis. This involves the multistep conversion of glucose (sugar) into two molecules of pyruvate. It can then enter the aerobic respiratory cycle to create energy or it can be fermented to produce energy and a waste product known as lactic acid. This former process (glycolysis) is much less efficient in producing energy. Our body uses this type of energy production when more than short bursts of energy are needed.

In 1924, German medical doctor, physiologist, and Nobel Laureate Otto Warburg made the discovery that cancer cells have a different metabolism from normal adult cells. He found that cancer cells rely on glycolysis even if oxygen is available. As a result, cancer cells are able to adapt and fuel themselves with enormous amounts of glucose compared to normal tissues in order to provide critical energy production for cell proliferation. In effect, Warburg felt that all cancers originated from dysfunctional cellular energy production (cellular respiration).[43] This is known as the Warburg Effect.

Over time this theory was abandoned in favor of the genetic causes of cancer.[44] But in recent years, there has been a renewed interest in Warburg's work. In 2012, Thomas Seyfried, a biochemical geneticist, published the book *Cancer as a Metabolic Disease,* which expanded on the work of Warburg. Seyfried's focus is on cancer as primarily a metabolic disease from mitochondria damage that requires unique treatments. Seyfried challenges the notion that genetic mutations are the primary causes of cancer.[45] Instead, he feels genetic mutations are often the result of damaged mitochondria.[46] Seyfried focuses on calorie restriction that reduces the production of lactate, reduces glucose and insulin, and produces ketones, which tumor cells cannot use for energy.[47] (This type of approach will be discussed later in this chapter using the ketogenic diet and intermittent fasting.)

As it turns out, cancer cells have an alteration in an enzyme known as hexokinase. This enzyme is expressed differently in cancer cells (known as hexokinase II), which results in cancer cells' uptake of glucose at a much higher rate than normal.[48] One of the results is the buildup of lactic acid, which is theorized to damage surrounding normal tissue and make invasion and metastasis easier.[49]

It is interesting to note that PET scans, the commonly used medical imaging to identify active cancer cells in the body, work on the premise that the active hexokinase II allows labeled glucose (a molecule that looks like glucose but has a single oxygen atom replaced by an isotope of fluorine) to concentrate inside cancer cells.[50] This then allows the PET scan imaging to pick up the metabolic activity of cancer cells.

It appears that Warburg was largely correct in his theory. A team of researchers from University of California, Los Angeles (UCLA) and collaborators from Memorial Sloan Kettering Cancer Center and Weill Cornell Medical College showed that depriving cancer cells of glucose does indeed cause them to die. When you take away glucose, your body responds by creating free radicals that destroy the cell.[51]

An excellent book reviewing the history of Warburg and his research and that includes modern understanding and studies is *Tripping Over the Truth: How the Metabolic Theory of Cancer Is Overturning One of Medicine's Most Entrenched Paradigms*, by Travis Christofferson.

NUTRITIONAL PREVENTION

We feel certain diets are credible for the nutritional prevention and integrative treatment of cancer. These include the Mediterranean diet, China diet, Kaufmann diet, ketogenic diet, and intermittent fasting.

MEDITERRANEAN DIET

Most people are familiar with the Mediterranean diet and its power to protect against cardiovascular disease. Yet this highly publicized diet has powerful anti-cancer properties.

The Mediterranean diet generally consists of fruits, vegetables, extra-virgin olive oil, fish, whole grains, legumes, moderate amounts of wine, and small amounts of red meat. It has been shown in large observational studies to be associated with lower cancer incidence.

One study of over 380,000 people from the United States found the Mediterranean diet decreased cancer mortality in men by 17 percent and in women by 12 percent after 5 years of follow up.[52] Other studies have demonstrated the anticancer properties of the Mediterranean diet for colorectal,[53 54 55] breast,[56 57] liver,[58] stomach,[59] prostate,[60 61] and esophageal cancers.[62]

One of the unique features of the Mediterranean diet is extra-virgin olive oil. A randomized, all female trial analyzed the effects of 1 liter (67 tablespoons) per week of extra-virgin olive oil consumed along with the Mediterranean diet, the effects of 30 grams of mixed nuts consumed daily along with the Mediterranean diet, and a control group. The average age of the women was 67.7 years. Approximately five years later, the women with the extra-virgin olive oil and Mediterranean diet were found to have a 68 percent lower relative risk of breast cancer compared to the control group. Women consuming the nuts and Mediterranean diet also had a lower risk than the control group but not as good as those who consumed the olive oil.[63]

We like the Mediterranean diet, especially for the prevention of cancer. However, due to the high glycemic index rating of North American grain products (breads, pastas, pastries, etc.), we recommend restricting or minimizing the grain portion of the diet.

CHINA STUDY DIET

In 2005, T. Colin Campbell, Ph.D., and his son Thomas M. Campbell II, M.D., co-authored the book *The China Study,* which reviewed nutritional data in relation to the risk of developing diseases, including cancer, in areas of rural China where people consumed locally grown food. It is one of the most comprehensive studies of health and nutrition that has ever been completed. The book's general conclusion was that a diet that has more than mild amounts of animal protein and dairy is a risk factor for cancer. A revised edition of *The China Study* published in 2016 concluded that a whole-food, plant-based diet decreases the risk of cancer and other chronic diseases.

KAUFMANN DIET

The Kaufmann diet has been developed over the years by researcher and mycotoxin expert Doug Kaufmann. The premise behind this diet is to consume foods that do not feed or perpetuate a pathogenic fungal infection, the root of many cancers.

The overuse of antibiotics, high-sugar diets (which include alcohol), and chemicals in the diet, such as GMOs, allow fungal overgrowth in the body. Fungal mycotoxins (metabolites of fungi) are common in the food supply in such foods as corn, peanuts, grains, milk, cottonseed, Brazil nuts, pecans, pistachios, and walnuts.[64]

Mycotoxins found in the environment are proven carcinogens. Many people are surprised to learn that mycotoxins are found in several medications, including penicillin. And besides their direct carcinogenic effects, mycotoxins suppress immunity.

Kaufmann has spent decades researching this matter and theorizes that "cancer begins when the DNA from Fungus and the DNA from our white blood cells merge to form a new hybrid 'tumor, or sac.' This hybrid attains a life of its own now, bypassing our immune defenses because it is 50% human, and therefore just enough to be recognized as 'self.'"[65]

Emerging evidence supports Kaufmann's hypothesis. For example, the p53 gene is the most commonly mutated gene in people with cancer.[66] Damage to this gene allows cells with damaged DNA to proliferate. Most p53 gene mutations are acquired mutations.[67] Research published in mainstream medical journals has demonstrated that the mycotoxin aflatoxin B1, made by *Aspergillus fungus,* is known to cause p53 mutations and liver cancer.[68]

Kaufmann has noted several similarities between cancer and fungi:[69]

- Each can thrive in a sac formation

- Each can metabolize nutrients in the absence of oxygen

- Each generates lactic acid

- Each depends on their hosts for sustenance, proliferation, and reproduction

- Each thrives in the presence of sugar and dies in the absence of sugar

- Both emit volatile organic compounds that dogs can detect

- Both respond to antifungal medications

Physicians are using the Kaufmann diet and program, which does not allow grains, alcohol, yeast, fungi/mushrooms, or peanuts and includes antifungal medications and supplements. The focus on protein sources and vegetables makes it similar to the ketogenic diet, although higher in protein.

There are two phases to this diet. The first phase is very strict, especially in terms of carbohydrate intake. The goal is to starve the fungi and simultaneously kill fungi. This reduces mycotoxin damage to cell DNA, reduces inflammation, and improves immunity, which allows cells to function normally in their cell division and energy production. The second phase allows for additional amounts of healthy carbohydrates. For more information, visit www.knowthecause.com.

KETOGENIC DIET

The ketogenic diet (KD) has been used by the medical profession for the treatment of seizures (especially for children) for many decades. In recent years, it has also been used for the treatment of Alzheimer's disease, Parkinson's disease, amyotrophic lateral sclerosis (Lou Gehrig's disease), traumatic brain injury, hypoxic/ischemic brain injury (stroke), autism, depression, headaches, narcolepsy, metabolic inherited diseases, various cancers, and cardiac ischemia.[70] It has also been used successfully to reduce body weight for those with obesity.[71]

The KD focuses on foods that are very low in carbohydrates and rich in natural fats, and which contain low to moderate protein. It is called a ketogenic diet since it causes the body to release ketone bodies (often referred to as ketones) by breaking down fat. This process is known as ketosis.

As discussed earlier with the Warburg Effect, the body uses carbohydrates broken down into glucose as the main sources of energy (glycolysis). When carbohydrates are restricted to a daily amount of approximately 50 grams or less, the body relies upon the liver for glucose. The liver contains glycogen, which is stored glucose. However, after 24 to 48 hours of carbohydrate restriction and the depletion of liver glycogen, the use of ketones is required as a fuel source (ATP). Ketones are derived from fatty acids in the diet or from the breakdown of fat in the body.

Research has shown that most tumor cells are unable to use ketone bodies for energy production due to changes in their mitochondria structure or function.[72] This results in metabolic stress for the tumor cells and creates an anticancer effect.[73] Furthermore, ketone bodies are toxic to some cancer cells.[74]

KD has been shown to have additional anticancer effects by increasing cancer cell oxidative stress;[75] being anti-angiogenesis, anti-inflammatory, and pro-apoptotic (pro-cell death);[76] and acting as an inhibitor of histone deacetylases[77] (which reduces the ability of cancer cells to proliferate). Since KD reduces insulin levels, it indirectly fights cancer through the reduction of cancer-supporting hormones such as TAF and IGF-1.[78][79]

One of the first KD studies was completed in 1987. Researchers found that mice with colon cancer on a ketogenic diet had a decreased tumor weight and improvement in cachexia.[80] Additional animal studies have shown reduced tumor growth and an increased survival rate in malignant melanoma, colon cancer, gastric cancer, and prostate cancer.[81] Animal research has found KD enhances the effects of radiation therapy.[82]

In terms of human studies, the published literature contains limited but encouraging data. In 1995, a case report described two female pediatric patients with advanced brain cancer (malignant astrocytoma) who were fed a ketogenic diet. In eight weeks, their FDG-PET scan showed a 21.8 percent decrease in glucose uptake, suggesting an anticancer effect. Also, both children showed improvements in function and nutritional status.[83] One of the children remained disease-free one year later and was still alive ten years later.[84]

In 2012, Dr. Eugene Fine at the Albert Einstein School of Medicine completed a four-week trial with 10 people with advanced-stage cancers. In nine patients with prior rapid disease progression, five achieved disease stabilization or partial remission based on PET scan. None of the patients had unsafe adverse events.[85]

And in 2016, Dr. Natalie Jansen of Germany treated 78 cancer patients in a private clinic setting for 10 months. The type and stages of the cancers varied. She reported, "In palliative patients, a clear trend was observed in patients who adhered strictly to a ketogenic diet. . . . those who adhere to it may have positive results from this type of diet."[86]

There are several clinical trials currently being funded by the National Institutes of Health using the ketogenic diet in combination with radiation and chemotherapy for various cancers.

Since KD has been shown in limited research to benefit some with cancer, it can be utilized in an integrative program under medical supervision. Formal studies did not find any serious adverse events. Side effects can often be resolved with diet changes.

A high fat intake may cause lethargy, nausea, and vomiting, especially in children.[87] Children may also be prone to hypoglycemia.[88] In our clinical experience, based on biochemical knowledge, we find the addition of supplemental L-carnitine (an amino acid) stops these side effects since carnitine increases fat metabolism at the mitochondria.

Adults may experience digestive discomfort due to the high fat intake and an increase in cholesterol levels.[89] They may also experience hypoglycemia, hunger and cravings, weakness, dizziness, fatigue, constipation, muscle cramps and dehydration, mild acidosis, ketone breath, weight loss, changes in blood pressure, heart palpitations, and nausea.[90] Kidney damage is a theoretical problem, although studies have not shown this to be a problem with KD.[91] Compared to results with children, ketogenic diets with adults result in fewer and more minor side effects.[92]

It is especially important to consult with a doctor before starting KD if you have a history of pancreatitis, active gallbladder disease, impaired liver function, impaired fat digestion, poor nutritional status, gastric bypass surgery, and abdominal tumors.[93]

Some studies have reported that KD depletes the body of minerals, such as selenium, copper, and zinc.[94] Supplementation of minerals during KD is recommended.

Some authors have raised concerns that the typical KD may be low in phytochemical-rich vegetables, but as described in *The Metabolic Approach to Cancer*, most people can achieve adequate phytochemicals with KD.[95]

A general KD guideline for the ratio by weight is 3:1 to 4:1 fat to (carbohydrate + protein).[96] This gives a calorie composition of about 8 percent protein, 2 percent carbohydrate, and 90 percent fat. A typical American diet typically consists of 15 percent protein, 50 percent carbohydrate, and 35 percent fat.[97]

Most people need to consume below 20 grams of net carbs (total carbohydrate amount in grams minus the grams of indigestible fiber) a day to achieve ketosis, although some people will achieve this at 30 grams.

KD removes sugars, all grain products, and starchy vegetables, such as corn, potatoes, peas, okra, artichokes, and most legumes. Fruits high in sugar are avoided except avocado, lemon, lime, and small amounts of berries, such as strawberries, blueberries, blackberries, and raspberries.

There are many non-starchy vegetables that can be consumed. Any of the leafy green vegetables and lettuces are good options. Other good choices include alfalfa sprouts, asparagus, beet greens, bok choy, broccoli, Brussels sprouts, cabbage, cauliflower, celery, chives, collard greens, cucumbers, fennel, garlic, kale, kohlrabi, leeks, mushrooms, olives, radishes, sauerkraut, scallions, snow peas, spinach, swiss chard, turnips, water chestnuts, and zucchini. Ensuring that you have an intake of these phytochemical-rich plants is critical to keeping the KD healthy beyond ketosis.

Proteins that contain more fat are best, such as wild-caught seafood, whole organic eggs, and grass-fed meat. Examples include meat (beef, pork, lamb, veal, goat, duck, venison, buffalo/bison); poultry (chicken, turkey); fish (anchovies, cod, halibut, herring, salmon, sardines, trout); shellfish and seafood (clams, crab, lobster, scallops, shrimp, mussels, oysters); nuts and seeds (macadamia, pecans, almonds, walnuts, flax, hemp, chia); and protein powders (those low in sugar).

Examples of fats and oils in KD include animal fats (ghee, butter), avocado oil, almond oil, avocado oil, cacao butter, olive oil, coconut oil, and coconut butter.

You should make sure you are in ketosis with the help of a home urine or blood ketone testing meter. You should test more frequently at the start of your program to make sure you are consistently in ketosis with your diet. One expert-recommended method is testing before breakfast, two hours after lunch, and two hours after the evening meal.[98] Once you become keto-adapted, you will need to use a blood meter to check ketones as the urine strips are only good in the early phases. Your nutritionist or integrative doctor will coach you on this aspect of KD, but it is critical to monitor if you are using KD as a specific cancer therapy.

Dr. Seyfried, one of the world's experts in KD and cancer, has developed a glucose ketone index calculator (GKIC) for cancer patients. It was researched in the treatment of KD and metabolic management of brain cancer.[99] The premise is that the glucose ketone index (GKI) is more reliable than glucose levels or ketone levels alone.[100] An optimal level is 1.0 or less.[101] The GKI is measured by dividing your blood glucose level (mmol/L) by your blood ketone level (mmol/L). You can convert your blood glucose reading from the typical mg/dL to mmol/L by taking your glucose number and dividing it by 18, or you can use a variety of websites for the conversion.

Seyfried recommends measuring blood glucose and ketone values two to three hours after a meal, preferably twice daily. The Precision Xtra meter is often recommended for measuring both glucose and ketones.

Again, if you are following KD, especially if you have cancer, make sure you do so under the supervision of a qualified medical professional. Typically, one follows KD intermittently along with other diets. For example, a modified Mediterranean diet, intermittent fasting, and KD can be rotated.

Several excellent books provide meal planning for KD, such as *The Ketogenic Kitchen* by Domini Kemp and Patricia Daly and *Fight Cancer with a Ketogenic Diet* by Ellen Davis. *The Metabolic Approach to Cancer* by Dr. Nasha Winters and Jess Higgins Kelley has a deep explanation of KD and metabolic-based therapies. The more broadly encompassing *Cooking through Cancer Treatment to Recovery* by Lisa Price and Susan Gins makes preparation and planning for healthy eating with cancer easy and accessible.

INTERMITTENT FASTING

One of the newer areas of integrative nutritional approaches to cancer is intermittent fasting, also known as periodic fasting.

With fasting, the same metabolic effects occur as with the ketogenic diet. After using glycogen released from the liver as the main energy source, amino acids turn into glucose, and the body breaks down fat to provide fatty acids that are converted into ketones as a fuel source.

Over 100 years ago, researchers demonstrated that calorie restriction associated with an antitumor effect in mice.[102] Since then, many animal studies have demonstrated that calorie restriction reduces the progression of tumors.[103] In addition, a 20-year study in rhesus monkeys found calorie restriction to decrease cancer incidence by 50 percent and lower the incidence of aging-related deaths.[104]

Periodic fasting can have beneficial effects on hormones and other factors that feed tumor formation, including IGF-1, insulin, glucose, IGFBP1, and the promotion of antitumor levels of ketone bodies. Experts state that periodic fasting creates "a protective environment for normal cells while creating a metabolic environment that does not favor precancerous and/or cancer cells."[105] And researchers have found in various studies that periodic fasting, lasting two days or more, can be "a highly effective strategy to protect normal cells and organs from a variety of toxins and toxic conditions while increasing the death of many cancer cell types."[106]

In a clinical trial, participants were prescribed a fasting mimicking diet (FMD) that lasted five days every month and provided between 34 percent and 54 percent the normal caloric intake with a composition of at least 9 percent to 10 percent proteins, 34 percent to 47 percent carbohydrates, and 44 percent to 56 percent fat. Patients were randomized to the FMD for five days every month for three months (three cycles) or to a control group that continued to consume their normal diet. Subjects were asked to resume their normal diet after the FMD period and were asked to not implement any changes in their dietary or exercise habits. Researchers found decreased risk factors and biomarkers for aging, diabetes, cardiovascular disease, and cancer without major adverse effects. Fasting blood glucose and IGF-1 levels were significantly reduced and remained lower than baseline levels even after resuming their normal diet following the final FMD cycle.[107]

In a different study, 10 patients with a variety of malignancies voluntarily fasted prior to (48 to 140 hours) and/or following (5 to 56 hours) chemotherapy. The patients received an average of four cycles of various chemotherapy drugs in combination with fasting. Common chemotherapy side effects, such as vomiting, diarrhea, fatigue, and weakness, were reduced. For the cases where cancer progression could be followed, there was no evidence that fasting had a growth-promoting effect on tumors or interfered with chemotherapy efficacy.[108]

In a pilot study, 7 out of 13 women diagnosed with HER2-negative stage II/III breast cancer were randomized to fast 24 hours before and 24 hours after receiving chemotherapy (docetaxel/doxorubicin/cyclophosphamide) or eat according to normal healthy nutrition guidelines. Short-term fasting was well tolerated with no differences between the two groups in terms of side effects. Additional benefits of fasting included significantly higher red blood cell count and platelets, as well as possibly less DNA damage in healthy cells compared to the non-fasting group.[109]

We can see that periodic fasting is an alternative to long-term calorie restriction for people with cancer, particularly when used strategically before and after chemotherapy treatments.

One strategy is to drink only water one to two days before and/or after chemotherapy. Another is to fast (drinking only water or vegetable juice or other modified versions) a few times a year for prevention purposes. We discuss this in more depth in Chapter 8.

MAINTAINING WEIGHT AND MUSCLE MASS

We have found diet to be critically important in preventing and treating cachexia, or major loss of skeletal muscle mass (which is usually accompanied by substantial weight loss), for those with cancer.[110] Up to 80 percent of advanced stage cancer patients have cachexia.[111]

Several factors can contribute to cachexia, such as chronic inflammation, pain and anticancer medications, cancer cell metabolism, and limited mobility. But certainly, one of the factors that can be addressed by you and your doctor right now is nutrition.

In the *Journal of Cachexia, Sarcopenia, and Muscle,* researchers concluded in a study of men with cancer that cancer stage, serum albumin (a protein), and weight loss predicted survival.[112] In other words, it is critical for people with cancer to optimize nutrition to prevent wasting of the body.

If cachexia is a problem for you, then work with your doctor and nutritionist on a diet to prevent or reduce it. This often involves the use of nutritional supplements that aid in digestion and absorption, as well as protein powders. For example, protein powders and amino acids can be used to support muscle mass. A review article in the journal *Biomedicine & Pharmacotherapy* recommends a nutritional regimen that provides 30 to 35 calories per 2.2 pounds of body weight per day; 1 to 1.2 grams of protein per 2.2 pounds of body weight per day, and a fat intake that can cover 30 percent to 50 percent of the non-protein calories. The article states, "In patients with chronic illnesses, oral nutritional supplementation has been shown to be beneficial in terms of physical function and weight gain."[113]

Omega-3 fatty acids have also been shown to be of benefit in several human studies for people with advanced cancer stages to stabilize weight loss, reduce lean tissue wasting, and increase survival in patients with advanced cancer.[114] [115] [116] [117] Of course, exercise is critical to incorporate along with nutritional support.

Cachexia is a primary reason why you need to work with a health professional to incorporate dietary changes such as KD, fasting, or intermittent fasting.

DIET ESSENTIALS

No matter what diet you follow under the guidance of your health professionals, there are a number of essential elements that most cancer nutrition experts agree on:

- Eat organic as much as possible

- Drink purified water

- Eat foods rich in fiber (plant foods)

- Eat foods rich in omega-3 fats (cold-water fish, some plant foods)

- Eat foods in their natural state

- Avoid hydrogenated vegetable oils, such as soybean, corn, and cottonseed

- Consume healthy oils, such as olive and coconut

- Minimize dairy

- Avoid artificial sweeteners and food preservatives

- Avoid deep-fried, grilled, or barbecued meats

- Avoid trans fats found in processed snack foods and fast foods

- Avoid excess salt (can use salt substitutes, such as those made with potassium chloride)

- Avoid soft drinks, excess fruit juice, and high fructose corn syrup

- Drink herbal teas, such as organic green tea

- Avoid rancid oils and excess polyunsaturated fats

- Use spices with your meals

- Minimize sugar and simple carbohydrate intake

- Avoid foods known to be contaminated with mycotoxins, such as peanuts

- Avoid preservatives, such as nitrates found in processed meats

- Minimize alcohol

- Eat in a relaxed atmosphere

Diet and nutrition are truly the base upon which all other cancer therapies build. We have seen time and time again that a patient's good response will fall away because the base of proper diet and nutrition is ignored. In many cases, diet is a difficult thing to change, but our experience has proven that it is critical and worth it. But more important than your diet, your attitude about your cancer treatment is a primary determinant of the success for your cancer treatment.

CHAPTER 6

SUPPLEMENTS FOR TREATING AND PREVENTING CANCER

S upported by published literature proving the safety and efficacy of nutritional supplements, an integrative doctor will usually prescribe nutritional supplements as part of a comprehensive program to improve a patient's quality of life and outcome. Many nutritional supplements can be incorporated into an integrative cancer program, including vitamins and minerals, herbal and other plant extracts, and homeopathic remedies. Conventional doctors are often unaware of the published literature proving the safety and efficacy of nutritional supplements, and most oncologists are not educated on the research involving supplements and integrative cancer therapy.

We acknowledge that research on nutritional supplements is for complementary or adjunctive therapy, not as a primary therapy for cancer. Therefore, supplement recommendations are generally used within integrative medicine (conventional and holistic) treatment plans. We feel strongly that a comprehensive strategy should include supplements (along with diet, exercise, stress reduction, and so on). These supplements are best used with the consultation of integrative medicine specialists.

It is important to note that many studies show a synergistic effect of supplements when used with conventional therapies in terms of reducing side effects, improving immunity, improving quality of life, and improving outcomes. There are also some studies demonstrating a cancer prevention benefit from specific nutritional supplements.

There are literally hundreds of supplements that could be reviewed in this chapter. We have included the ones that have the best research and that we have the most experience with. This summary of nutritional supplements can be used as a reference guide to enhance your health, to better understand what your integrative doctor is recommending, or as information to share with your oncologist to improve your therapy.

ACTIVE HEXOSE CORRELATED COMPOUND (AHCC)

WHAT IT IS: An extract from the mycelia of several species of basidiomycete mushrooms, including shiitake, which are cultured in a liquid medium with rice bran.

USES: Immune system activation, cancer prevention, integrative cancer treatment, and prevention of chemotherapy side effects.

HOW IT WORKS: Contains substances known as glucans that modulate the immune system. It has been shown to increase natural killer cell, T-cell immune response, and other immune factors.[1][2] Test-tube and animal studies and limited human studies have shown anticancer effects.[3][4][5]

KEY STUDIES: People with a history of liver cancer and subsequent liver surgery who were given AHCC supplementation had an increased overall survival rate compared to the control group.[6] Another study of patients with advanced liver cancer who were given supportive care were given AHCC or placebo. Those in the AHCC treated-group had a significantly prolonged survival compared to the control group.[7]

AHCC has been shown in studies to reduce the adverse effects of chemotherapy in people with advanced cancer,[8] and in those with pancreatic cancer (pancreatic ductal adenocarcinoma).[9]

SAFETY: Adverse effects are not common but may include diarrhea and itching. There is potential drug interaction with drugs metabolized by the CYP450 2D6 pathway (e.g., doxorubicin, ondansetron, selective serotonin reuptake inhibitors, tamoxifen), although this has not been shown in research.[10]

DOSAGE: 3000 to 6000 mg daily

ACETYL-L-CARNITINE (ALC)

WHAT IT IS: An amino acid that is produced in the body and is also available in supplement form.

USES: Mainly to reduce nerve pain known as neuropathy. This includes neuropathy caused by chemotherapy and diabetes. It may also help with memory.

HOW IT WORKS: ALC supports memory by enhancing the activity of the neurotransmitters acetylcholine and dopamine. It also transports fatty acids into the cell mitochondria for energy production. The mechanism of how it helps neuropathy is unclear but is likely multifactorial, including improved nerve transmission, structure, and function, as well as blocking pain signals.[11] It also has been shown to have a regenerative effect on nerve tissue.[12]

KEY STUDIES: A study involving 25 people with peripheral neuropathy induced by chemotherapy (taxane, 5 platinum) were given 1000 mg of ALC three times daily for eight weeks. At the end of the study, 23 out of 25 participants had significant improvement of their neuropathy.[13] Another study of 27 patients with chemotherapy-induced peripheral neuropathy from cisplatin or paclitaxel, or a combination of these two drugs, were treated with intravenous ALC. They were given 1 gram for at least 10 days and up to 20 days. The majority of those treated had at least minor improvement and the treatment was well tolerated.[14]

The use of ALC to improve cognitive function or slow cognitive decline in people with dementia are mixed. ALC was shown to improve cognitive functioning in patients with severe hepatic encephalopathy (brain disorder for those with liver disease).[15]

SAFETY: ALC is well tolerated. It may cause digestive upset and restlessness.

DOSAGE: Take 1000 mg three times daily, preferably on an empty stomach.

ARTEMISININ (QINGHAOSU)

WHAT IT IS: A substance derived from the plant known as Artemisia annua, also known as wormwood or sweet sagewort. It can be administered orally as a medication known as artesunate, or it can be given by intramuscular or intravenous injection.

USES: A treatment for malaria and other parasite infections.[16] It has also been studied as a potential treatment for cancer.[17][18]

HOW IT WORKS: Artemisinin has several mechanisms against cancer. It has been shown in multiple cell line studies to have a positive tumor kill effect.[19][20][21][22] It reacts with iron to form free radicals that can kill cancer cells.[23]

KEY STUDIES: Artemisinin was shown in an in vitro study to inhibit the cell proliferation and induce apotoposis (cell death) in human neuroblastoma cells.[24] A different in vitro study demonstrated antitumor activity against colorectal cancer cells.[25] Additional in vitro studies have shown artemisinin to have anticancer effects against prostate cancer,[26] breast cancer,[27] liver cancer,[28] leukemia,[29] and oral cancer.[30]

SAFETY: The oral form should not be used by those with ulcers.[31] It may cause digestive upset and rash.[32]

DOSAGE: Artemisinin is available in oral form, liposomal, and rectal suppository.

ASTRAGALUS (ASTRAGALUS MEMBRANACEUS)

WHAT IT IS: Astragalus has a long history of use in traditional Chinese herbal medicine and is popular in the West for immune system enhancement.

USES: Mainly used in the West for immune system support. It is commonly recommended for the prevention of upper respiratory tract infections and for supporting the immune system for those with cancer.

HOW IT WORKS: Contains a number of compounds, including polysaccharides, saponins, and flavonoids, all of which have immune enhancing, anti-inflammatory, antioxidant, and anticancer effects.[33]

KEY STUDIES: A study of 498 patients with acute myeloid leukemia (AML) found that the use of a multiherb product (including *Astragalus*, *Saliva miltorrhiza*, and *Spatholobus suberectus*) may prolong survival time.[34] Studies suggest that *Astragalus* (and formulas with *Astragalus* as the main compound) has benefits in reducing the adverse effects of chemotherapy.[35][36] Research has demonstrated that *Astragalus* has a suppressive effect on breast cancer growth and metastasis in assay studies.[37] Test tube studies have shown anticancer properties with *Astragalus* compounds for stomach,[38] colon,[39][40][41] and hepatic cancers.[42]

SAFETY: Very high doses may cause indigestion. It has a mild effect on blood thinning and blood pressure lowering.

DOSAGE: 1500 to 3000 mg daily

BEC (SOLASODINE RHAMNOSIDES)

WHAT IT IS: BEC, also known as Curaderm[BEC5], is a mixture of compounds known as solasodine rhamnosides. They are extracted from the fruit of *S. sodomaeum*, also known as *S. linnaeanum* (devil's apple), and *S. melongena* (eggplant).[43] The formula is used as a topical cream.

USES: Topical treatment of non-melanoma skin cancers, including actinic keratosis, keratoacanthoma, basal cell carcinoma, and cutaneous superficial squamous cell carcinoma.[44]

HOW IT WORKS: The solasodine rhamnosides in BEC, known as solamargine and solasonine, bind to the receptors of cancer cells and cause cell death (apoptosis).[45][46][47] This effect does not occur with normal cells.[48][49] Curaderm also contains 10 percent salicylic acid and 5 percent urea. These two substances are used to bring moisture to the area and break down the skin to allow BEC to penetrate the tumor.

KEY STUDIES: Actinic keratosis is a precancerous skin condition that can advance to squamous cell carcinoma. In one study, Curaderm[BEC5] was randomly assigned to people with actinic keratosis on the face, trunk, or extremities twice daily for three consecutive days. The rate of complete clearance at day 56 was 92 percent compared to 38 percent for placebo. The absolute success rates after one-year follow-up were 82 percent for solasodine glycosides and 18 percent for placebo.[50]

A double-blind, randomized study involving 10 centers in the United Kingdom looked at the effect of solasodine glycoside extract cream on basal cell carcinoma or placebo cream. The active compound was given to 62 subjects, and 32 were given a placebo. After eight weeks, the treatment group had a 66 percent cure rate compared to 25 percent for the placebo group. At the one-year follow-up, 78 percent of those receiving active treatment had no recurrence.[51]

An article citing case reports and the successful use of Curaderm[BEC5] published in the *Journal of Cancer Therapy* included two cases of squamous cell carcinoma and four cases of basal cell carcinoma. Treatments were supervised by dermatologists and oncologists.[52]

SAFETY: Serious adverse reactions are not common.[53] Local skin reactions can occur, such as burning, redness, itching, and ulceration.

DOSAGE: Curaderm[BEC5] is applied topically to the lesion, just enough to cover the lesion. It is applied twice daily (every 12 hours). After application, an occlusive dressing such as paper tape should cover each lesion until the next application. The treatment is stopped when the lesion has completely cleared and has been replaced with normal skin.[54]

BOSWELLIA SERRATA (INDIAN FRANKINCENSE)

WHAT IT IS: An extract from a tree known as *Boswellia serrata*. It has a long history of use in Ayurvedic medicine and is now popular as an anti-inflammatory compound in the West.

USES: Commonly used to treat arthritis but also has research showing it can benefit bronchial asthma and ulcerative colitis. It is also used as an adjunctive treatment for people with cancer, especially those undergoing radiation therapy.

HOW IT WORKS: *Boswellia* contains substances that have anti-inflammatory properties. This includes boswellic acid. More specifically, it inhibits 5-lipoxygenase[55] and cyclooxygenase-1,[56] and inhibits the signaling of inflammatory pathways through transcription factor, nuclear factor (NF-kappa B), and cytokine tumor necrosis factor (TNF-alpha).[57] Test tube and animal studies have demonstrated anticancer properties.[58 59 60 61]

KEY STUDIES: A prospective, randomized, placebo-controlled, double-blind trial was published in the journal *Cancer*. Researchers examined the effects of *Boswellia* for brain edema for people treated with radiation for brain tumors. People were either given radiation therapy plus *Boswellia* (4200 mg a day) or radiation and a placebo. Boswellia was found to significantly reduce brain swelling as measured by MRI as compared to placebo. A reduction of cerebral edema greater than 75 percent of those taking Boswellia was found in 60 percent of patients compared to 26 percent taking placebo.[62]

A different study examined the topical use of Boswellia for skin redness and other skin reactions for breast cancer patients undergoing radiation therapy. It was well tolerated and shown to reduce the use of topical corticosteroids and the severity of skin redness and other skin symptoms.[63]

SAFETY: Boswellia is well tolerated. Digestive upset is occasionally reported. It can have a mild blood thinning effect and caution should be used when on anticoagulant medications.[64]

DOSAGE: A general oral dosage can range between 1500 to 4500 mg daily of a Boswellia extract.

CANNABINOIDS

NOTE: It is possible that no other therapy used in cancer has more controversy than the use of medical cannabinoids. Some debate relates to the legal status of cannabinoids and social views on their use. Some is simply due to differences in the legal ability to obtain medical cannabinoids from jurisdiction to jurisdiction. Other controversies are based in simple ignorance of the facts.

Our goal is to present the best evidence-based information available so people can make a more informed decision regarding the use of medical cannabinoids in cancer care. As a practitioner with the legal right to authorize medical cannabinoid use in the state of Washington for many years, Dr. Anderson has had experience with hundreds of cancer patients using thousands of doses of medical cannabinoids. At the time of writing, the availability of cannabis-derived cannabinoids is very "jurisdiction dependent" (i.e., state or province rules differ) but hemp-derived cannabidiol (CBD) is available in all 50 U.S. states. We will be inclusive in the information below because rules and laws change, and we want patients to have the best information available should they have access to these potent agents.

WHAT IT IS: Medical cannabinoids are derived from common species, such as *Cannabis sativa* and *Cannabis indica*, that are members of the nettle family that have grown wild throughout the world for centuries. Both species have been used for a variety of purposes, including hemp to make rope and textiles, as a medical herb and as the popular recreational drug. Of note, "hemp" is a particular strain of *Cannabis sativa* that has very low psychoactive properties. There are over 70 cannabinoids, but the forms we normally refer to are CBD and delta-9-tetrahydrocannabinol (THC), which is the more psychoactive of the two.

Others include CBN, CBG, CBC, THCV, which are found in whole plants. There are other constituents, such as terpenes (aromatic oils) and limonene, with many nerve-calming, liver-supporting, and immune-helping effects. Other constituents include the flavonoids, which are anti-inflammatory and known as "cannaflavins."

HOW IT WORKS: The human body is made with an inter-cannabinoid system known as the endocannabinoid system. This system is well studied (although more is likely unknown than known).[65] The clinically important part of humans having an endocannabinoid system is that the use of medical cannabinoids enhances what the body already has the potential to do.

Medical cannabinoid can affect the following areas specifically important in cancer care by doing these things:[66][67]

- Lowering cancer-triggering inflammation

- Improving immune function

- Potentially improving some standard therapies

- Potentially lowering the need for pain medication

- Potentially lowering the need for sleep, muscle-relaxing, and anti-anxiety medications

- Decreasing nausea and improving appetite

- Balancing the immune system

- And many other potential benefits

KEY STUDIES: Medical cannabinoids have studied benefits in pain and anxiety and sleep medication reduction or replacement. Clinically, the lower the doses of opiate pain medications, the better the immune system works, such that people often want to be off of their prescription sleep or anxiety medications. We find medical cannabinoids assist in all these areas.[68][69][70]

In addition to the benefits for pain, sleep, anxiety, and quality of life, many direct anticancer potentials for medical cannabinoids are emerging in the research data.[71][72][73][74] It is for this reason, coupled with clinical experience, that we believe medical cannabinoids hold a significant place in integrative oncology.

SAFETY: Side effects of cannabinoids depend on the method of administration (e.g., smoking or vaporizing versus standardized extracts in capsule, liquid, or other forms) and the dose of the active compounds. The use of certain cannabinoids, such as CBD, have been well studied and considered to be well tolerated and safe in humans, even at high doses.[75] THC may cause a high, altered senses, mood changes, impaired body movement, impaired memory and focus, hallucinations (high doses), delusions (high doses), and psychosis (high doses).[76]

DOSAGE: Dosing is variable and depends on the amount of CBD and/or THC you are trying to achieve. CBD-only doses range from 25 mg to 200 mg daily from most sources. In cancer patients, we normally ramp up the CBD dose in four divided doses of 10 to 25 mg each. It should be noted that in the hemp-derived CBD products, a total dose of 250 mg hemp oil has only 25 to 65 mg actual CBD.

When using THC in the beginning of therapy, Dr. Anderson normally uses a standardized tincture (typically 20 to 30 percent THC) to allow for slow dose escalation, because people have such differing responses to THC. If a person is not a cannabis user, the THC dose needs to be small and ramped up slowly. Although studies are ongoing, it appears that CBD alone is helpful for most above-listed beneficial effects but that in cancer cell death, a mixture of THC and CBD is likely best (if one can obtain both). Clinical results seem to show a THC/CBD ratio of 1:1 to 1:4 as beneficial in the purely anticancer setting. In cases where we have patients who can legally obtain only CBD, we still use it, as benefits are significant.

If adding THC to the CBD, we continue the four divided doses of CBD during the daytime since those doses of CBD rarely have any "brain" effects (sleepiness and so on). Then the THC tincture is dosed after dinner and at bedtime as tolerated. A 20 percent tincture of THC has 200 milligrams in a milliliter (a small amount, as five milliliters = one teaspoon). Once tolerance is known, we attempt to match the milligrams of THC to the CBD dose for the day to get the 1:1 ratio to start for cancer care. Once dose tolerance is known, we may add suppositories of THC at night to increase THC dose.

GINSENG (*PANAX GINSENG, PANAX QUINQUEFOLIUS*)

WHAT IT IS: There are different types of ginseng. The two focused on in this book are *Panax ginseng*, also known as Asian ginseng. The other is American ginseng, also known as *Panax quinquefolius.*

USES: Historically used to treat fatigue and stress. Several studies have demonstrated anticancer properties[77 78 79 80 81 82] and a reduction in the side effects of conventional oncology therapies.[83 84]

HOW IT WORKS: Asian ginseng has been shown in animal studies to inhibit cell proliferation, angiogenesis (blood flow to tumors), and other mechanisms.[85] When *Panax ginseng* is consumed, a metabolite is formed by the intestinal flora known as compound K. This compound has shown in human colorectal cancer cell assays to have anticancer effects, such as inducing cell apoptosis.[86] American ginseng contains substances known as ginsenosides which have demonstrated anticancer properties.[87 88]

KEY STUDIES: A study of 1,455 Chinese breast cancer patients who took an average of 1300 mg of ginseng root material found that it "may improve both overall and disease-free survival and enhance the quality of life."[89] A different Korean population study found a reduction in the risk of endometrial cancer in breast cancer survivors.[90] A well-publicized study involving American ginseng and its potential benefits for cancer-related fatigue was published in the *Journal of the National Cancer Institute.* It was a multisite, randomized, double-blind trial that involved 364 participants. At eight weeks, those given 2000 mg of American ginseng had significant improvement over placebo.[91]

SAFETY: Both ginsengs are well tolerated. American ginseng can lower blood sugar levels in those with diabetes.[92] Both should be discontinued one week before surgery.[93]

DOSAGE: 1300 to 2000 mg daily.

GLUTATHIONE

WHAT IT IS: An antioxidant composed of the amino acids cysteine, glutamine, and glycine. It is found in fruits and vegetables and naturally produced in the body.

USES: In integrative oncology, glutathione is used post treatment to recover from the side effects of chemotherapy and radiation. It can also be used as part of a preventative program to improve antioxidant status, DNA repair, normal cell replication, immunity, and detoxification and to reduce DNA damage.

HOW IT WORKS: Glutathione is involved in energy production, drug detoxification, and DNA repair; neutralizes free radicals; and regulates cell proliferation and apoptosis (cell death), removal of environmental toxins and carcinogens (cancer-causing agents), and nerve regeneration.[94][95]

KEY STUDIES: A randomized, double-blind, placebo-controlled study involved 50 patients with advanced stomach cancer who were receiving cisplatin-based chemotherapy. People were treated with IV and intramuscular injections of glutathione or given a placebo. Those treated with glutathione showed no evidence of neuropathy (nerve damage) after the ninth week, whereas 16 patients taking placebo did. After 15 weeks, 4 out of 24 patients given glutathione suffered from neuropathy compared to 16 of 18 in the placebo group. Those receiving glutathione had a greatly reduced requirement for a blood transfusion compared to placebo.[96]

In another study, people with advanced colorectal cancer receiving oxaliplatin chemotherapy who were given intravenous glutathione had reduced problems with neuropathy. The activity of the oxaliplatin was not reduced.[97]

A separate study of women diagnosed with ovarian cancer treated with cisplatin found that patients receiving glutathione treatment had better kidney filtration and quality of life scores, including significant improvement in depression, emesis (vomiting), peripheral neurotoxicity, hair loss, shortness of breath, and difficulty concentrating.[98]

A study published in the *European Journal of Nutrition* demonstrated that a specific type of oral glutathione doubled the activity of natural killer cells compared to placebo.[99]

SAFETY: Glutathione is well tolerated. Even so, the use of glutathione during chemotherapy and radiation therapy is controversial, and it is generally used between or after conventional oncology treatments for recovery and prevention purposes.

DOSAGE: Oral glutathione is often used at doses of 500 to 1000 mg daily. The supplemental form is also available in the highly absorbable liposomal form. Glutathione is also administered by doctors in suppositories, transdermal (topical application to skin), intramuscular injection, and intravenous forms.

GERMANIUM

WHAT IT IS: Germanium, also called germanium sesquioxide or abbreviated CEGS, is a compound that can be given in supplemental and intravenous administration. This is the safe organic form that is used in supplements.

USES: Antioxidant, immune system enhancement, and antitumor effects.[100]

HOW IT WORKS: Animal studies have demonstrated that germanium has anticancer effects, including the enhancement of interferon-gamma and natural killer cell activity, and inhibiting tumor and metastatic growth.[101] [102]

KEY STUDIES: In one study, humans with cancer were given 1000 mg of germanium sesquioxide for 10 days. After three days, natural killer cell activity was significantly increased.[103]

Feeding or supplementing germanium sesquioxide has shown benefit in animal models for spontaneous leukemia, lung cancer, and chemically induced tumors of the digestive system.[104]

SAFETY: Studies have demonstrated that germanium sesquioxide, the type used in supplemental form, is safe even at large doses.[105] Other forms of germanium may be toxic.

DOSAGE: The oral form is normally 275 to 1000 mg daily in a pulsed fashion. Commonly taken two to three days per week, with four to five days per week not taking it.

RESVERATROL

WHAT IT IS: A compound produced naturally in foods, such as grape skins and berries.

USES: Often used as an antioxidant to protect against cellular free radical damage. It is also used for the integrative treatment and prevention of cancer.

HOW IT WORKS: Inhibits the proliferation of cancer cells through apoptosis (cell death) and possibly has estrogen blocking effects.[106] [107] [108]

KEY STUDIES: Several test tube and animal studies have demonstrated the inhibition of cancer cell proliferation.[109] [110] [111] [112] This also includes the inhibition of prostate cancer cell growth in test tube and human cell lines.[113] Research on mice with bowel cancer showed a 50 percent reduction in tumor size when given low dose resveratrol.[114]

SAFETY: Side effects are not common. Very high doses may cause digestive upset.[115] Those with hormone-sensitive cancers should check with their physician before using.[116]

DOSAGE: 250 mg to 1000 mg daily

MAITAKE (*GRIFOLA FRONDOSA*)

WHAT IT IS: An edible mushroom that has been long used in Japanese and Chinese medicine for a variety of health conditions. Extracts of maitake are popular for immune system enhancement.

USES: Treatment of hypertension, high cholesterol and triglycerides, diabetes, viral infections, cancer prevention, and integrative cancer therapy.[117]

HOW IT WORKS: Contains substances known as beta-glucans that stimulate different components of the immune system. Specifically, maitake extracts contain beta 1,6 glucan and beta 1,3 glucan.[118] Immune activity stimulated by maitake includes macrophages, natural killer cells, T cells, interleukin-1 and 2, interferon, lymphokines, and superoxide anions.[119] [120] [121] [122] [123] It also upregulates the expression of a gene known as BAK-1 that has antitumor activity.[124] Maitake extract has demonstrated in animal studies to protect healthy cells from becoming cancerous, help prevent metastasis, and slow or stop tumor growth.[125]

KEY STUDIES: A study of 18 people with myelodysplastic syndrome (MDS), a type of cancer where bone marrow cannot produce enough healthy cells, involved giving patients a maitake extract at a dose of 3 mg per 2.2 pounds of body weight for 12 weeks. Maitake was shown to increase immune parameters such as neutrophils and monocytes, and was well tolerated.[126]

In a preliminary, non-randomized clinic trial involving 33 people with advanced cancer, patients were given either oral maitake extract (MD fraction) or maitake extract in combination with chemotherapy. Cancer regression or significant improvement was observed in 11 out of 16 breast cancer patients, 7 out of 12 liver cancer patients, and 5 out of 8 lung cancer patients.[127]

In a survey of 671 patients undergoing chemotherapy, maitake was found to reduce adverse reactions and pain for those with terminal stage cancer.[128]

A study involving mice with breast cancer found that maitake extract (D-fraction) reduced the spreading of cancer and tumor formation.[129]

SAFETY: Maitake extracts are very safe. A small percentage of users may experience loose stool that may be alleviated with a lower dose. Those on immunosuppressive drugs should not use maitake without the consent of their physician. Maitake may reduce blood glucose levels.[130] However, we have not found this to be significant. There was one case report of a maitake user and a possible interaction with the medication Coumadin.[131] We have not found maitake to have a significant anticoagulant effect.

DOSAGE: The most well-studied maitake products are hot-water extracts. This includes maitake D-fraction and MD-fraction. For a therapeutic dose, the recommendation is 0.5 to 1 mg per 2.2 pounds of body weight per day, or 35 to 70 mg of maitake extract daily. Lower doses are recommended for maintenance or general immune support. It is best taken on an empty stomach.

FERMENTED WHEAT GERM EXTRACT (FWGE)

WHAT IT IS: A nutritional supplement that is used by cancer patients in Hungary to improve quality of life.[132] It is also available in North America and available under different marketing names, including Avemar, Avé, and AvéULTRA.

USES: Mainly as a dietary supplement for integrative cancer therapy. It is also used for autoimmune disorders.

HOW IT WORKS: Several of the anticancer effects from FWGE are thought to be due to high levels of a group of chemicals called benzoquinones.[133] FWGE blocks the glucose fuel supply of cancer cells.[134] It also enhances immune function with increased natural killer cell activity and intercellular adhesion molecule 1 (ICAM-1) expression[135][136] and causes cancer cell death (apoptosis).

KEY STUDIES: FWGE was tested with 66 people with colorectal cancer who received FWGE supplementation for more than six months, while 104 control patients received traditional anticancer therapies alone. By the end of the study, 23 percent of the patients receiving conventional cancer treatments had their cancer spread. In sharp contrast, only eight percent of the FWGE patients saw their cancer spread. Researchers noted that FWGE was beneficial in terms of overall and progression-free survival.[137]

In a randomized clinical trial, patients with melanoma were given standard chemotherapy or chemotherapy plus FWGE for one year. After a seven-year follow-up period, researchers found that patients who had taken FWGE were half as likely to die from melanoma during this time. The researchers noted that "the inclusion of Avemar (FWGE) into the adjuvant protocols of high-risk skin melanoma patients is highly recommended."[138]

In a smaller study, researchers followed 22 patients with oral cancer who took FWGE and compared them with 21 patients not receiving FWGE. Those who took FWGE reduced the risk for cancer progression by 85 percent.[139]

At the Los Angeles Biomedical Research Institute at Harbor-UCLA Medical Center, an open trial with 16 people with lung cancer who were receiving standard cancer therapy were supplemented with FWGE. Patients' symptoms and quality of life were monitored with a questionnaire. Researchers found a significant improvement in the overall state of health, including a reduction in fatigue and pain and an improvement in appetite and emotional state.[140]

In a study with human breast cancer cells, FWGE was combined with the estrogen blocking breast cancer drug tamoxifen, which led to an increased rate of cancer cell death.[141]

Furthermore, FWGE seems to have the ability to heal infections in children and teenagers undergoing chemotherapy. Researchers followed 22 kids and teens who were being treated for different types of cancer and found that those who had received FWGE had significantly fewer infections and fevers while receiving chemotherapy.[142]

SAFETY: FWGE is very well tolerated with occasional reports of digestive upset. If you are pregnant, a nursing mother, have had an organ or tissue transplant, are suffering from bleeding gastrointestinal ulcers, malabsorption syndrome, gluten-sensitive enteropathies (celiac sprue), or fructose intolerance, or have hypersensitivity to gluten or wheat germ, you should not use FWGE.[143]

DOSAGE: A typical dosage is 9 grams per day. It is available in powder or tablet form. It is best taken on an empty stomach. Vitamin C supplements or beverages containing high amounts of vitamin C should not be taken within two hours of ingesting FWGE.[144]

GREEN TEA (*CAMELLIA SINENSIS*)

WHAT IT IS: Made from the leaves of the plant *Camellia sinensis*, green tea is available in various forms, including tea, liquid extracts, capsules, tablets, and suppositories.

USES: Green tea is used for cancer prevention and treatment and cardiovascular disease, as well as other conditions.

HOW IT WORKS: Green tea contains compounds known as polyphenols. These include EGCG and ECG, which have powerful antioxidant properties that may protect against cell DNA damage.[145] In laboratory and animal studies, these polyphenols have been shown to inhibit tumor cell proliferation and induce apoptosis (cancer cell death). Compounds in green tea also inhibit angiogenesis (blood flow to tumors) and tumor cell invasiveness.[146] Other mechanisms include protection against ultraviolet B radiation,[147] immune system modulation,[148] and detoxification support.[149]

KEY STUDIES: Researchers from Vanderbilt-Ingram Cancer Center surveyed 75,000 middle-aged and older Chinese women. Most women reported drinking green tea. The researchers found that consuming tea at least three times a week for more than six months was associated with a 17 percent reduced risk of all digestive cancers combined. Those who consumed two to three cups per day had a 21 percent reduced risk of digestive system cancers. For those who drank tea regularly for at least 20 years, the risk for all digestive cancers combined was reduced by 27 percent. The most protective effect was for stomach, esophageal, and colorectal cancers.[150]

A review of 43 epidemiological studies, 4 randomized clinical trials, and 1 meta-analysis found that 58 percent of the included studies demonstrated a cancer prevention effect from long-term consumption of green tea. More than half of the studies (58 percent) suggest that long-term consumption of green tea may reduce the risk of certain types of cancer, particularly gastrointestinal cancers, such as esophageal, stomach, pancreatic, liver, and colorectal cancer.[151]

A study published in the *Journal of Clinical Oncology* looked at different doses of EGCG given to people with chronic lymphocytic leukemia (CLL). Doses ranged between 400 and 2000 mg twice daily. With this, 33 percent of patients had a reduction in absolute lymphocyte count and 92 percent of patients with lymph node swelling had at least a 50 percent reduction.[152]

A double-blind, placebo-controlled study followed 60 men taking 200 mg of green tea extract or a placebo three times daily for one year. The men had high-grade prostatic intraepithelial neoplasia, a precancerous condition of the prostate. Fewer prostate cancers occurred in the men taking green tea extract (one cancer in 30 men) compared with the placebo group (nine cancers in 30 men). No significant side effects were documented.[153]

Green tea extract has been shown to be synergistic and effective when combined with the taxane chemotherapy drugs against human prostate cancer cells[154] and to reduce the incidence of colonic adenomas (precancerous polyps) by 51 percent.[155]

SAFETY: The tea form is generally recognized as safe by the U.S. Food and Drug Administration. Since green tea contains caffeine, caffeine sensitivity reactions are possible but not common. The supplement form at higher doses may cause mild digestive upset, headache, dizziness, and muscle pain.[156] [157] There can be an elevation of liver enzymes, but it is reversible with a reduction in dosage or discontinuation of the supplement.[158] We have not found these adverse effects to be common. Green tea was shown to increase the oral bioavailability (or potency) of the cancer drug tamoxifen in one animal study.[159]

DOSAGE: Green tea extracts are often standardized by the amount of EGCG they contain. Supplemental amounts vary between 800 and 4000 mg daily, with higher doses used for active cancers and lower doses for prevention purposes.

TURMERIC (CURCUMA LONGA)

WHAT IT IS: A bright-yellow spice that is common in Indian food. It is also available as a nutritional supplement. Turmeric is a member of the ginger family. The root has long been used medicinally in Asia.

USES: For centuries, turmeric has been recognized as a healing agent in Ayurvedic and Chinese medicine. It is now commonly used by North American practitioners and holistic doctors for its anti-inflammatory benefits. It is also recommended for integrative cancer therapy, arthritis, depression, and digestive ailments.

HOW IT WORKS: Turmeric contains a group of compounds called curcuminoids known for their antioxidant and anti-inflammatory properties.[160] Curcumin is one of the most important curcuminoids and the focus of a great deal of research. In vitro studies have shown that curcumin has anti-inflammatory[161] [162] and anti-proliferative (anticancer) properties.[163] [164]

Curcumin regulates many cell-signaling pathways that are involved in cell proliferation, including Nrf2 and NF-kB.[165] It also inhibits compounds involved in the inflammatory response that can be involved in the initiation of cancer. This includes cytokines, chemokines, adhesion molecules, growth factors, cyclo-oxygenase, lipoxygenase, and inducible nitric oxide synthase.[166] In addition, it activates cancer cell death (apoptosis) and changes gene expression that is unfavorable to cancer growth.[167] It is often used as a sole extract in nutritional supplement form.

KEY STUDIES: In one study people with colorectal cancer were given oral curcumin supplementation for a time before surgery. Benefits included increased body weight and general health, and a number of favorable changes in biomarkers were measured, including increased tumor cell death.[168]

In another study lasting 30 days, a supplement of 1500 mg of curcumin was given to 16 chronic smokers and 6 nonsmokers. A significant reduction in urinary compounds that cause DNA damage was found with the smokers, whereas the control group had no change.[169] Research on curcumin with cancer is ongoing. The Mayo Clinic notes, "Laboratory and animal research suggests that curcumin may prevent cancer, slow the spread of cancer, make chemotherapy more effective and protect healthy cells from damage by radiation therapy."[170]

SAFETY: Side effects are minimal. Research has shown that people tolerate up to 8000 mg daily of curcumin for three months with minimal side effects.[171] Turmeric has antiplatelet properties, so lower doses may need to be used for those on anticoagulant therapies.[172]

DOSAGE: A typical oral dosage is 1500 to 8000 mg daily. Curcumin is also available in liposomal and suppository forms.

MODIFIED CITRUS PECTIN (MCP)

WHAT IT IS: An extract from the peel and pith (the white, threadlike part between a citrus fruit and its peel) of citrus fruits.

USES: Integrative treatment of cancer and toxic metal detoxification.

HOW IT WORKS: MCP has anticancer effects by binding and inactivating a protein known as galectin-3.[173] Galectin-3 is involved in the clumping and migration of cancer cells to tissue, the formation of blood vessels that feed tumors, the prevention of cancer cell death, and the metastasis (spreading) of cancer.[174] MCP targets all these pro-cancer effects of galectin-3. It also induces cancer cell death by interfering with important signaling pathways related to cancer cell proliferation and survival.[175] MCP improves immune cell activity,[176] helps certain chemotherapy drugs such as doxorubicin work more effectively,[177] and blocks galectin's ability to stimulate the formation of blood vessels in new tumors (known as anti-angiogenesis).[178]

KEY STUDIES: A 12-month trial of 15 grams daily of MCP supplementation was conducted with 10 men with prostate cancer. These patients never responded favorably to conventional treatment, such as prostatectomy, radiation, or cryosurgery. MCP was shown to significantly slow the rise of prostate-specific antigen (PSA) in 7 out of 10 men (using rising PSA as an indicator of cancer growth).[179] Studies done with human and mouse prostate cancer cells have shown that MCP can inhibit cell proliferation and apoptosis (cell death).[180]

A German study followed 29 patients with various solid tumors that in most cases had metastasized. Conventional treatments had been unsuccessful. The patients were given five grams of MCP daily and evaluated every four weeks. Quality of life improvements were found with physical functioning, global health status, fatigue, pain, dyspnea (shortness of breath), insomnia, and appetite loss compared with when they started supplementation.[181]

SAFETY: MCP is well tolerated. Digestive upset, such as abdominal cramps and diarrhea, may occur. Reducing or stopping MCP will eliminate these symptoms.

DOSAGE: For those with active cancer, the dosage is five grams taken with water three times daily. Prevention doses range between 5 and 10 grams.

MILK THISTLE (*SILYBUM MARIANUM, CARDUUS MARIANUM*)

WHAT IT IS: An herb that is commonly used in herbal and holistic medicine to support liver health. Milk thistle is native to the Mediterranean region. It gets its name from the milky white sap derived from crushing its leaves. It is a popular remedy in European herbal therapy for ailments of the liver, gallbladder, and kidney.

USES: To treat liver ailments, including those caused by alcohol, pharmaceuticals, mushroom poisoning, and viral infections such as hepatitis. This includes protection against liver damage for those taking medications for cancer therapy. Milk thistle extract, known as silibinin, is used for cancer prevention and treatment.

HOW IT WORKS: Milk thistle seeds contain a group of flavonoids collectively known as silymarin, which includes silibinin, silidianin, and silychristin. They are thought to repair liver cells that have been damaged, reduce inflammation, and have antioxidant properties.[182]

In terms of cancer, laboratory studies suggest that silymarin stops cancer cells from dividing and reproducing, shortening the life-span of cancer cells, and reducing blood supply to tumors.[183] Silymarin and its active constituent silibinin have the capability to potentiate (increase or magnify) the efficacy of known chemotherapeutic drugs.[184]

KEY STUDIES: Several studies, mainly done with animals, have demonstrated the anticancer effect of silymarin, including anticancer activity against breast, skin, prostate, cervical, liver, colon, ovarian, and lung cancers.[185]

SAFETY: Milk thistle is well tolerated. Side effects are often mild and may include digestive upset.

DOSAGE: A typical does of milk thistle extract is 500 to 1000 mg daily. Silibinin extract is available as a stand-alone supplement. Silibinin is used intravenously (see Chapter 7).

PROBIOTICS

WHAT IT IS: Probiotics refer to supplements that contain "friendly bacteria" that populate the digestive tract and other areas of the body.

USES: Probiotics are mainly used to support digestive health. They are also used for immune enhancement, anticancer properties, allergies, cardiovascular health, eczema, mood disorders, and many other conditions.

HOW IT WORKS: By supplying good bacteria, probiotics help the immune system function better so that it can detect and kill cells that can become cancer.[186]

Many studies have shown that probiotics enhance immune system response and reduce inflammation.[187] They also improve the detoxification of carcinogenic (cancer-causing) compounds in the colon and prevent cell DNA damage.[188]

KEY STUDIES: A 12 week, double-blind, randomized, placebo-controlled trial in colorectal cancer patients looked at the effect of probiotic supplementation. Probiotic supplementation significantly decreased the proportion of patients suffering from irritable bowel symptoms and improved cancer-related quality of life scores.[189]

A study published in the *Annals of Oncology* assessed published data consisting of 17 studies on the efficacy and safety of probiotics in cancer. Researchers concluded that probiotics may reduce the severity and frequency of diarrhea and the need for anti-diarrhea medications.[190]

A study of probiotic supplementation with people undergoing colorectal cancer surgery found that probiotic supplementation can reduce superficial incision infections and enhance immune response.[191]

A different study evaluating probiotic supplementation with patients undergoing colorectal cancer surgery found that supplementation significantly influenced the recovery of bowel function, including constipation and diarrhea.[192]

SAFETY: Overall, probiotics are extremely well tolerated. Rare cases of immune-compromised cancer patients developing infections possibly from probiotics have been reported.[193]

DOSAGE: Probiotic doses range from 5 billion colony-forming units (CFU) to several hundred billion. A typical preventative dose is 5 billion to 20 billion CFU per day.

LICORICE ROOT GLYCYRRHIZIN (*GLYCYRRHIZA GLABRA, GLYCYRRHIZA URALENSIS*)

WHAT IT IS: A commonly used herb in traditional Chinese medicine, Ayurveda, European herbal therapy, and naturopathic medicine.

USES: For immune enhancement, infections, digestive disorders, inflammation, hormone balancing, and many other conditions. It is also used for its anti-cancer properties.[194 195 196]

HOW IT WORKS: In vitro and in vivo research has demonstrated that two constituents of licorice root, isoliquiritigenin and naringenin, promote regulatory T cell activity.[197] Licorice root also reduces inflammation, induces cancer cell apoptosis (cell death), and may protect against DNA damage.[198]

KEY STUDIES: Research done on the Chinese species of licorice root (*Glycyrrhiza uralensis*) found that it inhibits cell proliferation in human breast cancer cells.[199] Research on the *Glycyrrhiza glabra* species has demonstrated anticancer properties for colon cancer cells.[200]

SAFETY: Licorice root is generally well tolerated. Excessively high doses may cause an elevation in blood pressure, water retention, and potassium imbalance,[201] but when regular doses have been prescribed in our clinical practice, it is rare that we have observed these side effects.

DOSAGE: Oral doses of licorice extract vary from 250 to 1000 mg daily. For those who are using licorice for digestive upset, such as mouth sores, acid reflux, and gastritis, the chewable form known as DGL (deglycyrrhizinated) is commonly used, which removes the substance that can elevate blood pressure or cause electrolyte imbalance. A typical dose is one to two tablets chewed two to three times daily. However, DGL is not the form to use for immune enhancement.

FISH OIL

WHAT IT IS: Omega-3 fatty acids derived from purified fish oil.

USES: The prevention of cardiovascular disease and cancer and to treat colitis, depression, psychiatric disorders, and skin conditions such as eczema.

HOW IT WORKS: Chronic inflammation is a known risk factor for cancer, and fish oil has natural anti-inflammatory effects. Studies demonstrate that omega-3 fatty acids decrease the inflammatory markers interleukin-6 (IL-6),[202] tumor necrosis factor-alpha (TNF-alpha),[203] and C-reactive protein.[204] Research has shown that the omega-3 fatty acids DHEA and EPA influence cancer proliferation, differentiation, and apoptosis (cell death) and inhibit angiogenesis (blood supply to tumors) and tumor cell invasion and metastasis.[205] They can favorably affect genetic expression related to cancer and DNA repair.[206]

KEY STUDIES: In a study, 22 people with leukemia or lymphoma were randomized to receive two grams of fish oil or no supplementation for nine weeks.

During the beginning of chemotherapy, those receiving fish oil had improvement in blood inflammatory markers and long-term survival.[207]

A study of patients receiving chemotherapy for advanced or recurrent gastrointestinal cancers and affected by cachexia (loss of skeletal muscle mass) found that fish oil supplementation significantly increased skeletal muscle mass and lean body mass over time, as well as improved chemotherapy tolerance and prognosis.[208]

A study of approximately 35,000 women living in western Washington State, ages 50 to 76 years, demonstrated that fish oil supplementation reduced the risk of invasive ductal carcinoma.[209]

Fish oil has been shown to improve the effectiveness of chemotherapy agents, including 5-fluorouracil (5-FU), paclitaxel, doxorubicin, and oxaliplatin.[210]

In a study of patients with non–small cell lung cancer receiving chemotherapy, patients receiving fish oil had an increased response rate and greater clinical benefit compared to those receiving only chemotherapy. Also, their one-year survival rate tended to be greater.[211]

SAFETY: Digestive upset may occur. Fish oil has an anticoagulant effect, so people on anticoagulant (blood thinning) medications should check with their physician before using.

DOSAGE: 300 mg of EPA to 2000 mg of EPA and DHA combined are typical doses. Fish oil is available in liquid and capsule formulas.

QUERCETIN

WHAT IT IS: A member of a group of plant pigments known as flavonoids. The primary sources are fruits and vegetables, especially citrus fruits, apples, onions, parsley, sage, tea, red wine, olive oil, grapes, and dark berries.[212]

USES: A supplement for the treatment of allergies, cardiovascular disease, prostatitis, inflammation, and cancer.

HOW IT WORKS: Quercetin has been shown in studies to exert the inhibition of cancer cell proliferation through multiple means. It has antioxidant, antitumor, and anti-inflammatory activity[213] and inhibits the genetic expression of genes, such as p21, that contribute to cancer growth and metastasis. It also causes cancer cell apoptosis (cell death).[214] Quercetin stimulates several detoxifying and antioxidant enzymes that can protect against environmental carcinogens.[215]

KEY STUDIES: In animal studies, quercetin has been shown to inhibit the proliferation of a wide range of cancers, including prostate, cervical, lung, breast, and colon.[216]

In vitro (test tube) and in vivo (animal) studies have demonstrated that quercetin inhibits pancreatic cancer growth.[217]

SAFETY: Quercetin is well tolerated. It should be used with caution if one is taking certain antibiotics, such as quinolone antibiotics,[218] anticoagulant medications, and possibly the chemotherapy medications doxorubicin and cisplatin.[219]

DOSAGE: A typical dosage is 1000 to 2000 mg daily.

IODINE

WHAT IT IS: A chemical element that is considered to be a trace mineral. The body requires small amounts of iodine but cannot make it. It must be consumed through the diet or supplementation.

USES: Mainly used by the body to make thyroid hormones.[220] It is also found in each cell of the body and is required to produce all hormones[221] and for proper immune system function,[222] has anticancer effects,[223] modulates estrogen response on breast cancer cells,[224] and is a potent antioxidant.[225]

HOW IT WORKS: Iodine is an antioxidant that protects against cell and DNA damage.[226][227] It also supports healthy immune function[228] and induces apoptosis in breast and thyroid cancer cells.[229] Iodine is formed into compounds called iodolactones that regulate breast cancer cell proliferation.[230]

KEY STUDIES: Studies on Japanese women have shown they have one of the lowest breast cancer rates in the world.[231] It is thought that the much higher consumption of iodine (25 times more than in the West) is a primary factor.[232] Iodine supplementation has been shown in animal and human studies to suppress the development and size of both benign and malignant breast cancers.[233]

A study of 22 women given iodine supplementation at 5 mg per day were found to have increased cancer cell apoptosis, decreased proliferation, and a decrease in the estrogenic effect on cells (most breast cancers are estrogen sensitive).[234]

The prostate gland is also sensitive to iodine uptake. Government nutritional studies have demonstrated that men with the highest levels of iodine compared to those with the lowest intake had a 29 percent lower risk of prostate cancer.[235]

The oral use of iodine for patients undergoing radiation therapy was found to reduce the incidence, severity, and duration of oral mucositis (pain and inflammation of the mouth).[236]

SAFETY: Iodine is considered to be safe when used at normal supplementation amounts. It may cause digestive upset or a skin rash.[237] Those on thyroid medication for hypothyroidism and hyperthyroidism or the use of the heart rhythm drug amiodarone should use iodine under medical supervision only.[238]

DOSAGE: Dosing depends on the health situation of the patient. Doses of 200 micrograms up to several milligrams may be prescribed and monitored by a doctor.

PROTEOLYTIC ENZYMES

WHAT IT IS: Enzymes derived from plant or animal sources. Proteolytic enzymes are proteins that break down protein and reduce inflammation.

USES: The treatment of cancer and cancer-related symptoms. They are also used to treat viral infections and inflammatory conditions such as arthritis. Proteolytic enzymes, when taken with food, are used as a digestive aid to break down protein. General pancreatic enzymes or plant-based enzymes can be used to break down protein, fats, and carbohydrates.

HOW IT WORKS: Cancer-fighting mechanisms include anti-inflammatory immune system modulation, and anti-angiogenic (reduced blood flow) to tumors.[239]

KEY STUDIES: In a two-year study, people with inoperable pancreatic adenocarcinoma followed a holistic treatment protocol involving pancreatic proteolytic enzymes; 8 of the 11 participants had stage IV disease. Nine survived one year, five survived two years, four survived three years, and two lived longer than four years. Compare this to a trial of 126 patients with pancreatic cancer receiving the chemotherapy agent gemcitabine where not one person lived longer than 19 months.[240]

In a collection of 31 case reports in *Alternative Therapies in Health and Medicine*, holistic treatment protocol included high-dose pancreatic proteolytic enzymes.

Beneficial effects for a variety of cancers were reported, including breast, colon, endometrial, non-Hodgkin's Lymphoma, pancreatic, renal cell (kidney), melanoma, sarcoma, ovarian, and lung.[241]

A study of one hundred patients with head and neck cancer examined the effect of supplementation of enzymes starting three days before radiation and continuing up to five days after completing radiation therapy. The results were positive, with the severity of acute radiation therapy side effects being significantly less for those patients receiving enzymes compared to the control group. This included symptoms such as mucositis, skin reaction, and throat pain.[242]

A study of 265 patients with multiple myeloma (stages I to III) demonstrated a significantly higher overall response rate and longer duration of remissions for those receiving chemotherapy and enzyme therapy than in those who received just chemotherapy.[243]

In a study of 2,339 breast cancer patients undergoing conventional cancer therapy, researchers gave 1,283 patients supplemental enzymes. Those receiving enzymes had significantly fewer side effects from conventional treatment compared with the control group. They also had improvements in the analysis of survival, recurrence, and metastasis.[244]

Oral enzyme therapy has been shown to benefit women undergoing radiation for locally advanced cervical cancer, where enzyme supplementation significantly reduced radiation therapy–related side effects.[245]

Patients with all stages of colorectal cancer were included in a review of controlled clinical trials using oral enzyme therapy. Patients receiving conventional cancer therapy and enzyme supplementation had diminished adverse reactions to chemotherapy and radiation in comparison with those receiving only conventional cancer therapy. The enzyme therapy was well tolerated.[246]

Pancreatic enzyme replacement has been shown to improve survival for those with cancer of the common bile duct who undergo pancreatic surgery.[247]

SAFETY: Proteolytic enzymes are quite safe.[248] They may cause digestive upset. Those with known gastritis or ulcers should take them with caution. Consult with a doctor if you have a bleeding disorder or are pregnant.

DOSAGE: The dosage of enzymes can vary depending on the product potency. For anticancer activity and to reduce the side effects of radiation and chemotherapy, a general dosage is three to five tablets/capsules three times daily, taken on an empty stomach. Those taking enzymes to reduce digestive symptoms typically take one to two tablets/capsules with meals. Patients with cancer should rely on their integrative doctor for dosage recommendations.

INDOLE-3-CARBINOL (I3C) AND DIM

WHAT IT IS: Plant chemicals derived from cruciferous vegetables, such as broccoli.

USES: Treatment of cervical dysplasia, breast cancer, and prostate cancer; detoxification; and estrogen metabolism.

HOW IT WORKS: I3C and some of its metabolites, such as 3,3'-diindolylmethane (DIM), have multiple anticancer effects. Both I3C and DIM inhibit the formation of estrogen from hormones such as testosterone and androstenedione.[249] This includes the metabolism of potentially cancer-causing estrogen metabolites and their ratios.[250] I3C and its metabolites promote the metabolism of xenobiotics (environmental hormone disrupters) that are potential carcinogens.[251] I3C inhibits estrogen-responsive genes that reduces cell proliferation in breast cancer.[252 253] I3C has been shown to inhibit angiogenesis (blood flow to tumors),[254 255 256] and I3C and DIM have both been shown to regulate inflammatory and immune responses that are important for normal cell division.[257] I3C has also been shown to have antiviral effects against human papillomavirus 16, which can cause cervical cancer.[258]

DIM has been shown to have several anticancer mechanisms, including the inhibition of multiple signaling pathways, restraining invasion, migration, and metastasis, as well as promoting apoptosis (cell death).[259]

KEY STUDIES: Population studies show an association between a diet high in cruciferous vegetables and a lower risk of cancer. In addition, I3C has been shown to have anticancer properties against a wide range of cancers.[260]

A study of women with cervical intraepithelial neoplasia (CIN 2 or CIN 3), also known as cervical dysplasia, were supplemented with I3C or a placebo for 12 weeks. Four of the eight women who took 200 mg per day had complete regression of CIN, and four out of the nine who took 400 mg per day had complete regression. None of the women who took a placebo had complete regression.[261]

A study of 78 women with cervical dysplasia (CIN 1-II) found that 100 to 200 mg daily for 90 to 180 days of DIM vaginal suppositories had a high rate of reversal of this condition.[262]

A trial of women with vulvar intraepithelial neoplasia, a precancerous condition of the vulva, found that supplementation of 200 mg or 400 mg per day of I3C for six months improved lesion size and appearance, as well as overall symptoms.[263]

A study of 95 women with a history of breast cancer who were taking the antiestrogen drug tamoxifen were given DIM (150 mg twice daily) or a placebo. Researchers found favorable changes in estrogen metabolism in the women taking DIM.[264]

Anticancer effects of I3C have been shown in human breast,[265][266][267][268] prostate,[269] endometrial,[270] liver,[271][272] melanoma,[273] and pancreatic cancer[274] cells. DIM was shown to have anticancer effects for human breast cancer cells.[275]

Animal studies have demonstrated that I3C has an anticancer effect against lung,[276] laryngeal,[277] and nasopharyngeal carcinoma.[278]

SAFETY: I3C and DIM are well tolerated, though with digestive upset occurring in some users.[279]

DOSAGE: Indole 3 carbinole has a typical dosage of 200 to 400 mg daily for women and 400 mg for men. DIM is often supplemented at 150 to 300 mg daily for women and 300 mg or higher for men.

INOSITOL HEXAPHOSPHATE (IP-6)

WHAT IT IS: Inositol hexaphosphate, also known as IP-6, myo-inositol hexaphosphate, and phytic acid, is a naturally occurring carbohydrate molecule that is present in plants and animals. It is available as a nutritional supplement.

USES: It is mainly used for cancer prevention and treatment. It is also used for high cholesterol and kidney stone prevention.

HOW IT WORKS: The exact mechanisms of IP-6 are not well understood, but it appears to reduce cancer cell proliferation through various means, such as cell signaling and genetic expression[280] and reduced tumor blood flow (anti-angiogenic).[281]

KEY STUDIES: In a study of patients with ductal invasive breast cancer being treated with chemotherapy, one group received IP-6 and inositol and the second group received placebo. Those in the treatment group had a significantly better quality of life and were better able to perform their daily activities in contrast with those taking placebo. Those receiving IP-6 and inositol did not have a drop in blood cells, including leukocytes and platelets.[282]

SAFETY: IP-6 may bind with minerals such as calcium, iron, magnesium, and zinc.[283] Therefore IP-6 should be taken several hours apart when supplementing these minerals. IP-6 has antiplatelet activity and should be used with caution with anticoagulants or antiplatelet drugs.[284]

DOSAGE: 3000 mg to 4000 mg twice daily

MELATONIN

WHAT IT IS: A hormone produced in the pineal gland.

USES: Melatonin is most commonly used to treat insomnia, jet lag, and seasonal affective disorder. It is also prescribed as part of integrative cancer therapy.

HOW IT WORKS: Melatonin stimulates immune cells, such as T-helper lymphocytes, monocytes, and natural killer cells.[285] It has potent antioxidant properties,[286 287 288] lowers the toxicity of several chemotherapy agents and reduces the side effects of chemotherapy,[289] exhibits antiproliferative effects,[290] activates p53 (a tumor suppressor gene),[291] is antimetastatic (prevents cancer spreading),[292] anti-angiogenic (reduces blood flow to tumor),[293] has anti-estrogen effects on cell receptors and genes that regulate their expression,[294 295] and inhibits telomerase activity (telomerase contributes to a cell's ability to survive).[296]

KEY STUDIES: A review of randomized clinical trials of melatonin supplementation was completed in patients with solid tumors. Melatonin supplementation provided substantial improvements in tumor remission, one-year survival, and alleviation of radiation and chemotherapy side effects such as fatigue, low platelets, and nerve toxicity.[297]

A study of women with metastatic breast cancer who were using the anti-estrogen drug tamoxifen without benefit were supplemented with 20 mg of melatonin in the evening. With this, 28.5 percent of the patients had a partial response in tumor reduction.[298]

A different study of women with breast cancer and melatonin supplementation was conducted. These women had received the chemotherapy agent epirubicin and had developed low platelets (thrombocytopenia). They were then given 20 mg of melatonin seven days before their chemotherapy treatment. There was a normalization of platelets in 9 of 12 patients after four cycles. There was also decreased tumor size in 5 of 12 patients.[299]

Melatonin supplementation at 20 mg each evening in addition to chemotherapy was found to improve tumor regression for patients with non–small cell lung cancer compared to a control group receiving chemotherapy only.[300]

The five-year survival rate of patients with metastatic non–small cell lung cancer patients treated with chemotherapy alone or the combination of chemotherapy and melatonin was studied. Researchers found overall tumor regression rate and the five-year survival results were significantly higher in those treated with melatonin.[301]

Patients with advanced cancers who were supplemented with 20 mg per evening of melatonin had a significantly lower frequency of cachexia, asthenia, thrombocytopenia, stomatitis, cardiac toxicity, neurotoxicity, and lymphocytopenia.[302] Additionally, the percentage of patients with disease stabilization and the percentage one-year survival were both significantly higher with a significantly better tumor response rate.[303]

Supplementing 20 mg of melatonin each evening was found to delay the onset of mucositis for patients receiving chemotherapy and radiation for head and neck cancer.[304]

A cream containing melatonin was shown to significantly reduce skin inflammation for women being treated for breast cancer with radiation therapy.[305]

SAFETY: Melatonin has been shown to have very low toxicity with a wide range of doses.[306]

DOSAGE: 10 to 40 mg each evening is a common dosage range, with 20 mg being the most common dose used in studies and in practice.

GARLIC (*ALLIUM SATIVUM*)

WHAT IT IS: A member of the lily family. It is available as a nutritional supplement in a variety of different commercial preparations.

USES: Commonly used to prevent and fight infections. It is also recommended for cardiovascular disease, including high cholesterol, atherosclerosis, and high blood pressure. Garlic is also recommended for the prevention and treatment of cancer.

HOW IT WORKS: Garlic may help prevent cancer by improving the immune response, such as macrophage activity against tumor cells,[307] natural killer cells,[308] and anti-inflammatory activity.[309] [310] [311]

Garlic also inhibits carcinogens from becoming metabolically active,[312] stimulates detoxifying enzymes that eliminate carcinogens from the body,[313] [314] and protects DNA from being damaged by carcinogens.[315] Garlic also has direct anticancer effects by inhibiting cancer cell replication and proliferation,[316] [317] inducing cancer cell apoptosis (cell death),[318] and inhibiting angiogenesis (blood flow to tumors).[319]

KEY STUDIES: A study published in *Cancer Epidemiology, Biomarkers & Prevention* found that the use of garlic supplements for four days or more a week for three years or more was associated with a reduced risk of hematological (blood) cancers.[320]

A trial of 37 patients with colorectal adenomas (noncancerous polyps in colon or rectum) found that high-dose aged garlic extract (2.4 ml per day) for 12 months significantly reduced adenoma size and number.[321]

Animal studies have reported that garlic and its constituents inhibit the development of chemically induced tumors in the liver, colon, prostate, bladder, breasts, esophagus, lung, skin, and stomach.[322]

SAFETY: Garlic supplements may cause digestive upset, bad breath, and body odor. Garlic decreases platelet aggregation and should be used with caution for patients on anticoagulant therapy.[323] Regular garlic supplements should be discontinued for one to two weeks before surgery. However, aged garlic extract has been shown in studies to be safe when taken along with anticoagulants (warfarin), aspirin, cholesterol-lowering statin drugs, or anticancer drugs (doxorubicin, 5-fluorouracil, methotrexate), and others.[324]

DOSAGE: The four main categories of garlic supplements are powdered (dehydrated) garlic, fluid extracts (such as Kyolic Aged Garlic Extract), steam-distilled garlic oil, and garlic oil macerates. A typical dose for powdered (dehydrated) garlic is 900 mg daily. Aged garlic extract is 2.4 ml of the liquid form or 3000 mg for the capsule form.

Consult with your integrative doctor for dosage recommendations.

COENZYME Q10 (COQ10, UBIQUINONE)

WHAT IT IS: A compound that is synthesized in the human body and is also found in small amounts in certain foods. CoQ10 is an antioxidant that protects against cell damage.

USES: Commonly used for the prevention and treatment of a variety of cardiovascular diseases. It is also used to enhance energy production and for cancer prevention and treatment, including the prevention of heart damage from chemotherapy.

HOW IT WORKS: CoQ10 is an important antioxidant that protects cell membranes and DNA from damage.[325] [326] The damage of cell membranes and DNA is a known risk factor for cancer. It also plays a significant role in boosting the immune system.[327]

KEY STUDIES: Two studies completed with female breast cancer patients demonstrated that CoQ10 supplementation resulted in tumor regression and metastasis for some patients.[328] [329]

Cancer patients treated with the chemotherapy drug doxorubicin who were supplemented with CoQ10 were shown to have a reduced incidence of cardiac dysfunction.[330] A different study of children with cancer being treated with a chemotherapy class of drugs known as anthracyclines who were supplemented with CoQ10 showed a protective effect against cardiac dysfunction.[331]

CoQ10 supplementation, along with a multivitamin/nutrient formula, was shown to provide significant protection against hearing disorders and tinnitus in patients undergoing cancer therapy with cisplatin chemotherapy.[332]

In a three-year trial, researchers found melanoma progressed more slowly if patients supplemented 400 mg daily of CoQ10 with low-dose interferon alpha as compared to interferon alpha–only treatment. There was also a significant reduction in the rate of recurrence of the tumor for those receiving the combination treatment compared to the drug-only treatment.[333]

An observational study found that people with lung, pancreas, and especially breast cancer were more likely to have low plasma CoQ10 levels.[334]

SAFETY: High doses of CoQ10 of up to 1200 mg daily have been shown not to have toxicity or significant adverse effects.[335] Side effects may include digestive upset. CoQ10 may interfere with the anticoagulant warfarin,[336] [337] although proper monitoring by a physician usually allows one to supplement CoQ10 without problem.

DOSAGE: 200 to 400 mg daily is a typical dosage range.

GLUTAMINE

WHAT IT IS: An amino acid manufactured by the body and also found in the diet.

USES: Mainly used for muscle growth and recovery, wound healing, inflammatory bowel disease, and to reduce the side effects of chemotherapy.

HOW IT WORKS: Glutamine supplies nitrogen and carbon for muscle and tissue healing. It also removes excess ammonia (a waste product) from the body.

KEY STUDIES: A study of supplemental glutamine was conducted with people undergoing radiation or chemotherapy for head and neck cancer. A dose of 10 grams taken three times daily or a placebo was given. Those who were supplemented with glutamine had a significant reduction of dermatitis (skin inflammation).[338]

A meta-analysis reviewed five clinical studies that included 234 patients with head and neck cancer who were undergoing radiation therapy. Researchers concluded that glutamine supplementation significantly reduced the risk and severity of oral mucositis (inflammation and ulceration of the mouth and throat) compared to placebo.[339]

Patients with lung cancer who were receiving radiation therapy and given glutamine supplementation had significant improvement in reducing inflammation and reduced toxicity. This included improvement in weight loss, esophageal movement, and markers of inflammation and toxicity.[340]

A study published in the journal *Nutrition and Cancer* evaluated 13 clinical studies for the safety and effectiveness of glutamine supplementation for patients with thoracic and aerodigestive (respiratory and digestive tract) cancers. In the review, 12 of the 13 studies showed a beneficial effect in the grade, duration of mucositis and esophagitis (inflammation of esophagus), gut permeability (absorption), and weight loss.[341]

In one study, women with breast cancer who had undergone breast surgery followed by radiation therapy were given either 15 grams of glutamine or placebo.

The treatment was started one week before radiation therapy and continued until one week after completion of the radiation. The women receiving the glutamine had a significant reduction in dermatitis compared to placebo.[342]

SAFETY: Glutamine is well tolerated. There is controversy about whether glutamine should be supplemented long term for those with active cancer, so consult with your physician.

DOSAGE: A total of 15 to 30 grams daily, taken in divided doses.

VITAMIN C

WHAT IT IS: An essential nutrient that the body does not manufacture and must be consumed through the diet or supplementation.

USES: To promote a healthy immune system to prevent and treat infections. It is supplemented as an antioxidant to protect cells against oxidative damage. It is also used for immune support for cancer patients. Anticancer activity of vitamin C is best achieved with intravenous vitamin C.[343]

HOW IT WORKS: Vitamin C stimulates the production and function of white blood cells.[344] It also reduces the damaging effects of oxidative stress in cancer patients.[345]

KEY STUDIES: Most studies on the cancer prevention properties of vitamin C have been demonstrated from dietary sources.[346][347][348][349]

Data from 13 studies determined the total intake of vitamin C from food and supplements was associated with a modestly reduced risk of colon cancer.[350]

The Women's Health Initiative study found that dietary and supplemental vitamin C was associated with a lower incidence of diffuse B-cell lymphoma.[351]

SAFETY: Excessive intake of oral vitamin C can cause digestive upset including diarrhea. Caution is recommended for those with a history of calcium oxalate kidney stones.[352]

DOSAGE: 1,000 to 10,000 mg daily.

ALOE (*ALOE BARBADENSIS, ALOE VERA*)

WHAT IT IS: *Aloe vera* is a plant that is used as a topical gel or lotion or internally when taken as liquid and capsule formulations.

USES: Topical use for the treatments of burns, wounds, infections, and other skin conditions. It is also used as an oral supplement for immune enhancement, cancer and cancer-related side effects, and digestive illnesses.

HOW IT WORKS: Aloe has a number of constituents that have immune modulating and anticancer effects.[353][354][355][356] It also contains a substance that inhibits cancer cell proliferation and causes cancer cell death through genetic expression.[357]

KEY STUDIES: A study involving 240 people with metastatic solid tumors had them randomized to receive chemotherapy with or without a species of aloe known as *Aloe arborescens*. The dose of aloe was 10 ml taken orally three times daily. The percentage of tumor regressions and disease control, as well as the percent of three-year survival, was significantly higher in patients treated with aloe than with chemotherapy alone.[358]

Patients with radiation-induced mucositis were found to have the same benefit from *Aloe vera* mouthwash as the conventional treatment of benzydamine mouthwash.[359]

SAFETY: Most commercial aloe products used for internal consumption have the bitter latex portion removed, which is a laxative. Aloe juice used for internal consumption is quite safe at normal dosages.

DOSAGE: For immune support take 10 ml three times daily or as directed by your integrative doctor. Also, aloe may be used as a mouthwash or it can be applied topically as a gel or cream.

OXALOACETATE (OAA)

WHAT IT IS: Oxaloacetate, also called oxaloacetic acid (OAA), plays a central and critical role in metabolism, including energy production. Low concentrations are found in oranges, apples, bananas, peas, and spinach.

USES: Treatment of brain injuries, such as concussion, and cancers of the central nervous system, such as glioblastoma.

HOW IT WORKS: Through removal of inflammatory (and tumor enhancing) glutamate and the improvement of the biochemical function of brain cells.

KEY STUDIES: In cancer, it is used as a glutamate scavenger that helps remove glutamate from the nervous system as well as the rest of the body. This removal process is more studied in brain trauma,[360][361][362][363][364][365] but the mechanism is the same in cancer. Glutamate is known to fuel cancer growth.[366][367] The reduction of glutamate and presence of OAA create a potential anticancer biological base in the brain in animal models.[368]

Dr. Anderson has used OAA in brain cancer patients and some other types of cancer as a synergistic therapy. It is especially useful in the metabolic approaches. In his clinical experience, it has improved outcomes in many tumor types as a part of a metabolic treatment protocol. OAA has been studied in humans,[369] but large scale human trials are not available.

SAFETY: OAA is considered to be very safe.

DOSAGE: A general dose is 300 mg daily. Some doctors prescribe 1500 mg daily for short-term use in the treatment of brain cancer.

POLY-MVA

WHAT IT IS: A dietary supplement containing a blend of the mineral palladium bonded to alpha-lipoic acid; vitamins B1, B2, and B12; formyl-methionine; N-acetyl cysteine; molybdenum; rhodium; and ruthenium.

USES: As a complementary therapy for people with cancer. It is also used for cardiovascular and neurodegenerative diseases,[370] diabetes and mitochondrial (cell energy) protection,[371] cell protection during and after radiation exposure,[372] and fatigue.

HOW IT WORKS: Poly-MVA supports mitochondria (energy factory of the cells) to produce more energy in healthy cells but weakens cancer cell metabolism by negatively affecting anaerobic cells.[373]

KEY STUDIES: Dr. James Forsythe, an integrative oncologist, has followed more than 1,000 patients using Poly-MVA. In one of his studies, 212 Stage IV cancer patients with multiple cancer origins were followed over a 26-month period. One group was given Poly-MVA and low-dose chemotherapy, and another group that refused chemotherapy was given Poly-MVA only. In both groups, Poly-MVA was first given intravenously and then switched to the oral form for up to six to eight months, after which a maintenance dosage of the oral form was continued. The overall response rate in people who received both chemotherapy and Poly-MVA was 61 percent. The overall response rate for Poly-MVA only was 39 percent. Both groups reported having significantly more physical energy.[374] Interestingly, this same research found that both treatments provided a six-year overall survival rate of 32 percent, while the average five-year survival rate is 2.1 percent in all stage IV cancers.[375]

Other research by Dr. Forsythe with Poly-MVA included 500 patients over a 40-month period and found the percent of survivors to be 59 percent.[376] The best responding tumors were prostate, breast, lung, head/neck, colorectal, and hematological (blood).[377]

Research published in the *Journal of Environmental Pathology, Toxicology, and Oncology* found that Poly-MVA enhanced the antitumor effect of radiation and had a protective effect against DNA damage and platelet count.[378]

A study published in the journal *Radiation Research* demonstrated that Poly-MVA reduced the inflammatory and mitochondria damaging effects of radiation in rats.[379]

SAFETY: Palladium is a chemical element that has various isotopes. There are six stable isotopes of palladium and an additional 25 that are radioactive. One type of palladium is used in an implanted seed for prostate cancer therapy. Also, palladium alloys are used in dentistry.[380] The type of palladium used in Poly-MVA is irreversibly bound to lipoic acid, which means the palladium is unavailable in a free form and therefore safely enters and leaves the body unchanged.

DOSAGE: A typical dosage for those with active cancer is four to eight teaspoons daily.

TOCOTRIENOLS

WHAT IT IS: Natural antioxidant compounds found in vitamin E. Examples of food sources include annatto beans, palm oil, and rice bran oil.

USES: To treat high cholesterol, improve nerve health, and help prevent cancer.

HOW IT WORKS: Tocotrienols have been shown to protect against radiation damage. They also reduce inflammation, including decreasing Nf-kB (inflammatory protein connected with cancer) and other inflammatory biomarkers. Tocotrienols help with apoptosis, cell cycle arrest, and angiogenesis; decreasing the expression of certain cancer genes; and increasing the expression of certain genes that suppress cancer.[381] The delta and gamma fractions have the most potent anticancer properties.

KEY STUDIES: Breast cancer research involving cell-line and animal studies has shown anticancer properties for delta and gamma tocotrienols.[382][383] Research has shown that a high concentration of tocotrienols was approximately 65 percent higher in the adipose tissues of patients with benign breast lumps compared to patients with malignant tumors.[384] And most importantly, in one study of 240 women with estrogen-positive breast cancer that who were given tamoxifen (20 mg) and tocotrienol (400 mg) for five years had a 70 percent decreased risk of dying compared to women taking only tamoxifen. Researchers found the risk of recurrence was 20 percent lower in those receiving both tamoxifen and tocotrienol compared to the control groups receiving tamoxifen plus placebo.[385]

Delta tocotrienol was shown to delay pancreatic progression and metastasis in animal research.[386] Research has also shown that delta tocotrienol enhances the effectiveness of the chemotherapy agent gemcitabine to inhibit pancreatic cancer growth and survival.[387]

SAFETY: Tocotrienols have been shown to be very safe.[388]

DOSAGE: 400 mg or more of delta tocotrienol or tocotrienol fractions as determined by your integrative doctor.

TURKEY TAIL (*CORIOLUS VERSICOLOR, TRAMETES VERSICOLOR*)

WHAT IT IS: The most well-studied medicinal mushroom in the world. It has a long history of use for immune enhancement in Chinese and Japanese medicine. The Chinese version is abbreviated PSP, and the Japanese is abbreviated PSK.

USES: For immune system support and as an integrative oncology therapy for the treatment and prevention of various cancers.

HOW IT WORKS: Turkey tail contains compounds known as beta-glucans that stimulate an immune response. Hot-water extracts of turkey tail have demonstrated increased white blood cell and antibody response (IgG, IgM).[389]

Other studies have shown to induce cell death,[390][391] reduce cell proliferation,[392][393] and significantly increase TNF-alpha and IL-8 gene expression.[394] Turkey tail extract has been shown to increase killer cell activity.[395]

KEY STUDIES: More than 400 published studies have demonstrated significant immune modulating properties of turkey tail and its anticancer activity.[396] Turkey tail has several published human studies as an adjuvant (complementary treatment) along with conventional oncology. In one study, researchers recruited 185 people with lung cancer who were being treated with radiation. Half of the group received a placebo and the other half received the turkey tail (PSK) extract. Those receiving the turkey tail did much better overall than those on the placebo. The five-year survival rates of the patients who got the extract were 39 percent for those who had stage I or stage II cancers, and 22 percent for those who had stage III. Those in the placebo group had survival rates of 16 percent and 5 percent. Lung cancer patients who were 70 years old or older who got the PSK had a much better chance of surviving than those that only received radiation.[397]

A ten-year study has shown that turkey tail benefits those with a history of colorectal cancer. The randomized double-blind trial divided a group of 111 volunteers with colon cancer into two. After surgery for colorectal cancer, the first group of 56 patients took a turkey tail extract (PSK). The second group of 55 was given a placebo. The rate of patients in remission (or disease-free) in the PSK group was more than double that of the placebo group. Researchers also found that the PSK patients' white blood cells showed "remarkable enhancement in their activities."[398]

Turkey tail may benefit those battling stomach cancers. One study published in *The Lancet* examined the effect of PSK in stomach cancer patients. All of the 262 volunteers had stomach surgery and were starting chemotherapy. The survival rate of the group using both turkey tail extract (PSK) and chemotherapy was 73 percent after 5 years. The group who got chemotherapy alone had a survival rate of only 60 percent. The researchers said that PSK had "a restorative effect in patients who had been immunosuppressed by both recent surgery and subsequent chemotherapy."[399][400]

There has also been research with esophageal cancer and turkey tail extract. A prospective, randomized, multicenter study of 158 esophageal cancer patients who underwent surgery, followed by radiation therapy, were divided into different groups. Two of the groups received chemotherapy, one with and one without turkey tail extract (PSK); the other two groups received no chemotherapy, with one of these groups receiving turkey tail extract. Researchers found that patients who received turkey tail extract (three grams per day) for three months beginning immediately after surgery had a significantly better survival rate at five years.[401]

There have been published trials demonstrating that turkey tail extract (PSP and PSK) improves disease-free and overall survival in breast cancer. In a study of 914 women with breast cancer who were undergoing conventional therapy, those who were given 3000 mg of turkey tail extract significantly extended survival in ER-negative, stage IIA patients without lymph node involvement.[402]

A five-year post-surgery study with 376 women with stage II ER-negative breast cancer compared the effects of chemotherapy (5-fluorouracil) to 3000 mg daily of turkey tail extract (PSK). The five-year overall and relapse-free survival rates were the same in both groups.[403]

In another study, women with breast cancer who were positive for HLA-B40 antigen (tumor-specific protein) who were given turkey tail extract (PSK) at a dose of three grams daily for two one-month courses each year in addition to chemotherapy had a 100 percent survival after 10 years compared to HLA-B40 negative patients who had approximately 50-percent survival.[404]

In a study involving 227 operable breast cancer patients with vascular invasion and/or metastatic lymph node involvement, turkey tail extract (PSK) was given at a dose of 3000 mg daily for 28 days as an adjunctive treatment in addition to combination chemotherapy. Researchers concluded that turkey tail extract improved the prognosis for breast cancer patients who had tumors that showed evidence of vascular invasion.[405]

A study at Shanghai University recruited 650 people with cancer who were undergoing chemotherapy and radiation and gave them either *Coriolus* extract (PSP) or a placebo. The volunteers who received PSP had fewer side effects than those that received placebo.[406][407]

SAFETY: Turkey tail is well tolerated.

DOSAGE: A typical dosage is 3000 mg daily.

VITAMIN D (CHOLECALCIFEROL)

WHAT IT IS: A fat-soluble vitamin that is found naturally in foods, such as salmon, herring, sardines, cod liver oil, butter, egg yolks, and shiitake mushrooms. Vitamin D is formed in the skin when it is exposed to sunlight.

USES: Vitamin D supplements are used in conventional medicine for the prevention and treatment of osteoporosis and rickets. In addition, many studies have demonstrated that vitamin D plays a role in many body processes, including cardiovascular, respiratory, blood sugar regulation, joint, cognitive, and muscular, while supporting a healthy functioning immune system and normal cell division.[408]

HOW IT WORKS: The liver converts vitamin D3 from foods, skin production from sunlight, and from supplements into a substance known as 25(OH)D, also known as 25-hydroxyvitamin D. It is then converted by the kidneys and other tissues into activated vitamin D ($1,25\ OH_2D_3$), also known as 1,25-dihy droxyvitamin D3, or calcitriol. This active form has several anticancer mechanisms, which include the suppression of cancer cell proliferation, stimulation of apoptosis (cell death), regulation of immune cell function, inhibition of angiogenesis (reducing blood supply to tumors), reduction of prostaglandin metabolism and action (reducing inflammatory compounds that stimulate cancer growth), antioxidant effects, DNA repair, interference with growth factors (such as IGF) that are involved in cancer cell growth, and influencing the expression of genes that control cell growth and other signaling factors involved with cancer formation.[409] The active form of vitamin D targets enzymes that break down vitamin D, making it more available to tissues for its antitumor effects.[410]

KEY STUDIES: Several population studies suggest that vitamin D deficiency increases the risk of adults developing cancer.[411] [412]

In a study of 790 female breast cancer survivors, 75.6 percent had low blood vitamin D levels.[413] A review of studies found that postmenopausal women with low levels of vitamin D had a higher risk of developing breast cancer compared to postmenopausal women with high levels of vitamin D.[414] In women with a history of breast cancer, vitamin D status has been strongly associated with better breast cancer survival.[415] [416]

Several studies have demonstrated high blood vitamin D levels associated with a lower risk of developing colon cancer, including a review in the *Journal of*

Clinical Oncology, which found that higher vitamin D intake and blood vitamin D levels were associated with a lower risk of colorectal cancer.[417] A review of studies involving people with colorectal cancer found that those who had normal vitamin D levels were more likely to survive than those with low levels of vitamin D.[418]

A study completed in the Unites States involved men with a diagnosis of low-risk prostate cancer who were supplemented with 4000 IU of vitamin D3 for one year. Of these men, 24 of the 44 (55 percent) showed an improvement in their biopsy results, 5 (11 percent) had no change, and 15 (34 percent) showed a worsening of their biopsy results.[419]

A study involving prostate cancer and vitamin D published in the *Journal of the National Cancer Institute* found that men with the highest blood vitamin D levels had less than half the risk of lethal prostate cancer compared to men with the lowest levels.[420]

A study published in the *British Medical Journal,* which followed men with prostate cancer who were receiving hormone therapy found that patients with medium to high blood vitamin D levels had a significantly better prognosis than men with low levels.[421]

SAFETY: Side effects are uncommon when blood levels of vitamin D are within the normal range. Vitamin D toxicity for prolonged periods of time may lead to high blood calcium levels, which can result in bone loss, kidney stones, and calcifications of organs.[422] Vitamin D toxicity is very unlikely in healthy people at daily intake levels lower than 10,000 IU.[423]

DOSAGE: There are two forms of supplemental vitamin D: D2 (ergocalciferol) and D3 (cholecalciferol). D3 is the type found in foods and manufactured in the skin from sunlight. It is the preferred supplemental form,[424] especially for cancer prevention. A typical daily dosage is 2000 to 5000 IU daily taken with food. The dosage will vary depending on one's blood levels. Current research suggests that a serum level of vitamin D (25-dihydroxyvitamin D) should be at least 40 ng/ml in order to reduce the risk of developing cancer.[425]

CHAPTER 7

INTRAVENOUS AND

INJECTION THERAPIES

O ne of the most common questions we are asked is "Why would I need an injection of something I can take by mouth?" Another is "Is it really better?" Both are excellent questions! The first consideration with regard to any agent used to help or heal in illness (natural or pharmaceutical) is "What is the best route of administration?" If there are multiple routes, then the question becomes "When would one route be preferred over another?" The common administration routes are: oral (PO), sublingual / below the tongue (SL), rectal (PR), inhaled (such as a nebulizer, spray or inhaler), and injected. Injections come in a few forms: intramuscular / in the muscle (IM), subcutaneous / in the fat (SQ), intradermal / in the dermis of the skin (ID), and intravenous (IV).

The first benefit of an injected agent is that it bypasses the digestive system where a great deal of potency can be lost. By avoiding the digestive system, you can often deliver more of an agent to the blood and then the cells than using an oral route. For example, urinary concentrations from intravenous vitamin C have been shown to be 140-fold higher than maximum oral doses.[1]

When a person is ill and run down, their natural digestive function can be very poor due to medications, chronic illness, cancer therapies, and many more factors. In these cases, an IV can get the agents needed into the person without losing impact in an inefficient digestive system. Thus these are the three main benefits of an injection over oral dosing:

- HIGHER POTENCY IN THE BLOOD AND TISSUES—Many drugs have higher potency in the blood and tissues when administered via injection. In the natural realm, one agent that reflects this effect is curcumin, which has poor absorption from the digestive tract in many forms. Infusing a pharmaceutical grade, pharmacy-prepared IV of curcumin makes 100 percent of it available for use by the cells at levels unable to be achieved via oral dosing.

- ABILITY TO DOSE HIGHER THAN IF GIVEN ORALLY—Some agents such as vitamin C are not absorbed after a certain dose has been taken orally. Many people have experienced loose bowels or diarrhea when taking too much vitamin C because it stops absorbing at a certain point and stays in the digestive tract (causing a lot of water to stay, hence the diarrhea). In an IV form, vitamin C can be given at many times the orally tolerated dose, which adds to the benefit of cells fighting cancer.

- BYPASSING AN ILL OR DAMAGED DIGESTIVE TRACT—In any chronic illness, in any absorptive disorder like celiac disease, and in most people who have had chemotherapy, the digestive tract can be so damaged it will not absorb much of what is eaten nutritionally, let alone vitamins or mineral supplements. One of the most crucial things we do in integrative oncology is to help people repair their systems during and after chemotherapy and radiation. This repair is crucial so that the body is strong enough to accept cancer-fighting support. The use of IV nutritional therapy, along with hydration and super antioxidants (such as glutathione), has literally saved patients' lives when critically ill and allowed healing so their bodies were ready to heal at deeper levels.

So what about IV and injections in the integrative oncology world—is this a really new thing? IV and injection therapies used in cancer care are not new at all. For example, the use of injectable curcumin, which Dr. Anderson has studied in the past decade for cancer, has reports dating back to 1937.[2] Many other examples can be given, but we will now turn to the information gained in what

Dr. Anderson believes is the greatest age of discovery in IV and injection therapies for cancer ever—the past 25 years.

OXIDATIVE THERAPIES

Oxidative therapies refer to various therapies that uses oxidants to stimulate body processes for fighting cancer as well as tissue healing.

IV VITAMIN C

The most well-known, and perhaps most controversial, IV therapy is high-dose intravenous vitamin C (HDIVC). The use of HDIVC was popularized largely by the work of Frederick Klenner, M.D., who used HDIVC in hospital practice from the 1940s through his passing in 1984, throughout which time he published case reports.[3][4][5] It is said he inspired Linus Pauling and Irwin Stone to expand their research on the benefits of vitamin C,[6] and he was a mentor to Dr. Anderson. Later, through the work of his estate and Dr. Lendon Smith, two books were published, keeping some of his hard-earned information alive.[7][8]

HDIVC is a very common therapy in integrative oncology. While lower doses of IV vitamin C are also used, HDIVC has particular potential benefits.

HDIVC does have the ability to become a *pro-drug* (meaning it becomes or triggers another chemical to have a drug-like effect) for hydrogen peroxide and also provides a host of nutrient and chemical manipulations that weaken cancer cells while strengthening normal noncancerous cells.[9][10][11] The pro-drug for hydrogen peroxide part of the mechanism cannot be effective with oral vitamin C because not enough will absorb.[12][13]

HDIVC also has potent anti-inflammatory effects. Like many chronic diseases, cancer is a disease of inflammation, which fuels abnormal cell division. Research at Riordan Clinic in Wichita, Kansas, has found that a series of IVC sessions can lower the blood inflammation marker CRP by approximately 75 percent.[14] Preliminary evidence shows that IVC activates a gene that suppresses tumor formation.[15] In addition, HDIVC has an anti-angiogenesis effect, as it gets into cancer cells and creates an inhospitable (aerobic) oxygenated environment.[16]

Paramount in the decision to include a particular therapy for any condition is the safety of that treatment. The bottom line with respect to HDIVC is that in properly screened patients, it is an extremely safe intervention. A 2010 review of over 50,000 HDIVC infusions found only five reported serious adverse events.[17] In a review performed personally by Dr. Anderson of the five cases mentioned, all could have been prevented with proper pre-HDIVC screening. Everyone should be prescreened for multiple conditions prior to any HDIVC, and particular attention should be paid to G6PD status (an enzyme that, if deficient genetically, does not allow the normal processing of hydrogen peroxide by your body). One should also have kidney function and blood mineral status monitored. Any trained provider of HDIVC will make sure to run all the necessary tests before they start the IV therapy.

One very common and important question is "What if I am on chemotherapy?" A great deal of confusing information regarding the appropriate place and timing for the administration of HDIVC with other chemotherapeutic agents exists, but Dr. Anderson has completed an up-to-date review of all available data in this arena.[18] A recent scientific paper shows the overall direction the data are pointing: "Clinical investigation of pharmacologic ascorbate should be considered as an addition to existing cancer treatments. Its mechanism of action as a pro-drug for $H2O2$ generation is distinct from most currently used agents. For this reason, there is potential for synergy, or at least an additive effect, in combination with other drugs. This strategy is similar to that used for treatment of many cancers, tuberculosis, serious bacterial infections, hepatitis, and HIV. Emerging data indicate that there are additive effects of ascorbate with other neoplastic agents."[19] A review of available data in 2008 summarized multiple existing cancer therapies and their effect in combination with ascorbate and found that all the agents were either not affected or enhanced by ascorbate. This review had one exception, which was the drug bortezomib,[20] but later clinical data showed that even this agent had synergistic effect with HDIVC.[21]

In a 2012 multicenter study, 60 people newly diagnosed with cancer and receiving conventional cancer therapy were administered HDIVC twice weekly for four weeks. Significant relief was noted in quality of life scores, including fatigue, pain, insomnia, and constipation.[22] And a study of 39 terminal cancer patients not undergoing chemotherapy and radiation therapy and given IV and oral vitamin C reported significantly lower scores of fatigue, pain, nausea/vomiting, and appetite loss. They also had higher scores for physical, emotional, and cognitive function.[23]

Data presented between late 2011 and 2012 from Dr. Anderson's NIH-funded research reveal only positive additive effects using HDIVC in combination with existing cancer treatments.[24] A 2014 published review of the effects of intravenous vitamin C on cancer and quality of life noted: "Several recent studies have indicated that intravenous (IV) vitamin C alleviates a number of cancer- and chemotherapy-related symptoms, such as fatigue, insomnia, loss of appetite, nausea, and pain. Improvements in physical, role, cognitive, emotional, and social functioning, as well as an improvement in overall health, were also observed."[25] This Bastyr Integrative Oncology Research Center (BIORC) study was funded by the NIH and operated at Bastyr University Research Center. Dr. Anderson was the chief of IV services and operated the IV therapy clinic. His patient group consisted of stage IV (four) cancer patients treated with HDIVC and many other IV therapies. Many findings that are reported in this book came from that work.

In this work, researchers found the three-year survival rates of stage IV colon, lung, and breast cancer patients and stage III ovarian cancer patients receiving HDIVC from BIORC were dramatically better than national statistics, based on the National Cancer Institute's SEER program.[26][27]

ARTESUNATE

Artemisia-based medications are used the world over for antimalarial activity, and artesunate is an IV medication derived from parts of artemisia. The pharmacology and safety of artesunate is well studied and published in the scientific literature. The use of these agents in the patient with cancer and the effectiveness of artesunate against cancer cell lines are published in the literature, though are newer areas of scientific research. Experience in our clinical research of over 4,000 IV doses of artesunate has shown this agent to be safe in patients with advanced cancers.

In adults, IV artesunate has a low side-effect profile when used in typical IV doses.[28][29] Toxicity in some cases (animal and human) was attributed to the oil-based forms of injectable artemisia products that are not recommended for use in humans, and these negative effects are not generally seen in the artesunate (water soluble) form of the drug.[30][31]

Studies assessing both the efficacy and safety of IV artesunate in children have noted similar positive profiles for safety. In safety studies of artesunate looking at groups of more than 200 children, no increased risk of adverse events was noted beyond the adult data (when dosed appropriately). This safety profile in the pediatric population has led to the World Health Organization recommending IV artesunate use in children infected with malaria.[32][33][34] The safety of this IV agent in children is critical, as Dr. Anderson has safely given hundreds of doses to children with cancer, both artesunate alone as well as with HDIVC.

In a study looking at the activity of artemisinin against human pancreatic cancer cells (placed in animals), it was shown to be similar in effect to that of gemcitabine (a potent chemotherapy) and proved to cause significant tumor regression.[35] Studies looking at cancer cells, animal models, and early preclinical human data show multiple anticancer benefits for artemisia agents like artesunate. These include direct tumor cell killing, internal tumor cell death, and the ability to slow the growth of pro-tumor blood vessels (anti-angiogenesis).[36][37][38][39][40][41][42]

Growing evidence shows that artemisinin and its derivatives also possess potent anti-inflammatory and immune-calming properties. This not only helps keep the immune system balanced but may also oppose some triggers of cancer metastasis.[43][44][45][46]

In addition to your physician being trained in the use of IV artesunate, they should know to watch for iron and copper depletion during therapy. One mechanism of action for artesunate is cyclic use of iron and copper for oxidant generation. In general, when using the oral form of artemisia (whole plant or artemisinin), we clinically see more iron depletion than when using the IV form. With either oral or IV use, iron and blood counts need to be monitored.

ARTESUNATE COMBINED WITH HDIVC

The combination of IV artesunate followed by HDIVC was brought to Dr. Anderson's attention during the NIH-funded integrative oncology study by a group of German oncologists. Originally it was thought to be synergy based on both agents being oxidative in nature. While this certainly is true, it also occurred to Dr. Anderson that the addition of the immune properties likely created added benefit from this unique combination. At present, the patient data collected shows a survival benefit over a three-year time period between two groups of stage-IV breast cancer patients (both using a full integrative oncology approach). In this group of 40 patients, the subgroup that added artesunate and HDIVC to their integrative oncology program had greater overall survival that was 16 percent higher than the non-IV group in year one, 22 percent higher in year two, and 11 percent higher in year three.[47]

HYDROGEN PEROXIDE

Hydrogen peroxide (H2O2) used as an IV agent may sound both interesting and scary. Most of us have used topical H2O2 to clean cuts or scrapes. So how can that work as an IV? Certainly a very specific type and strength of H2O2 is used for infusion, and it must be done under highly controlled conditions (as should all IV therapies). In the IV form, a pharmacy produces a sterile low concentration H2O2 (for IV use only), which is free of preservatives and stabilizers (such as those found in the topical forms). The concentration is added to a saline IV bag at a particular (even lower) concentration, which is slowly infused. The key to this dilute and slowly administered form of H2O2 working is that it has the similar ability to create chemical shifts also made by HDIVC administration.[48]

When we teach this to physicians in IV therapy classes, they logically often ask, "Then why not just use HDIVC?" which is a great question. The answer is that while HDIVC creates H2O2 at the tissue level (a good thing in weakening many cancer cells), it has a tiny production of immune messenger chemicals after that work is done. In contrast, H2O2 does not deliver any H2O2 to the cells but rather stimulates the same immune messenger chemicals in the bloodstream, allowing these messengers to be delivered all over the body,[49][50] stimulating the immune cells to "look at" and fight the cancer cells. This contrast between HDIVC and H2O2 is another reason that integrative physicians will often rotate these therapies.

OZONE

Ozone (O3) can be considered the "cousin" molecule to the oxygen (O2) we breathe in the air. It is naturally occurring in the environment and is relatively unstable, with the ability to easily donate a single oxygen molecule to reactions and become O2. Like H2O2, this reactivity provides a group of interesting benefits in the care of those with cancer. O3 has been shown in human studies in topical or rectal administration to greatly reduce the side effects from prostate cancer radiation therapy and has showed excellent safety in application.[51]

The use of O3 in the IV setting is similar in concept to our discussion of H2O2, and, of course, you should have O3 provided by trained personnel in a medical setting. It is the easy donation of one oxygen atom from the O3 (forming harmless O2) that generates many of its benefits (again similar to H2O2, but not the same). Many studies have been completed to discover the multiple effects O3 may have on the biochemistry. One such study lists over 10 critical biochemical changes O3 can make in the human body that move the immune system toward a more robust, but balanced, output.[52]

A study where O3 was given to cancer patients receiving radiation and chemo-therapies showed that the addition of O3 to their treatment both enhanced the actions of the chemotherapy and lowered many common chemotherapy and radiation therapy–related side effects while improving quality of life.[53] A similar animal model of metastatic cancer showed the same results.[54] In a study using data from outside human subjects (blood reactions in a petri dish) and inside humans (in vivo), it was found that medical ozone could be administered safely while modulating many critical immune messengers. The study concluded that "single ozone doses can be therapeutically used in selected human diseases without any toxicity or side effects" and lauded the potential for O3 therapy to improve medical care by improving the versatility and power of its biochemical and therapeutic effects.[55] Additional studies have shown the benefit of O3 therapy in radiation therapies with a combination of improved treatment outcome and lower side effects.[56]

The use of O3 is proposed to be augmented by other therapies, and in our experience works best in a well-rounded treatment approach. One such combination which shows promise as synergy with O3 is ultraviolet therapy.[57]

ULTRAVIOLET BLOOD THERAPIES

Ultraviolet Blood Therapy, or ultraviolet blood irradiation (UVBI), has been used in medicine for multiple purposes. Its use, like O3 and H2O2, has been widespread in the care of patients with cancer for decades. UVBI may improve outcomes in the cancer patient through its ability to both improve oxygen delivery and decrease the propensity for forming infections when one has cancer, especially when one has immune-depressing cancer therapies.[58][59]

People often ask us, "How does exposing my blood to UVBI help in my cancer care beyond potential quality of life improvements?" Many explanations are possible, but one shows much promise based on human research. One problem in the biology of many tumors is low oxygen, or hypoxia. In the hypoxic state, the tumor creates its own unique "local biology," which becomes part of its ability to resist therapies and prevent growing in an uncontrolled manner. Much like hyperbaric oxygen therapy discussed later in the book (page 243), as measured in a human study, UVBI shows promise to improve the tissue delivery of oxygen by the blood cells.[60] This improved oxygen transportation can reduce the tumor's ability to be hypoxic and its potential to weaken a part of the tumor's resistance to other therapies.

BIOLOGICAL, METABOLIC, AND PLANT-BASED THERAPIES

This group of IV therapies refers to mainly natural compounds that stimulate or support the body's immune system to fight cancer.

GLYCYRRHIZIN

Glycyrrhizin, or glycyrrhizic acid / glycyrrhizinic acid (GA), is a portion of the licorice plant. It has a great deal of potential in the treatment of patients dealing with cancer. Data in humans shows it to be a safe IV agent and beneficial in chronic viral infections.[61][62] Over a decade of clinical use has revealed no adverse events when used under standard dose and administration guidelines.[63] We have used GA in the IV setting for many years as a synergist in patient care with apparent benefits ranging from lower infections to improved quality of life and lower fatigue in the patient with cancer.

In one prostate cancer cell study, GA inhibited cancer cell proliferation and lowered the potency of the remaining cancer cells. The outcome was so impressive it led the study to state, "these studies suggest that glycyrrhizin has therapeutic potential against prostate cancer."[64]

As always with any IV therapy, safety is paramount and the provider should be properly trained in the use of IV GA. The most commonly reported side effect in higher IV doses is a rise in blood pressure.[65] In our experience, at lower doses, this is unlikely, but one should (as with any IV therapy) have their blood pressure monitored before, during, and after GA administration.

GLUTATHIONE

Antioxidants are molecules in the body that normally take a free electron or "radical" away from a substance and keep it from becoming a damaging "free radical." These free radicals create all kinds of damage in the body and are normally balanced out by antioxidants. Inflammatory triggers are necessary to parts of immunity and not all bad (see page 194), but here we will focus on the crucial role glutathione plays in maintaining antioxidant–free radical balance. Antioxidants are many in number, but the primary triplet of antioxidant activity between the plasma (water portion of blood), cell interior, and on cell and fatty membranes (coating of cells) consists of vitamin C—glutathione and tocopherols (the vitamin E family). Thus it is no surprise that glutathione (GSH) is a crucial factor in cancer therapy and healing.

GSH, and its precursors and co-factors, can be taken orally and often are. In the IV form, GSH is immediately available for use by the cells, as are all IV agents.

Many studies do show that GSH is lower in cancer patients and especially in those who are undergoing or have undergone conventional therapies such as chemotherapy, radiation, and surgery.[66] [67] [68] The importance of this is that with low GSH, we have less ability to balance antioxidant–free radical activity (redox), which can lead to cell damage and many potential ill health effects.

Safety with any IV therapy should be paramount. IV GSH has been used in studies and, more importantly, in tens of thousands of doses in our patient populations.[69] In our vast clinical experience, GSH is an incredible addition to many well-rounded treatment plans.

A common safety concern is, "Is GSH potentially damaging to the other therapies being given for cancer?" This is a question we dealt with in the HDIVC section, and the answer is similar: "It depends," but also "it isn't as problematic as one may think." The key considerations are potential synergy with or antagonism of the other therapy, timing of the infusion, and how GSH fits into the overall plan for the individual patient. We once thought that GSH would be antagonistic to oxidant chemotherapies, such as platinum-based drugs. This actually makes sense. But in two studies, and since then in many patients, we have seen only synergy when co-administered (or administered on the same day) with the chemotherapy.[70][71] Generally, unless there is specific data such as that mentioned for the platinum-based drugs, we will separate the GSH from any oxidative therapy by 12 to 24 hours. GSH is used very rapidly by the cells when given IV, and since it does not circulate long, it allows for close administration. As part of the original NIH study, Dr. Anderson published a clinical guideline for timing of IV therapies, which addresses this issue for GSH and many other IV therapies.[72]

DIMETHYL SULFOXIDE (DMSO)

DMSO is one of the most commonly known "alternative" therapies. Many people have used it for joint pain and other similar issues. It is noted for being absorbed through the skin and relieving pain. Stanley Jacob, M.D., a researcher at Oregon Health & Science University for decades, was the main originator of DMSO use in medicine. Research has shown immune system modulation,[73] improved healing, and improved drug delivery to the brain and into tissues with DMSO usage.

For decades, we have used IV DMSO clinically to help in pain and inflammatory conditions and to deliver other IV therapies into nervous system (including brain) tissues. In more recent years, it has been used for palliative care (helping control pain and improve quality of life), where DMSO and other nutrients such as magnesium and sodium bicarbonate were effective in reducing pain in different cancer therapy–related pain syndromes.[74][75][76][77]

DMSO can be helpful in pain reduction, as an anti-inflammatory substance, and as a drug delivery system, and emerging research indicates it can be a direct cancer-fighting agent.

GERMANIUM SESQUIOXIDE (GS)

Germanium sesquioxide (GS) has great potential in the treatment of patients with cancer and chronic illnesses. It has been studied in Asia and Russia for many decades and has had safe IV use in the U.S. for over 20 years. In studies, it has been shown to induce key immune chemistry, including interferon-gamma (IFN-gamma), and to enhance natural killer cell activity while inhibiting tumor growth and spread.[78][79] Our own clinical experience is that as an IV additive, it is safe when infused under standard dose and safety guidelines. We often add this powerful synergist to other IV therapies.

CURCUMIN

As an IV agent, curcumin is a promising adjunct to the care of the cancer patient population. Oral administration has been shown to provide some benefit, but oral absorption does not always allow maximum benefit.

A review of over 40 scientific publications, as well as clinical use of IV preparations of curcumin in well over 5,000 infusions that originally started as part of Dr. Anderson's research, have led us to see IV curcumin as potentially groundbreaking help for people with cancer. A drug version of IV curcumin (made patentable by changing the structure of curcumin, so it is not actually curcumin) is in clinical trials for approval as a cancer drug by the U.S. Food and Drug Administration.[80][81]

One limitation of IV curcumin is the different IV forms available.[82] IV curcumin is not a water-soluble product, so it requires special preparation to allow it to be infused into humans. There are four separate (and chemically distinct) forms of IV curcumin. Ultimately, at this point in time, an emulsion form of curcumin for IV use appears the most stable and safest form for higher doses, which was what Dr. Anderson used in his advanced metastatic cancer patients.

It should be noted that curcumin IV may be a short-term liver stressor at high dose, but is generally protective and restorative to the liver.[83][84] As for the kidneys, the same is true.[85][86][87][88][89][90][91] Dr. Anderson has seen many patients with low kidney function recover some lost kidney function after curcumin IV therapy. With regard to overall potential for curcumin to help in cancer care, the data is enormous. There are many mechanistic reasons for its healing capabilities, and we believe we have only scratched the surface of the potential.[92 93 94 95 96 97 98 99]

In a case series that he completed, Dr. Anderson found stabilization of disease progression or actual (radiology confirmed) disease regression in a group of stage-IV cancer patients who were resistant to all therapies (standard chemotherapy and radiation therapy, as well as natural therapies). This occurred in five of the six patients in the original group, and since then he has seen it in more patients. While there are some pharmaceutical considerations to be worked out for IV curcumin (especially at high dose), it is one of the most promising IV therapies on the horizon in cancer care.

SILYMARIN

Silymarin IV compounds (typically silibinin) have the potential for multiple mechanisms of action in oncology patients. Silibinin is a component of the milk thistle plant, a common oral supplement. In our clinical experience, silibinin IV is another synergistic agent in the treatment of people with cancer. It is well studied as a protector of liver function. More recently, it has also been shown to assist in the process of cancer cell death and immune system modulation.[100 101 102 103]

Much like curcumin, silibinin as an IV therapy shows great promise in cancer therapy. Also like curcumin, it is not a simple agent to make safe for IV use, but it is possible. From our experience, we predict it will likely be used in combination with other agents (such as curcumin and glycyrrhizin) in a well-rounded cancer IV care plan.

RESVERATROL

Resveratrol is produced by many plants when they are stressed or under attack. It gained fame as the constituent in red wine that provides antioxidant and other benefits. One type of resveratrol (trans-resveratrol) "has been reported to possess anti-oxidant, anti-inflammatory, anticarcinogenic, antidiabetic, anti-aging, cardioprotective and neuroprotective properties."[104] Although oral resveratrol is potentially well absorbed in studies, in humans it does not seem to have the actual benefit in cancer that it should (based on its potential cell activities).[105]

Much like curcumin, resveratrol has many excellent cancer-fighting abilities, but getting enough in a human to have those effects may be difficult. Given this, IV resveratrol has great potential in the treatment of patients who have cancer.[106] [107] Studies suggest multiple mechanisms of action in immune function regulation as well as balancing of the oxidant-antioxidant system, with both mechanisms having potential anticancer effects.[108] [109] IV use in humans has been limited due to IV-appropriate product availability, but in studies IV resveratrol has been shown to be tolerated and safe.[110] [111]

Plant-based compounds such as curcumin, silibinin, resveratrol, and curcumin all show potential synergy. In a recent study, scientists looked at resveratrol with curcumin in an animal model of prostate cancer. The study found the combination with plant-based compounds worked better in decreasing tumor size and modulating glutamine metabolism (a very "pro-cancer" process) and that four very key tumor promotor areas were "modulated to a greater extent by the combinations compared to the individual compounds."[112]

QUERCETIN

Quercetin is produced by many plants and chemically is a flavonoid that has protective and stabilizing effects, especially on the fruit and reproductive portions of the plant. It is often used orally in allergy therapies to calm histamine release. IV quercetin has studied potential for increased bioavailability and potent potential antitumor activity. Studies suggest multiple mechanisms of action in tyrosine kinase inhibition (a potent anticancer strategy) and tumor growth suppression. It has also been shown in humans to be safe for oral and IV administration.[113] [114] [115] [116]

In the years Dr. Anderson used it in cancer research, he and colleagues noticed that IV quercetin was well tolerated and, in some cases, showed positive effect in cancer stabilization or regression. IV quercetin is likely another candidate for use in synergistic application.

MISTLETOE

Most people think of mistletoe in connection with Christmas. As a cancer therapy, it was popularized about 20 years ago but has a history of use dating back many decades. It has two routes of administration: subcutaneous (SQ), which is the same method used to inject insulin, and IV. Both have benefits and your physician will help decide which is best. There are many forms used medically, and for the purposes of this chapter, we will refer to them collectively as "mistletoe." Should you look further into this therapy, a trained physician will be able to explain the differences in types and appropriate uses.

Mistletoe therapy has two primary effects born out in research. One effect is improved quality of life (QOL), and the other is direct immune stimulation and modulation to help the body fight cancer. As a natural cancer therapy, mistletoe has one of the most expansive research bases. To date, there are over 2,600 published scientific papers, over 250 of which reflect inclusion of modern North American scientific thought.

Mistletoe therapies have many potential mechanisms by which they can change the immune system and cancer cells to promote improved QOL, increased cancer cell death, improved "antitumor" immune activity, and other benefits. A subset of the QOL benefit is the ability for mistletoe to alleviate the side effects of chemotherapy and radiation therapy.[117] Additionally, it has been studied in, and shown to relieve, inflammatory triggers of cancer-related fatigue.[118]

Mistletoe is a true immunotherapy, meaning it has multiple actions on multiple portions of the native (your own) immune system, all of which have different outcomes. One mechanism that is crucial to tumor cell death and lowering cancer reccurrence is natural killer cell function. Mistletoe strongly affects natural killer cell function in an anticancer direction.[119] In addition, mistletoe can change the tumor cell biology in a manner that weakens the cancer cell.[120]

A concern that is often raised is the potential for reactivity with and inhibition of conventional chemotherapy drugs. In a study looking at the effect of mistletoe on multiple chemotherapy drugs (and in multiple different cancer cell types), the authors concluded that mistletoe "did not inhibit chemotherapy induced cytostasis and cytotoxicity in any of our experimental settings." And that "at higher concentrations [mistletoe] showed an additive inhibitory effect" with the chemotherapy drugs on the tumor cells. They concluded that their results "suggest that no risk of safety by herb drug interactions has to be expected from the exposition of cancer cells to chemotherapeutic drugs and [mistletoe] simultaneously."[121]

A recent overview of evidence-based findings found that mistletoe therapies "seem to be beneficial for the majority of cancer patients (85%) without serious side effects."[122] A second review consisting of a meta-analysis of survival of cancer patients treated with mistletoe conducted between 1985 and 2002, with a total of 3,324 patients, found a positive treatment effect.[123] A third recent review asserts that many derangements of immunity associated with cancer "can be counteracted by treatment with extracts derived from mistletoe." They conclude, "Although these drugs cannot replace conventional cancer treatment, they may improve the patient's quality and length of life."[124]

SALICINIUM

Salicinium is a unique natural anticancer agent that has effect on two potent cancer-promoting pathways: overproduction of lactic acid and use of the enzyme alpha-N-acetylgalactosaminidase (also known as nagalase).[125] The ability of salicinium to block both lactic acid production and nagalase can potentially remove two very pro-cancer processes with the use of one agent.

Salicinium provides this "double action" by manipulating a common enzyme in cancer cells called beta-glucosidase. Beta-glucosidase is an enzyme that is very active in most cancer cells and that is either not in normal human cells or of typically low activity.[126] [127] [128] Similar to HDIVC, this enzyme allows salicinium to be damaging to cancer cells while safe for normal human cells. Because salicinium is a complexed glycome molecule, it can rapidly enter cancer cells due to their hunger for simple sugars. The beta-glucosidase splits the glycome from salicinium and immediately attaches to the NAD+ enzyme, and this attachment stops both lactic acid production and nagalase. These two actions reduce the lactic acid export (a pro-cancer process) and allow the Gc-MAF to work and attract cancer-killing macrophage cells.

We have used salicinium in advanced cancer patients with excellent safety. If used in the context of a metabolic cancer program, in combination with dietary and other therapies, salicinium can be an excellent inclusion.

GC-MAF

Although not generally available in the U.S. as of publication, Gc-MAF has been used for many years in cancer and chronic infectious diseases in other countries. The enzyme alpha-N-acetylgalactosaminidase (also known as nagalase) blocks conversion of Gc protein to Gc-macrocyte activating factor (MAF) or "Gc-MAF," which prevents the macrophage of the immune system from killing cancer cells.[129] This blockade stops immune cells from "noticing" the cancer cell and killing it. The administration of Gc-MAF triggers the immune cells to "see" the cancer and potentially attack it.

Dr. Anderson used this agent with cancer patients in the early days of the IV research and found it to be very safe. It was always used as a synergist to other therapies since the improvement of immune action against the cancer cell coupled with another therapy to strengthen or stimulate the immune activity (such as oxidative therapies) go well together.

AMYGDALIN

Amygdalin (also known as Laetrile or "vitamin B17") has a long and confusing history in the integrative oncology world. The enzyme beta-glucosidase is over-expressed in cancer cells, which facilitates a chemical reaction that transforms amygdalin into hydrogen cyanide, which is toxic to cancer cells. Normal cells do not contain this enzyme in any great quantity, if at all, and therefore cyanide is not formed in normal cells.[130]

Several older studies have been conducted involving amygdalin, but a particular publication in 1982[131] was used as the basis to show "Amygdalin (Laetrile) is a toxic drug that is not effective as a cancer treatment," a conclusion that was widely accepted in the U.S. and Canada.

However, a more recent review publication[132] has demonstrated that not only is the toxicity issue very much overstated in the 1982 paper but the mechanisms against cancer are broader than originally thought. In addition to the aforementioned cell death mechanism (as a cancer cell toxin), amygdalin shows activity in improving natural programmed cancer cell death (apoptosis) and in slowing new blood vessel growth to tumors (angiogenesis) that the tumor uses to "feed" itself.

Dr. Anderson has never prescribed amygdalin alone, but rather has used it in a program involving multiple facets. He has administered thousands of doses outside of the U.S., and in some cases, amygdalin has stopped or slowed an aggressive cancer. Dr. Anderson and many integrative oncologists find amygdalin to be a beneficial resource in cancer care.

POLY-MVA

Poly-MVA ("Poly," also known as lipoic acid-palladium complex (Pd-LA) and lipoic acid mineral complex (LAMC)) is available as an oral and IV cancer support. Poly is a complex polymer molecule that can enter the cell and work in the mitochondria to create energy. It is unique in that in healthy cells, it supports the normal cell energy creation, but in many cancer cells, it forces the cancer cell into a metabolism that weakens the cancer cell. This is similar to, but not the same as, the way HDIVC and DCA create different effects in healthy versus cancerous cells.[133] [134] [135]

It differs from related free radical scavengers (e.g., alpha-lipoic acid) since there is no free lipoic acid or palladium. The lipoic acid and palladium are irreversibly bound together, resulting in a molecule that is both fat and water soluble with the ability to enter the mitochondria and act as an energy primer.

On a safety note, people sometimes become concerned because the palladium is in the formula. This would be an issue if the palladium were in a "free" form, but in the Poly-MVA, the irreversibly bound nature of palladium and lipoic acid makes palladium unavailable in a free form, and therefore it enters and leaves the body unchanged (and safely).

In treating patients who have cancer, it becomes important, when possible, to look for therapies that may have multiple avenues of benefit, as shown with IV vitamin C. In our clinical experience, Poly-MVA is another such therapy that brings the potential for an anticancer effect *and* improving the effects of standard therapies and (possibly most importantly) protecting and regenerating the normal cells. Published research addressing the potential use of Poly-MVA in various degenerative disease settings includes mitochondrial damage,[136] brain and heart protection,[137] diabetes and mitochondrial (cell energy) protection,[138] DNA repair,[139] and cell protection during and after radiation exposure.[140] [141] [142] [143] [144] [145] [146] [147] [148]

Poly-MVA has a long history of successful use in veterinary oncology,[149] and much of our initial interest in it for human cancer was based on the animal experience. In research areas (beyond the crossover from animal studies) with potential for human cancers, Poly-MVA has been studied in enhancing radiation therapy[150] and improving cell death in a brain tumor cell study.[151] While we will discuss the use of Poly-MVA in combination with DCA below, and in a global metabolic cancer program (Chapter 9), it should be noted that on its own, Poly-MVA has been of great help in improving the quality of life in many cancer patients.

DICHLOROACETATE (DCA)

DCA is a relatively small molecule which, in the past, was used as treatment for the metabolic disorder lactic acidosis. It inhibits lactate formation, and via a complex mechanism, switches cell metabolism away from lactic acid production (glycolytic) to mitochondrial energy metabolism (electron transport chain (ETC)).[152] Noncancerous human cells prefer this aerobic pathway for energy formation via ETC use, whereas cancerous cells experience the Warburg Effect, where most glucose is converted to lactate regardless of oxygen availability.[153] Forcing a cancerous cell into ETC use thereby increases damaging oxygen formation and oxygen consumption.[154]

Because of the differences in metabolism between most cancer cells and normal cells and through an intricate mechanism, DCA is able to cause cancer cell death via apoptosis and weaken the cancer cell in lowering its ability to proliferate. DCA also does this only in cancerous cells and not in normal cells.[155 156 157]

In earlier uses of DCA, it was often both overdosed and not administered with appropriate support factors. For example, DCA is both a consumer of and dependent upon (for metabolism) glutathione. Glutathione is an important detoxification molecule, and lowering its levels could slow detoxification and cause toxic side effects. The bottom line is that DCA is a potent agent in an anticancer strategy, but it must be used in very well-defined dosing parameters and always with support for the metabolic stressors it creates. While most DCA side effects are self-limited (such as dizziness and tingling in hands or feet), in earlier studies where DCA was used at high dose without any supportive therapy (for metabolism and detoxification), people did develop nerve inflammation. Dr. Anderson has administered over 10,000 doses of DCA to date with proper support therapies. He has not seen any cases of nerve inflammation, and any other side effects patients experienced were very short in duration and all resolved fully.[158][159][160]

Recently, many scientific papers have continued to explore the mechanisms and potentials of DCA in cancer therapies.[161][162][163][164][165] Multiple human scientific studies, including drug trials and case reports,[166][167][168][169][170][171][172][173][174][175] have been published with regard to DCA and several types of cancer. Currently, DCA is being tested with standard chemotherapy drugs as a synergistic agent.[176] It is our belief that DCA (with proper administration and supportive therapies) is an incredible tool in the battle against cancer, and truly is unique in its actions and efficacy.

THE COMBINATION OF POLY-MVA AND DCA

An excellent example of true therapeutic synergy was discovered in the earlier days of Dr. Anderson's IV research with the combination of Poly-MVA and DCA for both IV and oral use. We will discuss the next level of this therapy with regard to the global metabolic therapy approach in cancer (Chapter 9). For the IV section, we will describe the basis of the synergy and the initial case series that was compiled.

Due to the established side effect issues of DCA and considering its mechanism, Dr. Anderson and Dr. Gurdev Parmar postulated two synergistic effects could occur if Poly-MVA and DCA were used together: mutual anticancer benefit and improvement in the safety and tolerance of DCA. The first step was to have a cell line study done (where cancer cells in a petri dish are tested with each compound individually and then together) to see if the synergy seen "on paper" translated to cancer cell death. The short story is that both Poly-MVA and DCA had tumor kill, but together they had additive benefit, with less DCA being used with the same tumor kill.[177]

Due to these findings and from prior experience with DCA and Poly-MVA, Dr. Anderson and the IV team at the research center knew how to administer both agents safely so that we could provide the therapy without any risk other than those common to other IV therapies. We selected a group of people with advanced cancer who had failed all therapies (standard oncology therapies and natural therapies) and consented to this as a trial of unknown outcome (which is often referred to in oncology research as "salvage therapy"). Over the course of two years, we implemented the therapy. The original case series is summarized in the table below and was part of the original study, but has not been published separately since reported at the Society of Integrative Oncology,[178] as is the norm for many studies.

N (NUMBER OF PATIENTS) = 9	DISEASE PROGRESSION	STABLE DISEASE	IMPROVED QUALITY OF LIFE	DISEASE REGRESSION
66-year-old male, Non-Hodgkin's Lymphoma				XXX
5-year-old female, Mixed Acute Leukemia (MLL+)				XXX
71-year-old female, Multiple Myeloma				XXX
68-year-old female, Multiple Myeloma				XXX
72-year-old female, chronic lymphocytic leukemia (CLL)			XXX	
65-year-old male, Metastatic Melanoma	XXX			
3 GBM (high grade brain tumor) Post Surgery—one 46-year-old male, one 51-year-old female, and one 49-year-old female			XXX	

The goal of the DCA and Poly-MVA therapy is to attack the cancer cell where it is weakest via its unique (but impaired) metabolism relative to normal human cells.[179 180 181 182 183 184 185] We have used this therapy, and newer versions of it, many times in the years since this study and have had similar results. In some cases, the protocol involves dietary changes, a small group of oral supplements, and hyperbaric oxygen therapy.

Dr. Anderson has never seen these results when using DCA alone. Additionally the rate of side effects from the DCA was drastically reduced such that as of now, nobody has had to drop out of the therapy due to DCA-related side effects. The combined use of DCA and Poly-MVA has been one of the truly big advances in integrative cancer therapies in the past 20 years.

SUPPORTIVE, HEALING, AND PROTECTIVE IV THERAPIES

There are a number of other IV therapies that do not have an oxidative effect. They are used to promote tissue healing and to protect and support patients before, during, and after conventional therapies.

LOW DOSE IV VITAMIN C (LDIVC)

In the oxidative section at the beginning of the chapter, we discussed "high-dose" vitamin C and how it is an oxidative therapy commonly used in oncology. However, IV vitamin C has two different actions based on dose and the type of cell with which it interacts. A "low-dose" strategy is generally considered to be below the level needed to be an "oxidative" (HDIVC) therapy.

Generally speaking, a low dose is considered between 5 and 10 grams of IV vitamin C, though three scientific papers written on the dose threshold of LDIVC versus HDIVC are not in complete agreement (which is not uncommon in scientific papers).[186 187 188]

Two scientific papers are commonly cited as showing benefit with LDIVC,[189 190] and another presented at the Society for Integrative Oncology was a follow-up to show safety in the U.S. hospital setting.[191] All three studies used low-dose strategies and showed improved quality of life in patients with cancer.

In addition to the antioxidant support LDIVC offers, LDIVC has shown the ability to decrease gene mutations following oxidative stress (which is increased in cancer and by many cancer treatments).[192] Another paper shows LDIVC as augmenting natural killer cell function (mentioned in the germanium and mistletoe sections), which is incredibly important to remission and length of life in cancer patients.[193]

While these QOL studies used a simple formula (of a base IV solution such as normal saline) and a small dose of vitamin C (5 to 10 grams), the use of LDIVC offers many other potential benefits for broadening the therapeutic potential of the IV. High-dose strategies require specific mineral additives but are best not combined with other additives, such as many B vitamins and glutathione, to protect the oxidative properties of the HDIVC formula. However, when using the LDIVC doses, one can add other vitamins, minerals, and amino acids as well as follow the LDIVC with glutathion. This allows for patients with cancer to experience the full benefit in QOL and potentially other positive effects.

SPECIALIZED HYDRATION
WITH NUTRIENT SUPPORT

A landmark scientific paper in *Oncology Nurse Advisor* regarding the nutritional status of cancer patients states: "Malnutrition is the most common secondary diagnosis in cancer patients. Even patients who are eating can become malnourished because of specific biochemical and metabolic changes associated with cancer. These metabolic changes impair nutritional status and contribute to cancer-related malnutrition . . ."[194] The paper then cites studies showing that cancer-related weight loss, anorexia, and nutrient depletion is much more widespread than originally believed.[195][196] The bottom line, illustrated by multiple studies, is that cancer patients are depleted and the use of IV nutrients can extend life and improve QOL.[197][198][199][200][201]

"Specialized hydration with nutrient support" is a method that clinically emerged a number of years ago for use in an effort to help cancer patients with improved QOL and decreased side effects from their cancer and cancer therapies. IV hydration in and of itself is quite simple. If the person has good cardiac and kidney function, they can take a hydrating IV solution (such as normal saline and Ringer's lactate), which will build their fluid volume. Our idea was to use the principles of hydration IV therapy while using nutrients instead of simply saline or a similar fluid. The issue in the past was that most nutrient repletion solutions were actually dehydrating, which defeats the purpose of hydration in exchange for nutrient repletion. Over time, we were able to construct hydrating solutions that had broad nutrients, including vitamins, minerals, and amino acids. This way the patient has the benefit of both hydration and nutrient repletion.

We have seen these formulas rescue people from severe side effects from chemotherapy, improving mental function, reducing pain, and improving QOL at end of life. In our clinical experience, these specialized hydrating nutrient formulas are a critical part of IV therapy in patients who have cancer.

RADIATION AND CHEMOTHERAPY SIDE EFFECT FORMULAS

Nerve, joint, skin, and digestive damage are common following both chemotherapy and radiation. In our clinical experience, concurrent IV therapies with HDIVC, mistletoe, curcumin, and other IV therapies can diminish many of these side effects. (Hyperbaric oxygen therapy is another critical tool in this arena and is discussed on p. 243.) That said, it is common for people to have been through chemotherapy or radiation therapy and not have had such support; or even with that support, they may still have residual side effects.

Let's quickly review why tissues are damaged, giving rise to side effects (of radiation and chemotherapy) and what can be done about it. All cells, including neurological, are incredibly sensitive to mitochondrial damage, cell membrane damage, and other effects. Many oncologic therapies have deleterious effects on the cell matrix and nerve function, leading to significant decreases in quality of life. Supplementation and augmentation of glutathione function can aid in the regeneration of all damaged body tissues. These effects are especially seen in nerve, digestive, joint, skin, and other critical tissues.

We have already discussed general hydration and nutrient repletion support and the use of Poly-MVA and glutathione for cell repair. The use of an augmented glutathione support therapy can help the more severely injured tissues heal. Glutathione function is tied to oxidative stress, which leads (if unbalanced) to cell damage.[202] Glutathione status is depleted during chemotherapy,[203] while it is depleted by and required as a protectant for radiation therapy and exposure.[204][205]

And finally glutathione has been shown to be cell protective in some chemotherapy exposures.[206][207]

So the use of glutathione (along with Poly-MVA, vitamin C, nutrients, hyperbaric oxygen, and other treatments) for repair after cancer therapy is an easy case to make.

This leads us to Dr. Anderson's story about the clinical trial in patients with radiation damage after head and neck radiation therapy. Dr. Anderson's research center considered using glutathione IV alone, but we did not because glutathione is not a "lone ranger" acting without support. Glutathione, like all antioxidants supported by co-factors that assist it in returning to its useful "reduced" state, gets used once and becomes a non-beneficial nutrient.

A well-rounded protocol needed to be employed, which not only supplied the glutathione but also the necessary co-factors for glutathione recycling and nerve repair. Dr. Anderson started this therapy with radiation-damaged patients and assessed their nerve damage every four weeks. The protocol was an IV session (with this combination therapy) twice a week for four to eight weeks, and then weekly for eight weeks, followed by twice monthly for two to three months, if needed. Most patients recovered 90 percent or more of their nerve and other damaged function. It is crucial to note that the longer the time from injury (from radiation or chemotherapy) to use of the IV program, the the longer it took to have recovery. This study shows the incredible benefit to quality of life that a very specifically designed IV protocol can have.

CHAPTER 8

PROTECTION AND RECOVERY FROM SURGERY, CHEMOTHERAPY, AND RADIATION

While people may debate the merits of chemotherapy, radiation, surgery, or other interventions in cancer care, what cannot be debated is that people need to heal from (and often be protected during) such therapies. There are three primary issues around this topic and many ancillary issues to consider. First is the need for appropriate care before, during, and after standard therapies to decrease those therapies' side effects and to speed healing. Second is the potential during standard therapies to protect the healthy cells in the body and, if possible, augment the damage to the cancerous cells. And third is to use the benefits from such care to improve overall quality of life.

Concepts to consider are how each standard therapy (whether surgery, chemotherapy, or radiation) affects the body, how supportive therapies interact with standard therapies, and what the most efficient methods are in each case to promote healing.

SURGERY

In a scientific publication written by our colleagues Doctors Douglas MacKay and Alan L. Miller,[1] a clear outline of the steps in the surgical process is laid out in regard to supportive measures for healing. They are wounding, hemostasis, inflammatory phase, proliferative phase, and remodeling. Our only addition, based on our clinical experience, would be to add "surgical preparation" to the list.

The average person undergoing surgery is likely to be somewhat to greatly nutrient deficient. One study found that up to 40 percent of patients were nutrient depleted on hospital admission and almost all became nutrient depleted during their hospital stay![2] Another study found that preexisting malnutrition is largely unrecognized and may approach 50 percent in a hospital population, which has an increased correlation with surgical site infection and is related to nutrient and protein depletion.[3] This not only interferes with the biological response to wound healing, it also reduces immune function and causes increased surgical site infections.

We have been asked, "If we assume many people are nutritionally deficient, is there any information to say that supplementing the person's diet and nutrients has any benefit?" Several studies have explored if supplementing the diet and nutrients of a person who is nutritionally deficient has any benefits, and three in particular show that nutrient-supplemented patients in controlled trials significantly had reduced surgical site infection compared to the control (no supplement) group.[4][5][6] People having surgery need nutritional assessment and interventions. Using the stages of surgical process, we will outline our approach to support of patients having surgery.

PREPARATION

One of the most critical stages in having a positive surgical outcome is preparation. The healthier patients are entering surgery, the more likely they will experience a good outcome. Our general approach is to have people increase nutrients and be very careful with their food intake and dietary plan in the four to six weeks prior to surgery. This includes getting enough protein in the diet, but if insufficient, supplementing with amino acid or protein supplements. A presurgery diet also includes consuming a variety of colorful vegetables and anti-inflammatory fats, which provides maximum protection and "preloading" of the body to deal with the surgical experience. We will often add nutrient supplements to ensure that the nutrient preload is complete, including extra B-complex vitamins; vitamin C; trace minerals (especially zinc, chromium, and selenium); the fat-soluble vitamins A, D, E and K; and often specific botanical medicines as appropriate to the person's situation.

Two notes about preparation:

1. If a person cannot adjust their diet or supplement intake (or does not realize it is needed), they can still improve their healing with the other steps in the process.

2. For safety, we stop most nutritional supplements seven days prior to surgery so that there is no concern of altering or interfering with blood clotting, anesthesia, or other surgical parameters.

WOUNDING

Wounding is the actual process of surgery, which is a disruption of the body in order to gain the surgical result required. Depending on the surgery, this may be a small process or a very large one. In either case, the needs are overall the same with regard to healing. Wounding is a time where generally people are not receiving food or augmented nutrients, which is another reason why preparation is so critical.

HEMOSTASIS

Hemostasis is the process of beginning to heal following a surgical procedure. As humans, natural repair to skin and soft tissues in the body is preprogrammed. This process begins as soon as the wounding happens and requires a myriad of nutritional factors to operate. The early phases of this step are also not typically a time people are consuming food or outside nutrients, which, again, is why the preparation prior to surgery is critical to healing.

INFLAMMATORY AND PROLIFERATIVE PHASES

The inflammatory and proliferative phases are the next critical steps in promoting the natural repair process. We often believe inflammation is bad and should be avoided, but in reality, we would not survive without inflammation at proper times since it helps trigger immune and healing signals in the body. The proliferative phase is when the tissue heals and grows. These phases are dependent on proper amino acid intake (from proteins and amino acid supplements) as well as many vitamins and minerals, such as vitamins A and C and zinc.

These phases often occur in a time period where the patient is eating again and can take supplemental nutrients. If the patient is in the hospital, we often have a home-care plan ready with post-surgery meal ideas and nutrient supplementation prescriptions.

While most times the duration of stay in the hospital excludes or limits the ability to take supplements (or to eat healthfully), we would like to point out that in more integrated hospital settings, this time period is often augmented by specific food and nutrient supplement prescriptions. For example, Dr. Anderson's hospital patients are often given nutrient IV infusions during procedures and are prescribed oral supplements immediately after recovery. In addition, postsurgical targeted IV nutrient therapies, support supplements, and organic, fresh-made foods are given to speed healing.

As a personal example, Dr. Anderson chose to have a surgery at this hospital to see if our approach really made a difference. It was a surgical procedure he had undergone in years prior with a great deal of pain and complication. He was surprised that during the postsurgical healing days when he followed a specific food and nutrient supplement regimen, he needed absolutely no pain medication (opiate or otherwise), his swelling in the surgical area was minimal, and he healed much more rapidly than he had from the prior surgery.

REMODELING

The remodeling phase is the longer and slower process of the body reassembling the disrupted areas. It requires a great deal of amino acid availability (from protein in the diet and supplements), as well as many nutrient co-factors. Remodeling normally occurs when the patient is recovering at home and the postsurgical diet and nutrient plan mentioned above is already in effect.

A sample nutritional supplement regimen taken two to four weeks prior to surgery and for four to six weeks afterward with your doctor's consent may look similar to the following:

- High potency multivitamin and mineral, once daily

- Vitamin C, 1000 mg, twice daily

- Vitamin A, 5000 IU, daily with a meal

- Mixed vitamin E, 400 IU, daily with a meal

- Zinc, 25 to 50 mg, along with 2 to 3 mg of copper, daily with a meal

Supplements specific to post-surgery might include:

- Homeopathic *Arnica montana*, 30C or 200C, one to two times daily for two to three days (for bruising and swelling)

- Homeopathic *Hypericum perforatum,* 30C or 200C, taken one to two times daily for two to three days (for nerve pain)

- Bromelain or proteolytic enzyme product, 500 mg of bromelain or recommended dose of proteolytic enzyme formula, two to three times daily on empty stomach

- IV therapy: the use of IV nutrients is very effective in helping to prepare for and recover from surgery. Formulations often include vitamin C, B vitamins, amino acids, and minerals.

- Acupuncture is a great therapy in helping patients reduce their pain levels and quicken recovery time.

CHEMOTHERAPY

Supportive healing measures for chemotherapy usually involve consideration of three situations or phases: preparation before, support during, and recovery after chemotherapy.

These are the most common side effects from chemotherapy:[7]

- Fatigue.

- Loss of muscle mass and strength, weight loss, loss of desire to eat, and other related symptoms.

- Hair loss.

- Pain, including headaches; muscle, joint, and digestive system pain; as well as nerve pain (neuropathy).

- Digestive system effects also include nausea, vomiting, and diarrhea or constipation. This is usually related to mucus membrane inflammation (mucositis), dehydration, or a combination of other factors.

- Bone marrow and blood count / immune function changes.

- Other nervous system effects, including hearing, vision, or balance problems. Cognitive dysfunction (often called "chemo brain").

- Sexual and reproductive issues.

In conventional oncology, these side effects are not only well known but are also planned for and treated. Many of the side effects do not have curative treatments but instead have supportive or palliative measures available (such as anti-nausea or pain medications). In our clinical experience, this is an area where integrative oncology can really improve outcomes and quality of life for patients.

As a concept, the use of integrative oncology methods before, during, and after chemotherapy would appear to be reasonable. And over the past two decades, there has been an increasing, albeit slow, acceptance of this methodology in North America. Two of the very reasonable concerns that we believe have caused this slow adoption of integrative oncology are concern over interaction and potential decreased efficacy of the chemotherapy, and a lack of enough studies showing the efficacy of integrative oncology.

A great deal could be said regarding these two major concerns, but we will focus on the key points. First, concerns over negative interactions between chemotherapy and integrative therapies has been brought up for many decades. In the past, not a great deal of information was available and so the assumption that "nutritional and holistic therapies must interfere" was made in the absence of evidence, causing generations of oncologists to adhere to that axiom. One of the areas of greatest concern has been the use of IV vitamin C near the time of chemotherapy. This had been an area of great theoretical concern in the past and was almost universally discouraged by oncologists. In the early days of his NIH research, Dr. Anderson had to face this hesitation daily, which resulted in a yearlong project culminating in an almost 30-page summary of just the scientific citations organized by chemotherapy agent.[8] Dr. Anderson was actually surprised at the existence of the positive research on interactions between chemotherapies and vitamin C, as well as the amount of it. In all but three types of chemotherapy, the data showed that vitamin C would help improve the effect of the chemotherapy. In the three cases where there was any concern at all, the concern was removed by a simple separation of the chemotherapy from the vitamin C, usually by a day or two. Other scientific papers have shown the combination of IV vitamin C to be safe and effective during chemotherapy,[9] to have the ability to improve the activity of some chemotherapy,[10] and to improve the quality of life during chemotherapy and radiation therapy in patients with breast cancer.[11] One oncologist from these studies e-mailed Dr. Anderson and said, "When I challenged you to share any scientific data on vitamin C and chemotherapy, I never realized there was any, and moreover am shocked it is so positive. This will help me justify referring patients to your part of the study who desire IV vitamin C."

While the above examples are about a very common integrative therapy, the same can be said for other interventions researched in conjunction with chemotherapy, such as curcumin, melatonin, and naltrexone.

The second major concern regarding the lack of studies showing efficacy of integrative oncology is slowly fading as well. In one study again using IV vitamin C, researchers found improved quality of life in terminal cancer patients when IV vitamin C was included in an integrative protocol.[12] Another review showed safety and improved quality of life when integrative oncology was brought to a group of advanced pancreatic cancer patients.[13] Five other reviews all showed similar benefit and safety in the integrative oncology models studied.[14 15 16 17 18]

To maximize therapeutic effect while protecting the normal cells during chemotherapy, we will discuss the most useful efforts during preparation, active chemotherapy, and recovery.

PREPARATION

Much like preparation for surgery, the time before one begins chemotherapy can be critical to becoming as healthy as possible. This is a time where you should focus on nutritional support through diet and supplements and attempt to correct any imbalances that have existed prior to starting chemotherapy. During this phase, we also discuss the plan for treatment during the forthcoming active chemotherapy and the way we will work with side effects that might arise. If someone misses this phase, we can still work with them and help throughout any part of the process.

SUPPORT

We have been treating patients before, during, and after chemotherapy for two decades, and the only outcome we have seen is improved tolerance and quality of life.

The important thing to consider with integrative therapies during the chemotherapy period is your need for a trained integrative oncology professional. Chemotherapy is potentially very dangerous, and the side effects can be severe, so you need a provider experienced and versed in both the integrative approaches and the pharmacology of the chemotherapy with an understanding of the process you are in. The choice of therapies used in conjunction with chemotherapy will be specific to you as a person, as well as the type or types of chemotherapy you are having.

RECOVERY

The recovery period is often the first time we will see a patient, as they are often seeking relief from chemotherapy-induced side effects. While it is true that having integrative therapies during the preparation and active chemotherapy phases is best (and associated with the fewest side effects), you can begin at any time. One benefit in the recovery phase is that the oncologist is usually not at all concerned with interference with the chemotherapy because its job is over. And all oncologists want their patients with side effects to be treated and relieved of those effects.

Treatment during the recovery phase is aimed at two primary things: your specific side effects after chemotherapy and reducing cancer stem cell / tumor microenvironment activation, which can happen after chemotherapy.

RADIATION THERAPIES

Therapeutic ionizing radiation works by damaging the DNA of cancer cells, eventually causing cell death. The most commonly known form of radiotherapy is ionizing therapy, which is normally used in a focused manner (except for bone marrow transplant preparation) to avoid damage to local areas. It may be used for treatment of a tumor or tumor area, or it may be used for palliative purposes, such as therapy to stop a painful metastatic tumor. There are also implanted radiotherapy devices that deliver brachytherapy, or local radiation, which are used in prostate and other cancers.

Other forms of radiotherapy include fast neutron therapy, proton beam therapy, and gamma knife radiosurgery. All work in different ways with different specific targets, but all are in the radiotherapy family. They have varying side effects but generally, depending on the target of the therapy, may have similar effects to targeted ionizing radiation therapies.

Common side effects of radiation therapy include fatigue, skin damage, and local side effects based on the location of the radiation therapy (e.g., radiation to the abdomen often causes digestive symptoms and adhesions in internal organs, and radiation to the head may cause oral symptoms and dental issues). There is a specific but rare side effect following radiation therapy called radiation recall, which is a rash that looks like a severe sunburn. It happens when certain types of chemotherapy are given during or soon after external beam radiation therapy and appears on the body part receiving the radiation. It may appear days to years after radiation therapy.

A common therapy for radiation recall is the use of a topical steroid. Integrative methods discussed in other portions of the book are also used for radiation burns and radiation recall. The botanical medications *Aloe vera,* chamomile, calendula, and even turmeric have been used topically. A very effective therapy for radiation burns and mucositis (mouth and digestive inflammation secondary to radiation or chemotherapy) is medical honey, often referred to as manuka honey. Benefits include anti-infectious, anti-inflammatory, antiexudative, antioxidant, wound healing, wound debriding, and nutritional properties.[19] It is soothing with a nice taste, and if used internally, it is often added to a soothing herbal tea (such as chamomile) to enhance its effects.

There are often different approaches used in the preparation phase than during or after active radiotherapy. The common goals of an integrative approach are protection of normal cells, enhancement of radiation therapy, and recovery following therapies, but we also consider the goal of the radiation therapy. For example, if the traditional goal is localized radiation to a single tumor, the integrative treatment may be different than during palliative (i.e., for pain control) radiation therapies. The choice of therapies used with radiation therapy is very specific to the patient case, timing, and type of radiation and should be decided between you and your integrative oncology provider.

The radiation oncologist is the specialist in radiation therapies, and often during the preparation and post-radiation phases, they will be less concerned with other therapies than they would be during active radiation.

During active radiation therapy, depending upon the location and type of therapy and the individual radiation oncologist, their advice may be anywhere between "do not do any integrative therapies," and "the integrative oncology provider can guide the integrative therapies." This caution comes from their uncertainty regarding the potential for interference with radiation effect from integrative therapies.

One therapy gaining recognition is the manipulation of diet during radiation therapy to enhance radiation effects and potentially improve tolerance. This is accomplished by using a ketogenic diet, employing intermittent fasting, or both.

An excellent review[20] outlined five ways this approach can improve the outcome of radiation therapy. Although moderately technical in places, we will quote directly the mechanisms from the review to illustrate the significance of this therapy:

> Mechanisms . . . include (1) improved DNA repair in normal, but not tumor cells; (2) inhibition of tumor cell repopulation through modulation of the PI3K–Akt–mTORC1 pathway downstream of insulin and IGF1; (3) redistribution of normal cells into more radioresistant phases of the cell cycle; (4) normalization of the tumor vasculature by targeting hypoxia-inducible factor-1α downstream of the PI3K–Akt–mTOR pathway; (5) increasing the intrinsic radioresistance of normal cells through ketone bodies but decreasing that of tumor cells by targeting glycolysis.

This is an example of how a specific "prescription diet plan" can protect healthy cells and make cancer cells more sensitive to treatment.

While there may be a variety of integrative treatment goals during active radiation therapy that you and your integrative oncology provider decide upon, the most important part of the treatment is to stay in contact so that should a side effect arise, you can begin care immediately.

During the preparation and post therapy, the goals are to prepare your system for the stress of the therapy beforehand and then work on recovery afterward.

Beyond diet and some botanical medicines during or after radiation, one higher intensity therapy we may use is IV therapy. We will often use IV therapy at each stage (preparation, during radiation therapy, and in the follow-up phase) as an adjunctive therapy to help protect normal cells and improve healing and quality of life. Before radiation begins, we will often use IV nutrients, hydration, or IV vitamin C. During radiation therapy, we are more cautious about IV formulation and timing, but especially in cases where palliative radiation is being given, scientific data[21] supports our experience in the use of IV therapy to improve patient outcomes and quality of life.

The post-radiation therapy period is the most common time we have patients requesting more intensive therapies, such as IV procedures. This is because people often have side effects they need to relieve, and they are already doing more basic diet and oral therapies. In Dr. Anderson's NIH research, the IV service was provided to patients who were done with radiation and or chemotherapy and had no evidence of disease (were technically in remission) but had significant lasting side effects of treatment. The most common situation was a person who had radiation burns on the skin and in the deeper tissues, causing functional problems, often including nerve damage. A complication is that often people will not have nerve damage until later, after radiation therapy. The lag can be from less than a year to as much as 16 years after radiation.[22] In these cases, they may not seek therapy but prevention is still advisable.

The "radiation recovery" IV program used a unique biochemically derived formula to replenish the circulating glutathione (one of the body's most potent antioxidant and detoxification molecules) and the co-factors required for its use. Dr. Anderson had seen limitations in the use of glutathione alone in nerve damage or other side effects and knew that biologically, glutathione required a great deal of nutrient support to work properly. He went back to the science behind glutathione use in the body and how nature uses it to its best effect to create a well-rounded, complete formula.

The new formula was used in patients with nerve damage following radiation therapy, and overall they showed improved healing and nerve recovery.

It was an intensive program that involved two IV therapy sessions a week for eight weeks and then weekly for four more weeks, at which time a reassessment was made. If the nerve damage was healing at greater than 50 percent from baseline testing, the patient could choose to switch to an oral glutathione support program or continue IV therapy while starting the oral support. If the healing was less than 50 percent, improved IV and oral therapy was continued for eight more weeks. In every case during the research program, and a majority of cases in the years since, this approach provided nerve healing and recovery for patients. In cases where the injury was older or where the "latent onset" of nerve damage happened from past radiation therapy, the results were less dramatic than when the protocol was completed in the year following active radiation therapy.

While not everything from this research is published, Dr. Anderson has shared the information at scientific meetings and has published the presentation slides for reference and use by physicians.[23] The IV formula he used in the study contains vitamin C, calcium, magnesium, zinc, selenium, and B vitamins, which he would follow with glutathione. While most people can recover some or all nerve function following radiation therapy, it is best if the IV therapy can be implemented in the first year following completion of radiation therapy.

PROTECTION AFTER CHEMOTHERAPY AND RADIATION: CANCER SEEDING, THE TUMOR MICROENVIRONMENT, AND THE ACTIVATION OF CANCER STEM CELLS

A difficult topic in oncology is the long-term effects of standard cancer therapies beyond direct treatment-related side effects. The long-term effects of standard cancer therapies such as radiation and many chemotherapies can often include the strengthening of leftover cancer cells and creating an environment where cancer reccurrence and/or metastasis happen. Most people expect that with appropriate standard cancer treatment, they will have less or no cancer and will be better in the long run. This does happen, but more commonly, after being in remission, people will have new occurrences of cancer to deal with at some point. Scientific information has pointed to the cancer stem cell (CSC) and the tumor microenvironment (TM or stroma) as key players in cancer recurrence.

One sees headlines that, especially if having had standard therapy for cancer, are unsettling. They indicate chemotherapy and radiation can actually make stronger cells for later cancer growth.[24][25] Scientific publications have outlined the process for radiation[26] and chemotherapy,[27] with one group writing, "Although traditional chemotherapy kills a fraction of tumor cells, it also activates the stroma and can promote the growth and survival of residual cancer cells."[28] TM is involved in the strength of the CSCs and cross talk for tumor cell recruitment leading to regrowth, spread, or both in cancers.[29]

If the "bad news" is that conventional therapy, while being helpful initially, may strengthen future cancer cells and recurrences, then what would the "good news" be? The good news is that CSCs and TM can be modulated by many things to keep the potential for recurrence lower over time.

We are often asked by people who have had conventional therapy how to stay well. This is an excellent question and one we are considering all the time. We will discuss secondary prevention (staying well) in Chapter 9, but in the meantime, the following are some basic ways that you can keep the CSCs and TM "calm" to decrease the likelihood of activation leading to future cancers.

Dietary changes are always our first choice for therapy. One idea gaining popularity during and after chemotherapy and radiation is the use of intermittent fasting. Another diet change to consider is long-term periodic fasting to lower CSC triggering and decrease the chemical triggers that fuel active TM, causing less potential for cancer growth.[30][31] The use of a ketogenic diet (often with calorie restriction or intermittent fasting) is another possible approach to the CSC and TM problem.[32] We discuss dietary interventions in Chapter 5, and it is important to note that the same dietary changes that we recommend to help initially prevent or treat cancer also can potentially lower future cancer growth via decreasing CSC and TM activity.

Other basic ways to keep the CSC and TM less or inactive are through vitamin C (see page 156) and curcumin (see page 176). In addition to an appropriate diet, the use of curcumin and vitamin C as long-term oral supplements can potentially keep the CSC and TM activity quiet or inactive, thereby improving prevention of future cancer growth.[33][34][35][36]

Protection and recovery from standard therapies is a critical part of any well-rounded integrative oncology plan. As prevention is one of the oldest tenets of medicine, we see a large part of our job relating to preventing side effects and future cancer growth. We also know that in the real world of oncology, some things cannot be prevented, so we need to have strategies for healing and recovery as well. The therapies you consider in the setting of recovery, healing, and prevention can have an important impact on the cancer journey.

CHAPTER 9

COMMON CANCERS AND
INTEGRATIVE APPROACHES

In this chapter we will outline the frequency of common cancers, their differences based on staging, and the way we think about treatment based on the cancer and its progress. Our goal is to outline the thought process in formulating a specific cancer care plan based on individual factors that are unique to each person. In addition to cancer frequency, we will describe our process in considering active cancer therapies based on "addressing the foundations" or working with the whole body to oppose the cancer and return health and balance. We will also look at the incredibly important topic of "secondary prevention" or the process of stopping a return of cancer once you have been diagnosed with "no evidence of disease."

Cancers of different types occur in differing amounts across the population. In North America and the United Kingdom, the four most common cancers are breast, lung, prostate, and colon.[1][2] In this chapter we will outline our common approaches to these and other cancer types. To set the stage for this discussion, it is important that we give some background regarding the thought process and more specific factors that enter into our integrative oncology approaches.

In describing our therapeutic approaches we also need to talk about the things that modulate our thought process so that we can offer the best possible care for each patient by meeting them where they are in their individual cancer journey.

A primary consideration is "What are the chances of survival with standard cancer therapies for this type of cancer?" If there is a very high survival rate, then often it is wise to seriously consider following the standard protocols while adding a well-rounded integrative oncology program. If, on the other hand, the survival chances are low, we often carefully consider the potential for side effects, lower of quality of life, and other negative effects in balance with the low potential for remission.

Another consideration beyond the type of cancer and the likelihood of survival is the actual stage of the cancer and your specific survival potential given that stage. A lower stage cancer generally has a much higher survival rate than a higher stage cancer of the same type. We will often highly recommend standard cancer therapies in a "high survival" cancer (with a well-rounded integrative oncology program), even though it may be similar for a low stage cancer. On the other hand, in a high-stage cancer where survival is much lower and effects of standard treatment would more likely cause harm than remission, we will often tip the balance in the other direction and focus on an aggressive integrative approach.

A common question from patients and families is "If I'm in the middle, what's best for me?" The thought process is similar in that we must consider the cancer itself, the stage, and potential survival, as well as the patient's wishes regarding therapy. In cases "in the middle," there are even more subtle considerations that include the ability of the person to tolerate therapies, their immune function, and overall vitality. Other factors may include age, prior health concerns, and location. The final decision is always up to the person with cancer and their family and support network. Certainly, one needs good information and expert opinions to inform any decision, and the input of an integrative oncology specialist is crucial to this process. But no one can decide the best pathway through the cancer journey for you.

Below are two charts to illustrate some of these concepts:

OVERALL PERCENT SURVIVAL AT 1, 5, AND 10 YEARS:[3]

TYPE	SURVIVAL AT 1 YEAR	5 YEARS	10 YEARS
BREAST	96	87	78
LUNG	32	10	5
PROSTATE	94	85	84
COLON	76	59	57
TESTICULAR CANCER	99	98	98
HODGKIN'S LYMPHOMA	91	85	80
LEUKEMIA (ALL)	69	52	46
PANCREATIC	21	3	1
BRAIN (ALL)	40	19	13
OVARY	72	46	35

BREAST CANCER 5-YEAR SURVIVAL BY STAGE:[4]

BREAST CANCER STAGE	5 YEAR SURVIVAL
0/I	100
II	93
III	72
IV	22

Integrative approaches to common cancers are in one sense very specific, but also have basic core foundations that we use to inform our approach in any specific case. The major foundations to consider are diet, metabolism and nutrition, immune system function, mental and emotional factors, your physical body, and side effects and quality of life.

SPECIFIC THERAPIES FOR THE MOST FREQUENT CANCERS

Breast, lung, prostate, and colon are the most common types of cancers, but our recommendations may apply for the other cancers as well. In instances where a type of cancer has a known specific therapy, we will discuss it at the end of each section. However, we wanted to summarize our top treatment thoughts in the beginning of the chapter so that you would have a place to start, which can then be added to or modified. You will notice that some supplement recommendations are used in most, if not all, types of cancers. This is because we have found them to be not only well studied but also clinically reliable.

The following are the most commonly diagnosed non-skin cancers and our top starting therapy ideas based on tumor type. Please note that we customize these plans based on tumor stage, patient vitality and health, and many other factors. (All statistics are sourced from the American Cancer Society.[5])

BREAST CANCER

One in eight women in the United States will be diagnosed with breast cancer in her lifetime, which makes it the most commonly diagnosed cancer in women. It is also the second leading cause of cancer death among women of all ages. Male breast cancer is rare, but an estimated 2,500 men will be diagnosed with breast cancer and approximately 460 will die each year. One reason we see many breast cancer patients in remission for prevention is that over 3.3 million breast cancer survivors are alive in the United States alone.

Breast cancer is often diagnosed by receptor type; and terms such as *estrogen receptor positive, progesterone receptor negative, HER-2 positive, triple negative,* and *triple positive* are used to denote these receptor types. These diagnoses (made after a biopsy or examining tissue extracted from surgery) are helpful in identifying the aggressiveness, hormone sensitivity, and many other factors in breast cancers.

Hormone receptor status refers to breast cancer cells that have certain proteins that are estrogen or progesterone receptors. Breast cancer cells can have one, both, or none of these receptors. If you are hormone receptor positive, then hormone therapy such as estrogen that blocks these receptors or lowers hormone levels is used.

About one in five women with breast cancer has tumors with a higher level of a protein known as human epidermal growth factor receptor 2–positive (HER2/+), often referred to as HER2. This is known as HER2-positive breast cancer. HER2 is a growth-promoting protein that promotes more aggressive cancer growth. Drugs such as Herceptin are often used as part of conventional treatment for HER2-positive breast cancer.

Triple-positive breast tumors are estrogen positive, progesterone positive, and HER2 positive.

The term *triple-negative breast cancer* means that breast tumors are not HER2 positive and do not have estrogen or progesterone receptors. This type of breast cancer grows and spreads more quickly than hormone-positive breast cancers. Hormone therapy and HER2 drugs are not indicated, although other treatments can be used.

It should be noted that many tumors start with one type and actually over time can develop other types as well,[6] so this method of identification only applies to the biopsy it was made on.

Treatment

- DIET
  - In addition to the dietary considerations on page 90, the diet should include organic vegetables from the cruciferous (also known as brassica) family. These include kale, cauliflower, Brussels sprouts, broccoli, kohlrabi, turnips, collard greens, mustard greens, bok choy, and cabbage. Another food to consume daily is mushrooms. Button and other mushroom types are an excellent immune boost and addition to breast cancer therapy. Sources of "clean" protein and fat should be included to balance macronutrients.

- SUPPLEMENTS

  - Diindolylmethane (DIM) at a dose of 300 mg and indole-3-carbinol (I3C) at a dose of 300 to 400 mg are recommended to support cruciferous vegetables in the diet for hormone metabolism.

  - Mushroom extracts are excellent for adding natural cancer-fighting power. Maitake and *Coriolus* forms are commonly used (although some formulas with mixed mushroom extracts are excellent as well). Doses of 3000 to 9000 mg of *Coriolus* have been used in active breast cancer; for maitake extract, take 35 to 70 mg daily. If using mushroom supplements in combination with other therapies, we clinically see a need for lower doses.

  - Fermented wheat germ extract has been studied in combination with chemotherapy. Take 9 g daily.

  - Tocotrienol: 400 mg daily for women taking tamoxifen to reduce risk of dying and recurrence.

  - Modified citrus pectin: 5 g three times daily.

  - Iodine is used to block estrogen receptors. Doses of 500 mcg up to 12.5 mg daily may be used.

  - These "basics" are helpful across several cancer types:

    » Curcumin: 1000 to 2000 mg two to three times daily

    » Melatonin: 5 to 20 mg at bedtime

    » Low-dose naltrexone (LDN): 2 to 4.5 mg four mornings per week (Rx)

    » Berberine: 250 mg twice a day

    » Vitamin D: 5000 IU daily with a meal (blood testing should confirm a blood value of at least 50 ng/ml)

» Vitamin K2 (MK-4): 50 mg once to twice daily

» CBD: 25 to 50 mg of the active component two to three times daily

» Probiotic: 20 billion colony forming units (CFU) or higher daily

- IV / INJECTION THERAPIES

  – Artesunate followed by high dose IV vitamin C (HDIVC): 50 to 100 grams

  – Mistletoe

  – Curcumin or quercetin

  – Ozone

- OTHER

  – Intermittent fasting (page 117)

  – Copper chelation with tetrathiomolybdate (TM) - (Rx)

  – Vitamin A (as retinyl palmitate): 5,000 to 10,000 IU per day

  – Poly-MVA: two to four teaspoons twice daily

  – THC (if legal): to go with the CBD, as directed by your prescriber

  – Hyperthermia (page 243)

Prevention

Prevention of breast cancer is critical once you are in remission. Maintaining an active remission (i.e., actively doing things to prevent activation of the cancer stem cells) is critical. Continuing the dietary interventions, supplements (usually at lower doses), and lifestyle therapies (mind-body, exercise, and so on) are critical steps to follow. Continuing on a high vegetable, clean food, and low glycemic diet plan is critical as well. Foods rich in iodine have preventative effects; and fermented soy foods such as miso, tofu, natto, and tempeh have been shown in population studies to have breast cancer protective properties.

Working with a practitioner on appropriate digestive function, detoxification, and hormone balance (to the degree possible) and assuring there are no latent infections (which are common after cancer therapies) will keep the rest of the system as healthy as possible.

Physical activity can reduce breast cancer mortality by about 40 percent.[7] We recommend at least 30 minutes of moderate-intensity physical activity at least five days of the week, or 75 minutes of more vigorous exercise, along with two to three weekly strength-training sessions.

OVARIAN CANCER

Ovarian cancer is often discovered in more advanced stages due to having very few symptoms that women will notice in its early stages. In our experience and emerging research regarding integrative methods to help ovarian cancer, many of the approaches are the same as those discussed in the breast cancer section. There is one difference:

- IV VITAMIN C (before, during, and after standard therapies): While we recommend IV vitamin C in most cancers, it has been studied in ovarian cancer specifically in concert with standard therapies and was shown to improve outcomes in ovarian cancer patients.[8] This research matches our personal experience in using IV vitamin C in ovarian cancer. Our other common recommendation of using artesunate with the IV vitamin C is supported by a separate study[9] showing synergy of artesunate and common therapies for ovarian cancer. We normally recommend this as a high-level therapy to begin as quickly as possible in our ovarian cancer patients. A typical dosage is 50 to 100 grams per IV.

LUNG CANCER

Lung cancer is very common and is normally divided into the cell type seen on biopsy. Non–small cell lung cancer (NSCLC) is the most common type of lung cancer, making up 80 to 85 percent of all cases. It typically grows and spreads more slowly than small cell lung cancer (SCLC), which is much deadlier than NSCLC. Some lung cancer tumors are composed of cells from more than one type of NSCLC. Many cancers from other parts of the body metastasize to the lungs, so one may have a "lung tumor," but it is the original tumor type and neither NSCLC or SCLC.

Treatment

- DIET
  - Because lung cancer can be diagnosed later in its progression and needs an aggressive approach, using a combination of intermittent fasting (12 to 16 hours with noncaloric liquids and then 12 to 8 hours where one eats) with a high vegetable, clean food (organic), and low glycemic (no grains or starchy vegetables) diet plan is useful. If your physician agrees, we would suggest potentially using a ketogenic diet as a step up in intensity.

- SUPPLEMENTS
  - Artemisinin[10] (part of the wormwood plant): 200 to 400 mg twice a day on an empty stomach three days weekly. (If a liposomal form of artemisinin is used, the dose is 150 to 200 mg once a day, three days weekly.)
  - Fish oil containing 2500 mg of EPA and DHA combined daily may improve chemotherapy efficacy[11]
  - Astragalus root:[12] 1000 to 1500 mg twice daily
  - These "basics" are helpful across cancer types:
    - » Curcumin: 1000 to 2000 mg two to three times daily

> » Melatonin: 5 to 20 mg at bedtime

> » Low-dose naltrexone (LDN): 2 to 4.5 mg four mornings
> per week (Rx)

> » Berberine: 250 mg twice a day

> » Vitamin D: 5000 IU daily with a meal (blood testing should con-
> firm a blood value of at least 50 ng/ml)

> » Vitamin K2 (MK-4): 50 mg once to twice daily

> » CBD: 25 to 50 mg of the active component two to three
> times daily

- IV / INJECTION THERAPIES

  - HDIVC: 50 to 100 grams

  - Mistletoe

  - Curcumin or quercetin

  - Ozone

- OTHER

  - Intermittent fasting (page 117)

  - Copper chelation with tetrathiomolybdate (TM) - (Rx)

  - Poly-MVA: two to four teaspoons twice daily

  - THC (if legal): to go with the CBD, as directed by your prescriber

  - Hyperthermia (page 243)

Prevention

- Clean diet and fluids / remove environmental toxins

- Exercise and mind-body work

- Low glycemic / very low sugar diet

- Quit smoking

- Mediterranean diet, which is associated with a much lower risk of lung cancer[13]

- Green tea and green tea extract

PROSTATE CANCER

Prostate cancer is the most common non-skin cancer in men. In fact, about one man in seven will be diagnosed with prostate cancer during his lifetime. Prostate cancer develops mainly in older men. Approximately 60 percent of prostate cancers are diagnosed in men aged 65 or older, and it is rare before age 40. The average age at the time of diagnosis is about 66. Prostate cancer is the third leading cause of cancer death in American men, behind lung cancer and colorectal cancer. About 1 man in 39 will die of prostate cancer.

Although prostate cancer can be a serious disease, most men diagnosed do not die from it. Close to three million men in the United States who have been diagnosed with prostate cancer at some point are still alive today. We find it one of the most survivable and treatable of all cancers.

Treatment

- DIET
  - The Mediterranean diet is associated with lower overall mortality in men diagnosed with nonmetastatic prostate cancer[14] and is protective against prostate cancer.[15] In addition to the dietary considerations on page 110, the diet should include organic vegetables from the cruciferous (also known as brassica) family. These include kale, cauliflower, Brussels sprouts, broccoli, kohlrabi, turnips, collard greens, mustard greens, bok choy, and cabbage. Another food to consume daily is mushrooms. Button and other mushroom types are an excellent immune boost and addition to prostate cancer therapy. Food sources of lycopene have prostate

cancer–protective properties. Tomato-based foods such as tomato sauce and juice are the primary sources. Sources of "clean" protein and fat need to be included to balance macronutrients.

- SUPPLEMENTS
  - Modified citrus pectin (MCP): 5 grams three times daily
  - Green tea extract: 400 mg two to three times daily
  - Reishi mushroom: 1000 mg two to three times daily
  - *Boswellia serrata:* 1500 mg two to three times daily
  - Pomegranate extract: 500 mg one to two times daily
  - Grape seed extract: 150 mg twice daily
  - Broccoli seed extract: 100 mg two to three times daily
  - Resveratrol: 500 mg two times daily
  - These "basics" are helpful across cancer types:
    » Curcumin: 1000 to 2000 mg two to three times daily
    » Melatonin: 5 to 20 mg at bedtime
    » Low-dose naltrexone (LDN): 2 to 4.5 mg four mornings per week (Rx)
    » Berberine: 250 mg twice a day
    » Vitamin D: 5000 IU daily with a meal (blood testing should confirm a blood value of at least 50 ng/ml)
    » Vitamin K2 (MK-4): 50 mg once to twice daily
    » CBD: 25 to 50 mg of the active component two to three times daily

- IV / INJECTION THERAPIES

  - Artesunate – HDIVC: 50 to 100 grams

  - Mistletoe

  - Ozone

- OTHER

  - As with all cancer, exercise is critical to patients with prostate cancer. Within tolerable limits, exercise five times weekly is recommended.

  - Hyperthermia (page 243)

  - Dietary interventions

Prevention

A plant-based diet that avoids or restricts red meat and dairy products is recommended. Some studies have shown that approximately eight ounces of pomegranate juice or the use of pomegranate extract slows the rise of PSA levels.[16]

Three hours or more of vigorous physical activity per week has been shown to result in a 61 percent reduced risk of dying from prostate cancer.[17] One example would be brisk walking.

COLORECTAL CANCER

New cases of colon and rectum (colorectal) cancer were approximately 40 per 100,000 men and women per year. The number of deaths was approximately 15 per 100,000 men and women per year. Approximately 4.3 percent of men and women will be diagnosed with colon and rectum cancer at some point during their lifetime. In 2014, there were an estimated 1.3 million people living with colorectal cancer in the United States.

Early detection is critical for improved survival as evidenced by an approximate 90 percent five-year survival (relative) at stage I and 14 percent five-year survival (relative) at stage IV.

Treatment

- DIET
  - If a person has had surgery, they need to be on a postsurgical diet until the digestive tract heals. Once the healing is complete, diet is crucial in colon cancer and may need to be altered in regard to what is tolerated. Some of the cruciferous vegetables may not be tolerated, but often digestive enzymes and probiotics will help. Good sources of prebiotic foods (cabbage, onion, and so on) are needed, along with soluble fiber (found in the vegetables listed below). In addition to the dietary considerations on page 90, the diet should include organic vegetables from the cruciferous (also known as brassica) family, as tolerated. These include kale, cauliflower, Brussels sprouts, broccoli, kohlrabi, turnips, collard greens, mustard greens, bok choy, and cabbage. Another food to consume daily is mushrooms. Button and other mushroom types are an excellent immune boost and addition to colorectal cancer therapy. Sources of "clean" protein and fat should be included to balance macronutrients.

- SUPPLEMENTS
  - In GI cancers, and especially colorectal cancer, oral therapies that have "access" to the GI cells are critical to success.
    - » Artemisinin[18] (part of the wormwood plant): 200 to 400 mg twice a day on an empty stomach, three days weekly
    - » Fermented wheat germ extract: 9 grams daily
    - » Turmeric root: 1000 mg three times daily
    - » Quercetin: 500 mg twice daily

>» DIM: 75 to 150 mg once to twice a day

- These "basics" are helpful across cancer types:

    >» Curcumin: 1000 mg two to three times daily (note this dose is lower due to the addition of turmeric root, which is used for its topical effect in the GI tract above)

    >» Melatonin: 5 to 20 mg at bedtime

    >» Low-dose naltrexone (LDN): 2 to 4.5 mg four mornings per week (Rx)

    >» Berberine: 250 mg twice a day

    >» Vitamin D: 5000 IU daily with a meal (blood testing should confirm a blood value of at least 50 ng/ml)

    >» Vitamin K2 (MK-4): 50 mg once to twice daily

    >» CBD: 25 to 50 mg of the active component two to three times daily

- **IV / INJECTION THERAPIES**

    - Artesunate – HDIVC: 50 to 100 grams

    - Mistletoe

    - Ozone

- **OTHER**

    - As with all cancers, but especially in colorectal cancer, attention to the digestive system and its health is essential. Proper microbiome support (removal of any GI pathogens and restoration of beneficial bacteria) is critical.

    - Intermittent fasting (page 117)

    - Copper chelation with tetrathiomolybdate (TM) - (Rx)

— Poly-MVA: two to four teaspoons twice daily

— THC (if legal): to go with the CBD, as directed by your prescriber

— Hyperthermia (page 243)

Prevention

Adequate vitamin D and K intake are critical. The maintenance of the microbiome is also critical to prevention. Because the GI tract is a common entry point for toxins, a clean, organic diet and detoxification strategies during remission are key. Green tea and green tea extract have cancer preventative properties.

KIDNEY AND BLADDER CANCER

About 64,000 new cases of kidney cancer will occur annually, and men develop it almost two to one over women. Annually, about 14,400 people will die from it. Most people with kidney cancer are older, with the average age at diagnosis being 64, and it is very uncommon in people younger than age 45. Kidney cancer is among the 10 most common cancers in both men and women.

Bladder cancer has almost 80,000 new cases annually, and about 17,000 will die yearly from it. Men develop it three to one over women. The rates of new bladder cancers and of cancer deaths and have been dropping slightly in women in recent years. In men, incidence rates have been decreasing and death rates have been stable. Bladder cancer accounts for about 5 percent of all new cancers in the U.S. It is the fourth most common cancer in men, but it is less common in women.

Although the two are different cancer types, we find they generally respond to similar integrative approaches.

Treatment

- DIET

    — A plant-based diet rich in whole foods is recommended. People with poor kidney function require specialized diets from a health professional.

- SUPPLEMENTS

    - EGCG (grean tea extract): 200 to 400 mg twice daily

    - Mixed tocopherols / tocotrienols: 150 to 250 mg per day

    - Milk thistle: 250 mg twice daily

    - DIM: 75 to 150 mg twice daily

    - These "basics" are helpful across cancer types:

        » Curcumin: 1000 to 2000 mg two to three times daily

        » Melatonin: 5 to 20 mg at bedtime

        » Low-dose naltrexone (LDN): 2 to 4.5 mg four mornings per week (Rx)

        » Berberine: 250 mg twice a day

        » Vitamin D: 5000 IU daily with a meal (blood testing should confirm a blood value of at least 50 ng/ml)

        » Vitamin K2 (MK-4): 50 mg once to twice daily

        » CBD: 25 to 50 mg of the active component two to three times daily

- IV / INJECTION THERAPIES

    - Artesunate – HDIVC: 50 to 100 grams

    - Mistletoe

    - Poly-MVA

- OTHER

    - Hyperthermia (page 243)

    - Intermittent fasting (page 117)

    - Copper chelation with tetrathiomolybdate (TM) - (Rx)

- Vitamin A (as retinyl palmitate): 5,000 to 10,000 IU per day

- Poly-MVA: two to four teaspoons twice daily

- THC (if legal) to go with the CBD: as directed by your prescriber

Prevention

Although critical in any cancer, being extremely aware of and avoiding environmental toxins is primary in kidney and bladder cancer. Consumption of clean filtered water and organic foods and reducing any other toxic exposures should be a priority.

BRAIN CANCER

Brain tumors come in many types, but the most deadly and aggressive are the astrocytomas with the higher grade glioblastoma (GBM) type being the most difficult to treat. The GBM represents about 15 percent of all primary brain tumors and about 60 to 75 percent of all astrocytomas. They increase in frequency with age, affect more men than women, and are rare but not unheard of in children.

With standard treatment, median survival for adults with an anaplastic astrocytoma is about two to three years. For adults with more aggressive GBM treated with concurrent temozolomide (Temodar) and radiation therapy, median survival is about 15 months and two-year survival is 30 percent. However, a 2009 study reported that almost 10 percent of patients with glioblastoma may live five years or longer. Children with high-grade tumors (grades III and IV) tend to do better than adults; five-year survival for children is about 25 percent.

There are multiple "survival factors" for GBM, one of which is the gene MGMT. Patients who have had their MGMT gene shut off by a process called methylation also have prolonged survival rates.

Treatment

NOTE: GBM is such an aggressive and deadly cancer that treatment is best started as soon as possible, as opposed to phasing things in.

- DIET

  - Although beneficial in most cancers, a very low carbohydrate diet approach is critical in GBM.[19]

  - Second choice is a high-fiber, vegetable-based, low-carbohydrate diet supplemented with MCT Oil (4 to 8 tablespoons daily)

  - All organic sources of food and filtered water

  - Ketogenic diet is preferred

  - If possible, daily intermittent fasting (16 hours water only / 8 hours eating time period)

- SUPPLEMENTS

  - Support oxidative (normal cell) metabolism / oppose glycolytic (lactate) metabolism:

    » Poly-MVA: 8 teaspoons divided through the day, four to five days weekly

    » *Boswellia* extract (may reduce brain swelling for those receiving radiation therapy): 4200 mg a day

    » Oxaloacetate: 100 to 300 mg twice a day

    » Berberine: 250 to 500 mg twice a day with food

  - Synergy for metabolic therapy / direct brain tumor activity:

    » CoQ10: 100 to 200 mg twice a day

    » Retinyl palmitate: 5000 IU daily

    » *Boswellia:* 250 to 500 mg three times daily with food

    » Ketone supplement: ketone salt form, drink 2.5 to 10 grams daily

  - These "basics" are helpful across cancer types:

> » Curcumin: 1000 to 2000 mg two to three times daily

> » Melatonin: 5 to 20 mg at bedtime

> » Low-dose naltrexone (LDN): 2 to 4.5 mg four mornings per week (Rx)

> » Vitamin D: 5000 IU daily with a meal (blood testing should confirm a blood value of at least 50 ng/ml)

> » Vitamin K2 (MK-4): 50 mg once to twice daily

> » CBD: 25 to 50 mg of the active component two to three times daily

- IV / INJECTION THERAPIES

  - Poly-MVA + DCA protocol

  - Curcumin and quercetin

- OTHER

  - Hyperbaric oxygen therapy: two to three times weekly as a trial if available

  - THC added to CBD if legal

Prevention

- Clean diet and fluids / remove environmental toxins

- Exercise and mind-body work

- Low glycemic / no sugar diet

MELANOMA

Melanoma accounts for less than one percent of skin cancer cases, but the vast majority of skin cancer deaths. An average of one person dies of melanoma every hour. An estimated 87,000 new cases of invasive melanoma will be diagnosed in the U.S. in 2017, and an estimated 9,700 people will die of melanoma in 2017.

As with all cancers, early detection at lower stages is critical to achieving better outcomes. The estimated five-year survival rate for patients whose melanoma is detected early is about 98 percent in the U.S. The survival rate falls to 62 percent when the disease reaches the lymph nodes, and 18 percent when the disease metastasizes to distant organs.

Regardless of the stage it is diagnosed, therapies normally include surgical resection, some chemotherapies in particular cases, and other standard interventions. Melanoma at any stage is a cancer that requires an aggressive "waste no time" approach.

Treatment

- DIET

    – Melanoma is often a very aggressive tumor and therefore needs an aggressive approach. Using a combination of intermittent fasting (12 to 16 hours with noncaloric liquids and then 12 to 8 hours where one eats) with a high vegetable, clean food (organic), and low glycemic (no grains or starchy vegetables) diet plan is useful. If your physician agrees, we would suggest potentially using a ketogenic diet as a step up in intensity as well.

- SUPPLEMENTS

    – Fermented wheat germ extract: 9 grams daily

    – Modified citrus pectin (MCP): 1000 to 2000 mg three times daily

    – Poly-MVA: two to four teaspoons twice daily

    – Vitamin A (retinyl palmitate): 10,000 to 15,000 IU daily

    – CoQ10 (ubiquinone): 200 mg daily

    – Thyroid Rx: To keep the TSH between 0.5 and 1.0,[20] as determined with a physician

- These "basics" are helpful across cancer types:

  » Curcumin: 1000 to 2000 mg two to three times daily

  » Melatonin: 5 to 20 mg at bedtime

  » Low-dose naltrexone (LDN): 2 to 4.5 mg four mornings per week (Rx)

  » Berberine: 250 mg twice a day

  » Vitamin D: 5000 IU daily with a meal (blood testing should confirm a blood value of at least 50 ng/ml)

  » Vitamin K2 (MK-4): 50 mg once to twice daily

  » CBD: 25 to 50 mg of the active component two to three times daily

- IV / INJECTION THERAPIES

  - Mistletoe

  - Poly-MVA

  - HDIVC

  - Curcumin or quercetin

  - Ozone

- OTHER

  - Intermittent fasting (page 117)

  - Copper chelation with tetrathiomolybdate (TM) - (Rx)

  - THC (if legal) to go with the CBD: as directed by your prescriber

  - Hyperthermia (page 243)

  - Azelaic acid[21] (This is a common topical dermatology drug but has promise in oral and IV forms for melanoma. Outside of research, however, these non-topical forms are not currently available.)

Prevention

- Clean diet and fluids / remove environmental toxins

- Exercise and mind-body work

- Low glycemic / very low sugar diet

- Adequate blood vitamin D levels, possibly through supplementation

LEUKEMIA AND LYMPHOMA

There are multiple forms of leukemia and lymphoma, and all have differing characteristics and aggressiveness. They fall under the category of hematological malignancy, where they are divided by cell abnormality and characteristics. Some are slower in progression with higher relative survival, and some are much more aggressive and deadly. Of course, every type must be assessed in regard to how it is affecting the patient, its known aggressiveness, and other personalized factors. But regardless of the type, we have seen clinically that the hematologic cancers have some unity in the integrative oncology therapies they respond to.

Treatment

- DIET

  - Of all the cancers we have seen, the hematologic variety is one of the most positively responsive to carbohydrate restriction. With the more aggressive forms, we would suggest immediately using a ketogenic diet as a step up in intensity if possible. In the early treatment time period, we often combine this with intermittent fasting (12 to 16 hours with noncaloric liquids and then 12 to 8 hours where one eats). If the cancer type is less aggressive, we may start with a high vegetable, clean food (organic), and low glycemic (no grains or starchy vegetables), low carbohydrate diet with at least 12 hours intermittent fasting, adjusting as necessary.

- SUPPLEMENTS

  - Artemisinin (part of the wormwood plant): 200 to 400 mg twice a day on an empty stomach, three days weekly. (If a liposomal form of artemisinin is used, the dose is 150 to 200 mg once a day, three days weekly.)

  - Poly-MVA: two to four teaspoons twice daily

  - EGCG (green tea extract): 400 to 2000 mg twice daily

  - Mixed tocopherols / tocotrienols: 150 to 250 mg per day

  - *Coriolus:* 1000 mg two to three times daily

  - Fish oil may help those undergoing chemotherapy. Take 2000 mg fish oil daily.

  - These "basics" are helpful across cancer types:

    » Curcumin: 1000 to 2000 mg two to three times daily

    » Melatonin: 5 to 20 mg at bedtime

    » Low-dose naltrexone (LDN): 2 to 4.5 mg four mornings per week (Rx)

    » Berberine: 250 mg twice a day

    » Vitamin D: 5000 IU daily with a meal (blood testing should confirm a blood value of at least 50 ng/ml)

    » Vitamin K2 (MK-4): 50 mg once to twice daily

    » CBD: 25 to 50 mg of the active component two to three times daily

- IV / INJECTION THERAPIES

  - Poly-MVA + DCA protocol

  - Mistletoe

  - Curcumin or quercetin

- OTHER

  - Hyperbaric oxygen therapy once to twice weekly

  - THC (if legal) to go with the CBD, as directed by your prescriber

  - Consider hyperthermia (page 243)

- PREVENTION

  - Clean diet and fluids / remove environmental toxins

  - Exercise and mind-body work

  - Low glycemic / very low sugar diet

LIVER CANCER

The liver is a common site of metastasis, but primary cancer of the liver is a different process and requires some different treatment than metastatic liver cancer. A positive aspect of primary liver cancer is that the liver processes most of what we eat or have in an IV very quickly, so helpful agents (such as those listed below) are highly available to the liver for healing and protection.

Treatment

- DIET

  - Primary liver cancer (but not metastatic liver cancer) is one of the few cancers where a ketogenic diet should *not* be used. A modification is mentioned below, and if appropriate, we recommend considering intermittent fasting. In addition to the dietary considerations listed on page 91, the diet should include organic vegetables from the cruciferous (also known as brassica) family. These include: kale, cauliflower, Brussels sprouts, broccoli, kohlrabi, turnips, collard greens, mustard greens, bok choy, and cabbage. Another food to consume daily are mushrooms. Button and other mushroom types are an excellent immune boost and addition to liver cancer therapy. Sources of "clean" protein and fat should be included to balance macronutrients.

- SUPPLEMENTS

  - Mushroom extracts are excellent when adding natural cancer-fighting power. Maitake and *Coriolus* forms are commonly used. Doses of 3000 to 9000 mg are recommended for *Coriolus*, 35 to 70 mg daily for maitake extract. If using the mushroom supplements in combination with the other therapies mentioned, we clinically see a need for lower doses.

  - Active hexose correlated compound (AHCC): 2000 to 3000 mg once to twice daily

  - Artemisinin: 200 to 400 mg twice a day on an empty stomach, three days weekly. (If a liposomal form of artemisinin is used, the dose is 150 to 200 mg once a day, three days weekly.)

  - Fermented wheat germ extract (studied in combination with chemotherapy): 9 grams daily

  - For liver glutathione support: selenium (200 mcg daily), zinc (10 to 20 mg daily with food), methylated B-vitamin complex, Poly-MVA (2 to 4 teaspoons twice daily) or alpha-lipoic acid (300 mg once to twice daily), silymarin (milk thistle) 400 to 500 mg twice daily, and reduced glutathione 500 mg daily

  - These "basics" are helpful across cancer types:

    » Curcumin: 1000 to 2000 mg two to three times daily

    » Melatonin: 5 to 20 mg at bedtime

    » Low-dose naltrexone (LDN): 2 to 4.5 mg four mornings per week (Rx)

    » Berberine: 250 mg twice a day

    » Vitamin D: 5000 IU daily with a meal (blood testing should confirm a blood value of at least 50 ng/ml)

» CBD: 25 to 50 mg of the active component two to three times daily

» Probiotic: 20 billion colony forming units (CFU) or higher daily

- IV / INJECTION THERAPIES

  – Artesunate followed by high dose IV vitamin C (HDIVC): 50 to 100 grams

  – Mistletoe

  – Curcumin or quercetin

  – Ozone

- OTHER

  – Intermittent fasting (page 117)

  – Copper chelation with tetrathiomolybdate (TM) - (Rx)

  – Vitamin A (as retinyl palmitate): 5,000 to 10,000 IU per day

  – THC (if legal) to go with the CBD: as directed by your prescriber

  – Hyperthermia (page 243)

Prevention

Prevention of liver cancer is critical once one is in remission. Maintaining an active remission (i.e., actively doing things to prevent cancer stem cell activation) is critical. Continuing the dietary interventions, supplements (usually at lower doses), and lifestyle therapies (mind-body, exercise, and so on) are critical steps to follow. Continuing on a high vegetable, clean food, and low glycemic diet plan is critical as well.

Working with a practitioner on appropriate digestive function, detoxification, and hormone balance (to the degree possible) and assuring there are no latent infections (which are common after cancer therapies) will keep the rest of the system as healthy as possible.

PANCREATIC CANCER

Pancreatic cancer is often diagnosed later in the process, making it a very aggressive cancer and needing aggressive and encompassing therapy (similar to brain cancers).

In our experience, it is very similar to primary liver cancer. Thus the therapies are the same in pancreatic cancer as in primary liver cancer with the following exceptions:

- QUERCETIN: This is a potent flavonoid found in many plants. It has many immune activities that are similar to some found in mushrooms and curcumin, but unique to quercetin. Doses of 1000 mg three times a day with meals are common for pancreatic cancer.

- PROTEOLYTIC ENZYME THERAPY: As it is complex and requires personalization, we recommend seeking an integrative oncology practitioner who can help you manage this therapy (see page 147).

- CURCUMIN: While curcumin is mentioned in the primary liver cancer section, we wanted to point out it is the "top of the list" priority supplement for pancreatic cancer. The doses are the same as discussed in the liver section at 1000 to 2000 mg two to three times daily.

- DELTA TOCOTRIENOL: 400 mg daily

THYROID CANCER

If diagnosed at earlier stages, which is common, thyroid cancer is one of the very curable cancers using standard oncology therapies. In some cases there are success rates above 95 percent with standard therapies. In these instances, we recommend completing the standard therapies first, having integrative oncology support before and during these therapies, and working diligently on healing and secondary prevention after standard therapy.

Treatment

- DIET

  - For people receiving radioactive iodine ablation after thyroid cancer surgery, a low iodine diet is recommended for one to two weeks before radioiodine therapy and one to two days afterward.[22] This includes the avoidance of iodized salt, sea salt, seafood and sea products, dairy products, egg yolks or whole eggs, bakery products with iodine, chocolate, soybeans, and supplements with iodine. After this period of time, a plant-based diet or Mediterranean diet is recommended.

- SUPPLEMENTS

  - IODINE: In some studies, the role of supplemental iodine following thyroid cancer therapy has shown a benefit and stabilizing effect to the healing and hormonal recovery people require.[23] [24] Iodine supplementation for this preventative phase can safely be achieved using 200 to 500 micrograms daily of iodine. Occasionally larger doses are required, but it should be dosed and monitored by your integrative oncology professional.

  - CHAMOMILE: The common tea herb chamomile has been shown in a small study to be of assistance in thyroid cancer.[25] The authors of this study saw a correlation between consumption of chamomile tea and lower rates of thyroid cancer and other thyroid diseases. While this is more of a preventative strategy, it is clear that support during and after cancer treatment can also help with the repair and healing required once that cancer is present and being treated. Chamomile tea is readily available, has a nice calming effect, and can be consumed through the day.

- OTHER

  - DENTAL: Oral health, including infections in and around the teeth and gums, tonsils, and the "ear, nose, and throat" region are important to consider in thyroid cancer. Likewise, dental toxicity from amalgam fillings should be assessed. This connection is made because the lymphatic drainage (the body's natural removal system for infectious and toxic material) from the mouth, ear, nose, and throat areas is shared with the thyroid tissues. Having less inflammatory material (either toxic or infectious) creates less stress and more immune balance in the area, improving healing and prevention. We often recommend seeing a biological dentist for an assessment.

  - DETOXIFICATION AND HEALING (for both the surgery as well as to detoxify, for those who receive radioactive iodine therapy).

  - FOR LIVER GLUTATHIONE SUPPORT: selenium (200 mcg daily), zinc (10 to 20 mg daily with food), methylated B-vitamin complex, Poly-MVA (2 to 4 teaspoons twice daily) or alpha lipoic acid (300 mg once to twice daily), and silymarin (milk thistle) 400 to 500 mg twice daily, and reduced glutathione 500 mg daily.

  - These "basics" are helpful across cancer types:

    » Curcumin: 1000 to 2000 mg two to three times daily

    » Melatonin: 5 to 20 mg at bedtime

    » Low-dose naltrexone (LDN): 2 to 4.5 mg four mornings per week (Rx)

    » Berberine: 250 mg twice a day

    » Vitamin D: 5000 IU daily with a meal (blood testing should confirm a blood value of at least 50 ng/ml)

    » Vitamin K2 (MK-4): 50 mg once to twice daily

- » CBD: 25 to 50 mg of the active component two to three times daily

- » Probiotic: 20 billion colony forming units (CFU) or higher daily

- IV / INJECTION THERAPIES

  - Artesunate followed by high dose IV vitamin C (HDIVC): 50 to 100 grams

  - Mistletoe

  - Curcumin or quercetin

  - Ozone

CHAPTER 10

OTHER ALTERNATIVE THERAPIES FOR CANCER

I n the past 10 years, we have seen a growth of potential alternative, integrative, and complementary therapies for cancer; and by the time this book is published, there will likely be even more. In this chapter, we will outline some additional "alternative" therapies we have clinically seen be of benefit to patients over the years.

It is important to remember that many of the therapies discussed here may not be "alternative" at all in much of the world and that we are basing the determination of "alternative" on the more conservative Western, and specifically North American, view of oncology therapies. We have both received some critical feedback for using the term *alternative* because many people believe that the alternatives should have the same place in cancer therapy all the other "standard" therapies have. We certainly understand this and are merely using the term to denote "not standard of care in North America."

The primary job of integrative oncology is to push the boundaries of care into areas that yield better and better outcomes for people who have cancer. Conventional cancer therapy, while holding a place in cancer care, is not enough. To quote a recent paper looking at the effectiveness of recent cancer therapies:

> This systematic evaluation of oncology approvals by the EMA in 2009–13 shows that most drugs entered the market without evidence of benefit on survival or quality of life. At a minimum of 3.3 years after market entry, there was

still no conclusive evidence that these drugs either extended or improved life for most cancer indications. When there were survival gains over existing treatment options or placebo, they were often marginal.[1]

Our ability in integrative oncology to keep searching for and testing new and broader therapies is critical to outcome improvement. We are certainly cautious and take into serious consideration safety data, patient responses, and clinical outcomes. But a patient with cancer today simply does not have the luxury of time to wait for all therapies to be approved in every avenue of discussion. They need to work with their trusted integrative physician to find the right method of therapy for them.

Another reason for inclusive therapy is the need to have multiple avenues into the cancer patient's system in order to treat them in the most broad and effective manner possible. We find this need best expressed by a colleague who is a naturopathic oncologist and one of the founders of the American Board of Naturopathic Oncology:

> "I have maintained the opinion that naturopathic oncology, as a whole, is not very good at killing cancer cells. What we are good at is causing the cancer cells to die.
>
> The focus of the naturopathic doctor is on the person with cancer and the stroma within which the cancer cells live; whether we are talking about cancer cells living within the confines of a tissue-based mass (tumor) or circulating freely in the blood or lymphatic system (circulating tumor cells). As it goes, cancer cells arise from oneself, they are inherently not different than one's other (normal) cells; in fact they start out with the same genetic code as all other cells in the body. To become cancerous, normal cells must sustain some type of damage or injury, then find a way to survive in the body. Therein lies the question posed by naturopathic oncology: what is it about the environment that allows the cancer cells to survive?
>
> It is the challenge and duty of the naturopathic physician to engage this concept, then to design an appropriate treatment plan. This philosophy is what sets naturopathic oncology apart from conventional medicine, yet allows for an integrative approach. Even with the remarkable advances that have been made in the medical sciences, we still have only glimpses into the wonderful and intricate workings of the human body. Treatments which attempt to attack disease from without remain, despite their increasing sophistication, blunderings about in a

place of marvels. Cancer is a disease that requires individualized treatment that is as physiological as we can attain, with constant reverence for the mystery and beauty of the human body, even in illness."

— Dan Rubin, ND, FABNO,
founder of Naturopathic Specialists, LLC, in Scottsdale, Arizona

In our practices, we have seen patients use and gain benefit from the following therapy types over time. In some cases, the therapy is only available outside the U.S., and in some cases, patients can access it within the U.S.

DETOXIFICATION THERAPIES

Cancer can be stimulated by toxicity in the body either directly (due to a known carcinogen like cigarette smoke) or indirectly (by secondary effects of toxicity, such as mitochondrial dysfunction and antioxidant imbalance). Cancer therapies can also cause toxicity on multiple levels. Some are toxicities causing a significant side effect (such as vomiting, hair loss, or heart disease) and some are direct toxicities (such as platinum toxicity or glutathione depletion).[2][3][4] In considering detoxification in the setting of cancer, there are some critical decisions to make regarding timing and application of depuration (promoting whole-body toxin elimination) and detoxification (specific removal of specific toxins). The main factors to consider are timing (whether the person is in active chemotherapy or radiation therapy or having surgery), past therapies and their potential contribution to the level of toxicity, overall health (whether the person can safely depurate or detoxify), and prior toxic exposure history.

TIMING

We need to assess if the person is in active chemotherapy, radiation therapy, aggressive natural anticancer therapies, or having surgery and the appropriateness and potential stress on the body any depuration or detoxification may cause. A primary benefit is that all the basic interventions we will work on with a patient (e.g., diet, hydration, clean foods and water, movement, and mental and emotional support) are already supporting depuration. So regardless of the other therapies one may or may not include at a particular time, our patients are already consistently helping the whole body eliminate toxins naturally. Often if a person is undergoing radiation, chemotherapy, or having surgery, their system is under so much stress that additional detoxification strategies may not be appropriate. Aftercare detoxification is an appropriate consideration in these cases.

PAST THERAPIES AND THEIR POTENTIAL CONTRIBUTION TO THE LEVEL OF TOXICITY

Have you had a platinum-based chemotherapy? Or have you had a mitochondrial toxin therapy such as radiation therapy or many chemotherapies? Other factors we consider at this point are how potentially imbalanced the antioxidant system may be (your primary aid in both detoxification and protection from toxic insults). Many standard cancer therapies significantly stress the antioxidant system and, just as general depuration is critical, this system must be repaired and rebalanced.

OVERALL HEALTH

A critical assessment of the overall health of the patient should be completed to see if they can safely depurate or detoxify. In many cases, aside from the general baseline depuration measures previously mentioned, we will wait and build up a patient's reserves and energy before adding detoxification strategies. Our general approach is to not initiate extra detoxification while a person still has a very active cancer process in an attempt to prevent overwhelming the system. Some patients may be concerned that they will just continue to be toxic and ask why we may wait. We often explain the depuration aspect of their baseline plan and how helpful that is and that some therapies we use during either recovery or active cancer therapy (such as IVC[5][6] or curcumin[7][8][9]) are actually detoxifying therapies in addition to offering other benefits.

PRIOR TOXIC EXPOSURE HISTORY

Since it is possible for metal and chemical toxins to be carcinogenic,[10] it is not uncommon for a person with cancer to carry a significant toxic burden with them into the cancer journey. And while all the previously mentioned considerations apply to all people with known or suspected past exposure, we will often make sure that the basic depuration strategies and multiple-benefit therapies (e.g., IVC and curcumin) are part of the entire cancer treatment time. In people with high body burdens, we will begin specific detoxification strategies (e.g., chemical detoxification via sweating, liver and kidney support, and metal detoxification via chelation therapies) if applicable and as soon as practical.

While it is often said that "you can't detox your cancer away," we do find that you also cannot ignore the role of toxins as a cause of cancer and illness in general. A well-thought-out approach with reasonable timing and implementation has been the most clinically effective in our oncology practice.

ELECTROTHERAPIES

Electrotherapies in medicine have been available in some form since electricity became available. If one looks at historical uses, some seem very odd and potentially scary. That said, electrotherapies have evolved just as all other medical modalities have in the years since their inception. Generally they can be seen as falling into three categories in cancer care: cancer side effect therapies, general quality of life (QoL) therapies, and direct cancer treatments.

One common use of low-intensity, low-frequency electrotherapies is the reduction of swelling (lymphedema) secondary to breast cancer. One study found that this therapy supplementary to manual lymphatic drainage significantly enhanced pain alleviation and swelling reduction in patients with lymphedema compared with manual lymphatic drainage alone.[11] Another study (not using lymphatic massage) found no significant edema improvement but did find a significant improvement in QoL in those receiving the electrotherapy.[12]

General QoL therapies may include, but are not limited to, electrotherapies, some hydrotherapy procedures, many physical therapy procedures, and other interventions. In these cases, the goal of the electrotherapy may be aimed at pain reduction, muscle relaxation, or immune support.

Lesser known direct cancer therapies involving electrotherapy are making a resurgence. These involve either direct therapy to the tumor or therapy in the area over a tumor. They are beginning to be used more in North America, as well as in Europe and Asia. One elaborate study concluded that "electrotherapy of low-level direct current is promissory for cancer treatment," and that the "use of this mathematical approach and the theorem provide a rapid way to propose different optimum electrode arrays in dependence of location, depth, shape and size of the solid tumors with the purpose of obtaining the higher antitumor effectiveness and as a result to implement the electrotherapy in the Clinical Oncology."[13] As sophistication around these therapies increases, we believe more will be available in overall cancer care.

HYDROTHERAPY

Hydrotherapy is a very old natural therapy. It is also a broad term that can mean many things. Entire clinics in many parts of the world are set up to support hydrotherapy for patients, though they are most popular in Europe. In modern research, many explanations of the scientific basis by which hydrotherapy works have been supported, which only validate what physicians have seen clinically for hundreds of years.[14]

The process of hydrotherapy generally involves changes in temperature to cause stimulation of immune, vascular, and other physical processes. In turn, these processes can help to increase and focus the healing forces of the immune system to help the person with cancer maintain health, heal, or improve QoL.[15] [16] [17] [18] [19]

In clinical practice, a trained practitioner can employ various types of hydro-therapy and match them to a patient's physical capacity, health needs, and many other parameters. Some can even be prescribed for home use, which becomes an excellent self-care strategy. In our experience, the use of hydrotherapy can have a spectrum of benefits from QoL to immune support and even in the anti-cancer arena.

HYPERBARIC OXYGEN THERAPY

Hyperbaric oxygen therapy (HBOT) is the use of oxygen under pressure to super-saturate the fluid portion of the blood (plasma) with oxygen. Doing so delivers a higher concentration of oxygen to the tissues and triggers many immune and repair processes. HBOT does this in a manner that regular oxygen therapy cannot, and so it is an important tool in many parts of cancer care.

Some people reading this may have heard that HBOT is contraindicated in cancer patients. This idea comes from a dated notion that the oxygen would "feed the cancer" and make it worse., despite scientific evidence to the contrary. A number of scientific reviews have outlined the ways in which HBOT is not only beneficial in cancer therapy but also in helping to control side effects of standard therapies.[20][21][22] Some research is now starting to outline the potentials for synergy between HBOT and standard therapies as well.[23]

Dr. Anderson has had the unique opportunity to work with patients in both an outpatient setting with HBOT and a hospital with HBOT available. In these settings, he has personally seen benefits for patients with cancer in the active treatment, recovery, and healing phases. HBOT can only be appropriately assessed by a qualified practitioner trained in the use of hyperbaric medicine in cancer.

HYPERTHERMIA

The use of hyperthermia as a support to cancer immunotherapy is supported by an increasing number of scientific studies. Scientific results have demonstrated improved antitumor immune responses with the addition of mild hyperthermia.[24] In addition to the benefit hyperthermia provides in tumor fighting through the immune system, it also can sensitize tumor cells to be more likely to die during radiation therapy and chemotherapy.[25]

Dr. Anderson has hyperthermia facilities in both the hospital and outpatient centers he works with and has seen very positive benefits for cancer patients. In an effort to provide the best information about cancer hyperthermia, we have asked our colleague Dr. Gurdev Parmar to describe his experience using hyperthermia in cancer care in North America:

"I have been using the Oncotherm modulated electro-hyperthermia device for providing loco-regional hyperthermia (LRHT) for solid tumours since June of 2010. We have now administered over 15,000 of these treatments at our clinic, treating over 25 solid tumour types, and only five cases of superficial burns, and four cases of subcutaneous fibrosis (relatively minor side effects). I have also gained experience in using the Heckel HT2000 device for providing fever-range whole body hyperthermia (FR-WBHT) treatment, having administered over 1,000 of these treatments at our clinic. The mechanisms of action of hyperthermia include heat-induced cytotoxicity, vasodilation for drug delivery, improved oxygenation for radiosensitization, and induction of heat shock proteins that result in an in-vivo tumor vaccine-like response. In fact, the Oncotherm device holds a U.S. patent with this description:

"'The present invention relates to a vaccine composed of at least one immune stimulant and radiofrequency waves using capacitive coupling and to a method, especially an in-situ and in vivo vaccination method for treatment of primary cancer and its metastases even in disseminated cell-states, which cannot be detected by presently available imaging methods or for prevention of relapse of the cancer disease, and especially for enabling and supporting the patient's own immune system to recognize and kill the cancer cells and to build up a memory to prevent relapse of a cancer disease' (US 20150217099 A1).

"We have collected data on every patient treated with hyperthermia in our clinic thus far, first retrospectively in 2015 looking back the first five years, and prospectively since then. I have attached a few of the KM curves from this retrospective study, comparing the outcomes of our clinic's patients who included LRHT and/or FR-WBHT in their treatment, versus the same cohort in the SEER database, who presumably used standard of care alone. All 10 of the most commonly treated cancer types in our clinic over those first five years showed a significant improvement in survival. As I have been treating patients with cancer since the year 2000, 10 years before adding hyperthermia, I have observed an improvement in the outcomes of my patients with hyperthermia, both in terms of quality of life and overall survival. Our retrospective data represents the largest data set on the subject matter I am aware of in North America, and supports my observations. We are constantly working toward starting a well-designed prospective trial to further investigate what seems to be a promising approach.

"Our clinic has an experienced team of naturopathic physicians in our cancer care center, surrounded by an incredible support staff. We have hosted patients from every continent, and regularly host patients from across the lower mainland;

B.C., Canada; and the U.S. We provide full laboratory services, numerous IV and injection therapies, pharmaceutical prescriptions, botanical medicines, acupuncture, nutritional supplements, dietary and lifestyle advice, and all other manners of intervention with evidence and history of safe and effective use in an integrative naturopathic setting. We provide consultation for patients just being worked up for a potential cancer diagnosis by biopsy, through primary therapy, and into secondary prevention, survivorship and palliative care."

— Gurdev Parmar, ND, FABNO,
founder and medical director, Integrated Health Clinic,
Fort Langley, British Columbia, Canada

The extensive experience of Dr. Parmar is in line with what we have seen clinically ourselves. Hyperthermia is an incredible addition to the tools of integrative oncology for optimal cancer care.

IMMUNOTHERAPIES

Immunotherapy technically includes any method that augments or changes a person's immune system to fight or kill cancer, including HBOT, hydrotherapy, and hyperthermia, as well as cancer vaccines and viral therapies. Immunotherapies are some of the oldest therapies in cancer care. In 1891, William B. Coley injected streptococcal organisms into a patient with inoperable cancer. He thought that the infection he produced would have an effect of shrinking the malignant tumor, and he was correct. Dr. Coley was head of the Bone Tumor Service at Memorial Hospital in New York and injected more than 1,000 cancer patients with bacteria or bacterial products. These products became known as "Coley's Toxins." Dr. Coley is generally considered the "Father of Immunotherapy."[26]

Since the time of Dr. Coley, our understanding of the way the immune system works has taken leaps and bounds forward. In modern times, immunotherapy is a promising treatment that is gaining acceptance for the management of several cancers, including melanoma, renal cell carcinoma, prostate cancer, and lung cancer.[27]

One active area of immunotherapy is the development of "cancer vaccines." Cancer vaccines are different from traditional vaccines (for infectious disease) in that they focus on clearing active disease (cancer) rather than preventing disease (infection).[28]

Another active area of cancer immunotherapy is the development of viral therapies to trigger an anticancer immune response. Similar to Dr. Coley's work, the use of viral stimulation of the immune system to fight cancer is another "way in" to the immune system. One example is Rigvir, a therapy used in Europe and Mexico with varied results.[29][30] Like any cancer therapy, it is not a cure but shows some promise in the areas of QoL, likely lowering cancer stem cell activity and in some cases creating synergy with other therapies. Although early in their evolution, viral therapies show promise in a well-rounded cancer approach that wishes to involve immunotherapy.

INSULIN POTENTIATION THERAPY

Insulin potentiation therapy (IPT) is a treatment that involves using insulin injections combined with low-dose chemotherapy agents. The theory is that insulin potentiates the effects of chemotherapy, allowing the use of much lower doses of chemotherapy. In this therapy, a patient with cancer is given 75 to 90 percent reduction of typical chemotherapy doses, thus reducing the risk for side effects. There are a limited number of doctors in the United States who offer IPT.

There have been two clinical studies published in peer-reviewed journals. The larger study utilized one controlled, randomized clinical trial, 30 women with metastatic breast cancer who did not respond to chemotherapy and hormone therapy were treated with IPT. Patients were divided into three groups of ten: one group received the anticancer drug methotrexate, another group received only insulin, and a third group received a combination of methotrexate and insulin. Researchers found that progressive disease was less frequent in the group receiving both treatments (IPT) and the median increase in tumor size was significantly lower in the IPT group.[31]

MIND-BODY

In some ways, it would seem everyone has a sense that the body and mind are interconnected and that connection can affect health and healing. In our experience, however, this can become an area of confusion or contention when misunderstandings arise. One example is reflected by a person asking, "So you are saying the cancer is all in my mind?" Another may be, "So I can think my cancer away?" And another may be, "I'm a scientist, and there is nothing in my health that my mind really has any control over!"

In the NIH-funded research Dr. Anderson was involved in, one part of the holistic integrative oncology model included a mind-body intervention. As part of the study design, every cancer patient had this intervention available, but not all availed themselves of it. In those who did work with the mind-body practitioners (physicians and counselors), we would see an interesting opening up of communication, often dealing with long-suppressed issues and hurts. End-of-life patients who worked closely with the mind-body practitioners often experienced mental and emotional healing and breakthroughs, which helped them become more peaceful for themselves and loved ones. Those who were still in the cancer journey would often experience the same breakthroughs, which helped a spectrum of issues. Improved pain management, energy, happiness, family relationships, and other factors were potentially affected.

Research has looked into two primary areas of benefit from mind-body approaches in cancer: quality of life (QoL) improvement and immune-based improvements likely improving cancer outcomes.

In the area of improved QoL, guidelines have been published integrating mind-body approaches and perspectives in the care of people who have cancer.[32] Studies have been completed, including mind-body interventions to reduce pain, anxiety, insomnia, hot flashes, anticipatory and treatment-related nauseas, and to improve mood. Mind-body treatments evaluated for their utility in oncology include relaxation therapies, biofeedback, meditation and hypnosis, yoga, art and music therapy, tai chi, and qigong.[33] In many studies mind-body techniques such as meditation, yoga, tai chi, and qigong have been found to lower distress and lead to improvements in different aspects of quality of life.[34] We have also had patients specifically ask about prayer as a mind-body modality. In fact, there are studies on this subject, and in one recent paper, prayer was found to improve both blood pressure and anxiety in those undergoing chemotherapy.[35] In our practices, we routinely see improved QoL in people who are mindful, involved in their own process, and proactive in seeking the mind-body help they need.

Another area of study is improvement in actual cancer outcomes beyond QoL. Interventions that provide emotional and social support and improve stress management at the end of life might have a positive impact on physiological stress-response systems that affect survival. The line connecting psychosocial factors to oncology can help to align better stress management and social support with enhanced resistance to tumor growth. Mind-body medicine is a discipline that helps cancer patients mobilize all their resources to live well with cancer.

In a wide review of publications on the topic, 8 of 15 published trials indicated that psychotherapy enhanced cancer survival time. No studies showed an adverse effect of psychotherapy on cancer survival. There is evidence from the trials reviewed that effective psychosocial support improves quantity as well as quality of life with cancer. There is evidence that chronic depression predicts poorer prognosis with cancer. Dysregulated circadian cortisol patterns predict more rapid cancer progression. Inflammatory processes affect cancer growth and progression. Sympathetic nervous system activity, telomere length, telomerase activity, and oncogene expression are affected by stress and can affect cancer growth.[36] One paper states, "We know that it is not simply mind over matter, but mind matters."[37]

PHOTODYNAMIC / LASER THERAPIES

Photodynamic therapies (PDT) and laser therapies (LT and LLLT) have been used in medicine for well over 100 years. They have enjoyed a resurgence in use and research due to advances in technology allowing more specific use and accurate testing. Both PDT and LT/LLLT have applications in direct tumor therapy and in therapy for side effects and QoL.

In the arena of therapy, PDT is increasingly being recognized as an attractive alternative treatment modality for superficial cancer.[38] Treatment consists of two relatively simple procedures: the administration of a photosensitive drug and illumination of the tumor to activate the drug. Efficacy is high for small superficial tumors and, except for temporary skin photosensitization, there are no long-term side effects if appropriate protocols are followed. Healing occurs with little or no scarring, and the procedure can be repeated without cumulative toxicity. Examples of well-studied cancers where PDT is used for treatment include non-melanoma skin cancer and Barrett's esophagus.[39]

PDT and LLLT are becoming known for improving QoL by lowering side effects such as inflammation in the mouth and throat (mucositis) during and after standard cancer therapies.[40 41 42]

In the arena of improving survival and outcome, a study suggests that LLLT may improve survival of head and neck cancer patients treated with chemo- and radiotherapy.[43] Additionally, the use of direct blood irradiation is making a resurgence in cancer care. In our clinical practices, we have seen these types of therapies improve QoL and life span. Publications are forthcoming regarding these therapies, and a textbook by Dr. Michael Weber[44] is available for a broad and in-depth review of the topic. The clinic, hospital, or physician you see will need both equipment and training to provide these services. In the setting of cancer care, phototherapies can be an incredible help.

PLASMAPHERESIS

Plasmapheresis is also categorized as therapeutic plasma exchange. In therapeutic plasma exchange, an automated centrifuge is used to discard filtered plasma and return red blood cells and replacement colloid, such as donor plasma or albumin, to the patient. In membrane plasma filtration, secondary membrane plasma fractionation can selectively remove undesired macromolecules, which then allows for the return of the processed plasma to the patient instead of donor plasma or albumin.

In the 1970s, immunosuppressive factors in the plasma of cancer-bearing patients were described. Plasmapheresis has been widely applied to many human malignant diseases for immunosuppressive factors being removed with new plasma separating methods. Plasmapheresis is known to improve the performance status or quality of life in advanced cancer patients.[45] In one study, plasmapheresis was used to remove cancer-promoting factors in 25 advanced cancer patients who did not respond to immune-chemotherapy. The improvement of subjective symptoms was seen in 60 percent of patients, and reduction of tumors was observed in

28 percent of the patients.[46] Other studies have shown similar mechanisms and results in critically ill people and those with cancer.[47] [48]

Plasmapheresis is not common in oncology settings outside Asian and European countries at this point. There are some centers offering it in North America, Mexico and South America as well. This therapy has a place in the treatment of people with cancer and should only increase both in research regarding its efficacy and availability for patients.

THE TAKEAWAY

In the fight against cancer and the need to support the person who has cancer to the fullest extent possible, there really should be no limit to the avenues used to effect such support. Some of these therapies are slowly gaining entry into the "mainstream" of oncology. Some are unlikely to gain such acceptance quickly. The bottom line is that if the physician can be trained to safely and effectively use these therapies, they will have more to offer the patient who has cancer. It is, in our experience, only when we can offer broad-based therapies in cancer care that we have the greatest positive outcomes possible in the most people who have cancer.

ENDNOTES

INTRODUCTION

1. "Cancer Stat Facts: Cancer of Any Site," Surveillance, Epidemiology, and End Results Program, National Cancer Institute, accessed November 13, 2016, http://seer.cancer.gov/statfacts/html/all.html.

2. "Cancer Facts & Figures 2016," American Cancer Society, accessed November 13, 2016, https://www.cancer.org/content/dam/cancer-org/research/cancer-facts-and-statistics/annual-cancer-facts-and-figures/2016/cancer-facts-and-figures-2016.pdf.

3. "Cancer Facts & Figures 2016," American Cancer Society.

4. "Cancer Facts & Figures 2016," American Cancer Society.

5. "Cancer Facts & Figures 2016," American Cancer Society.

6. "Survey: Bankruptcy Worries for One-Third of Cancer Patients," Medscape.com, accessed November 13, 2016, http://www.medscape.com/viewarticle/842718.

7. "Cancer Facts & Figures 2016," American Cancer Society.

8. "Cancer: In Depth," National Center for Complementary and Integrative Health, National Institutes of Health, last modified July 2014, accessed November 13, 2016, https://nccih.nih.gov/health/cancer/complementary-integrative-research.

9. Grace K Dy et al., "Complementary and alternative medicine use by patients enrolled onto phase I clinical trials," *Journal of Clinical Oncology*, 2004 Dec 1, 22(23):4810–5, https://doi.org/10.1200/JCO.2004.03.121.

10. Alex Sparreboom et al., "Herbal remedies in the United States: potential adverse interactions with anticancer agents," *Journal of Clinical Oncology*, 2004, 22(12):2489–2503, https://doi.org/10.1200/JCO.2004.08.182.

11. Sparreboom et al., "Herbal remedies in the United States."

12. Roxanne Nelson, "Can Integrative Oncology Extend Life in Advanced Disease?" last modified October 25, 2013, accessed November 14, 2016, http://www.medscape.com/viewarticle/813217.

CHAPTER 2

1. Vincent T DeVita, Jr.; Theodore S Lawrence; and Steven A Rosenberg, *DeVita, Hellman, and Rosenberg's Cancer: Principles & Practice of Oncology*, 10th ed. (Wolters Kluwer Health, 2016), 24.

2. KW Kinzler and B Vogelstein, "Lessons from hereditary colon cancer," *Cell*, 1996, 87:159–170, PMID: 8861899.

3. V Vinnitsky, "The development of a malignant tumor is due to a desperate asexual self-cloning process in which cancer stem cells develop the ability to mimic the genetic program of germline cells," *Intrinsically Disordered Proteins*, 2014,2(1), http://dx.doi.org/10.4161/idp.29997.

4. "The Stem Cell Theory of Cancer," Stanford Medicine, accessed November 5, 2017, https://med.stanford.edu/ludwigcenter/overview/theory.html.

5. AR Burleigh, "Of germ cells, trophoblasts, and cancer stem cells," *Integrative Cancer Therapies*, 2008 Dec, 7(4):276–81, https://doi.org/10.1177/1534735408326454.

6. CA Ross, "The trophoblast model of cancer," *Nutrition and Cancer*, 2015, 67(1):61–7, https://doi.org/10.1080/01635581.2014.956257.

7. Burleigh, "Of germ cells, trophoblasts, and cancer stem cells."

8. JP Medema, "Targeting the colorectal cancer stem cell," *New England Journal of Medicine*, 2017 Aug 31, 377(9):888–890, https://doi.org/10.1056/NEJMcibr1706541.

9. Otto Warburg, Franz Wind, and Erwin Negelein. "The metabolism of tumors in the body," *The Journal of General Physiology*, 1927, 8(6):519–530.

10. TN Seyfried et al., "Cancer as a metabolic disease: implications for novel therapeutics," *Carcinogenesis*, 2014, 35(3):515–527, https://doi.org/10.1093/carcin/bgt480.

11. DS Wishart, "Is cancer a genetic disease or a metabolic disease?" *EBioMedicine*, 2015, 2(6): 478–479, https://doi.org/10.1016/j.ebiom.2015.05.022.

12. TN Seyfried et al., "Press-pulse: a novel therapeutic strategy for the metabolic management of cancer," *Nutrition & Metabolism*, 2017, 14:19, https://doi.org/10.1186/s12986-017-0178-2.

13. BW Stewart and CP Wild, editors, "World cancer report 2014," Lyon: International Agency for Research on Cancer.

14. GBD 2015 Risk Factors Collaborators, "Global, regional, and national comparative

risk assessment of 79 behavioural, environmental and occupational, and metabolic risks or clusters of risks, 1990–2015: a systematic analysis for the Global Burden of Disease Study 2015," *The Lancet*, 2016 Oct, 388 (10053):1659–1724, https://doi.org/10.1016/S0140-6736(16)31679-8.

15. M Plummer et al., "Global burden of cancers attributable to infections in 2012: a synthetic analysis," *Lancet Global Health*, 2016 Sep, 4(9):e609–16, https://doi.org/10.1016/S2214-109X(16)30143-7.

16. "Risk Factors for Cancer," National Cancer Institute, accessed November 5, 2017, https://www.cancer.gov/about-cancer/causes-prevention/risk.

17. J Ferlay et al., "GLOBOCAN 2012 v1.0, Cancer Incidence and Mortality Worldwide: IARC Cancer," Base No. 11, Lyon, France: International Agency for Research on Cancer, 2013.

18. Stewart and Wild, "World cancer report 2014."

CHAPTER 3

1. "Understanding Cancer Prognosis," National Cancer Institute, National Institutes of Health, accessed June 25, 2017, https://www.cancer.gov/about-cancer/diagnosis-staging/prognosis.

2. "Understanding Cancer Prognosis," National Cancer Institute.

3. "NCI Dictionary of Cancer Terms," National Cancer Institute, National Institutes of Health, accessed June 25, 2017, https://www.cancer.gov/publications/dictionaries/cancer-terms?cdrid=45849.

4. "Understanding Cancer Prognosis," National Cancer Institute, National Institutes of Health, accessed June 25, 2017, https://www.cancer.gov/about-cancer/diagnosis-staging/prognosis.

5. "Understanding Cancer Prognosis," National Cancer Institute.

6. JH Rowland and A O'Mara, "Survivorship care planning: unique opportunity to champion integrative oncology?" *Journal of the National Cancer Institute Monographs*, 2014, (50):285, https://doi.org/10.1093/jncimonographs/lgu037.

7. K Bell and S Ristovski-Slijepcevic, "Cancer survivorship: why labels matter," *Journal of Clinical Oncology*, 2013 Feb, 31(4): 409–11, http://ascopubs.org/doi/full/10.1200/jco.2012.43.5891.

8. Susan Leigh, "Cancer Survivorship: A Nursing Perspective," accessed July 16, 2017, http://eknygos.lsmuni.lt/springer/566/8-13.pdf.

9. LL Wu et al., "Urinary 8-OHdG: a marker of oxidative stress to DNA and a risk factor for cancer, atherosclerosis and diabetics," *Clinica Chimica Acta*, 2004 Jan, 339(1–2):1–9.

10. JT Thornthwaite, "Anti-malignin antibody in serum and other tumor marker

determinations in breast cancer," *Cancer Letters*, 2000 Jan 1, 148(1):39–48. PMID: 10680591.

11. SM Harman et al., "Discrimination of breast cancer by anti-malignin antibody serum test in women undergoing biopsy," *Cancer Epidemiology Biomarkers & Prevention*, 2005 Oct, 14(10):2310–5. PMID: 16214910.

12. RD Blumenthal, "An overview of chemosensitivity testing," *Methods in Molecular Medicine*, 2005, 110:3–18.

13. RD Blumenthal and DM Goldenberg, "Methods and goals for the use of in vitro and in vivo chemosensitivity testing," *Molecular Biotechnology*, 2007 Feb, 35(2):185–97.

14. Publications relating to CTCs and ctDNA may be found at https://biocept.com/technology/publications.

15. MG Krebs et al., "Circulating tumour cells: their utility in cancer management and predicting outcomes," *Therapeutic Advances in Medical Oncology*. 2010 Nov, 2(6): 351–365, https://doi.org/10.1177/1758834010378414. PMCID:3126032.

16. LA Cole, "HCG variants, the growth factors which drive human malignancies," *American Journal of Cancer Research*, 2012, 2(1):22–35.

17. X Sun and X Liu, "Cancer metastasis: enactment of the script for human reproductive drama," *Cancer Cell International*, 2017, 17:51.

18. N Yamamoto et al., "Immunotherapy for prostate cancer with Gc protein-derived macrophage activating factor (GcMAF)," *Translational Oncology*, 2008, 1:65–72.

19. M Korbelik et al., "The value of serum alpha-N-acetylgalactosaminidase measurement for the assessment of tumour response to radio- and photodynamic therapy," *British Journal of Cancer*, 1998, 77:1009-1014.

20. AL Reddi et al., "Serum alpha-N-acetylgalactosaminidase is associated with diagnosis/prognosis of patients with squamous cell carcinoma of the uterine cervix," *Cancer Letters*, 2000, 158:61–64.

21. N Yamamoto et al., "Deglycosylation of serum vitamin D3-binding protein leads to immunosuppression in cancer patients," *Cancer Research*, 1996 June 15, 56(12):2827–2831. PMID: 8665521.

22. H Ikushima and K Miyazono, "TGFβ signalling: a complex web in cancer progression," *Nature Reviews Cancer*, 2010 Jun, 10(6):415–24, https://doi.org/10.1038/nrc2853.

23. J Foekens et al., "Thymidine kinase and thymidylate synthase in advanced breast cancer: response to tamoxifen and chemotherapy," *Cancer Research*, 2001 Feb 2, 61(4):1421–1425.

24. M Gulaboglu et al., "Blood and urine iodine levels in patients with gastric cancer," *Biological Trace Element Research*, 2006 Dec, 113(3):261–71, PMID: 17194926.

25. JF Håkonsen Arendt et al., "Elevated plasma vitamin B12 levels and cancer prognosis: A population-based cohort study," *Cancer Epidemiology*, 40:158–165, http://dx.doi.org/10.1016/j.canep.2015.12.007.

26. JFB Arendt et al., "Elevated plasma vitamin B12 levels as a marker for cancer: a population-based cohort study," *Journal of the National Cancer Institute*, 2013 Dec 4, 105(23):1799–805, https://doi.org/10.1093/jnci/djt315.

27. DeVita, Lawrence, and Rosenberg, *Cancer: Principles & Practice*, 24.

28. "Definition of Naturopathic Medicine," The American Association of Naturopathic Physicians, accessed June 25, 2017, http://www.naturopathic.org/content. asp?contentid=59.

29. Rowland and O'Mara, "Survivorship Care Planning."

30. Staff, National Cancer Institute. Accessed July 16, 2017, https://cancercontrol.cancer. gov/ocs/about/bio_rowland.html.

31. Rowland and O'Mara, "Survivorship Care Planning."

32. SJ Sohl et al., "Characteristics associated with the use of complementary health approaches among long-term cancer survivors," *Supportive Care in Cancer*, 2013 Nov 22, 22(4):927–936, https://doi.org/10.1007/s00520-013-2040-z.

33. SC Bischoff et al., "Intestinal permeability—a new target for disease prevention and therapy," *BMC Gastroenterology*, 2014, 14:189, https://doi.org/10.1186/ s12876-014-0189-7.

34. Bischoff et al., "Intestinal permeability."

35. Bischoff et al., "Intestinal permeability."

36. Bischoff et al., "Intestinal permeability."

37. C Resnick, "Nutritional Protocol for the Treatment of Intestinal Permeability Defects and Related Conditions," *Natural Medicine Journal*, 2010 March, 2(3), http://www.naturalmedicinejournal.com/journal/2010-03/ nutritional-protocol-treatment-intestinal-permeability-defects-and-related.

38. Bischoff et al., "Intestinal permeability."

39. C Resnick, "Nutritional Protocol for the Treatment of Intestinal Permeability Defects."

40. Suzanne Reuben, "2009–2009 Annual Report President's Cancer Panel. Reducing Environmental Cancer Risk," National Cancer Institute, National Institutes of Health, U.S. Department of Health and Human Services, accessed October 24, 2017, https://deainfo.nci.nih.gov/advisory/pcp/annualReports/pcp08-09rpt/PCP_ Report_08-09_508.pdf.

41. Markham Heid, "How stress affects cancer risk," The University of Texas MD Anderson Cancer Center, accessed July 18, 2017, https://www.mdanderson.org/ publications/focused-on-health/december-2014/how-stress-affects-cancer-risk.html. html.

42. Y Chida et al., "Do stress-related psychosocial factors contribute to cancer incidence and survival?" *Nature Reviews Clinical Oncology*, 2008 Aug, 5:466–475, https://doi. org/10.1038/ncponc1134.

43. Brian Lawenda, "Stress and Cancer 101: Why Stress Reduction Is Essential," *Integrative Oncology Essentials*, accessed July 18, 2017, https://integrativeoncology -essentials.com/2012/04/anticancer-lifestyle-stress-reduction-101.

44. Vicki A Jackson and David P Ryan, with Michelle Seaton, *Living with Cancer* (Baltimore, MD: Johns Hopkins University Press, 2017), 101–104.

45. "Tips for reducing stress," Cancer.net, accessed July 18, 2017, http://www.cancer.net/ coping-with-cancer/managing-emotions/managing-stress.

46. BL Andersen et al., "Biobehavioral, immune, and health benefits following recurrence for psychological intervention participants," *Clinical Cancer Research*, 2010, 16(12):3270–3278, https://doi.org/10.1158/1078-0432.CCR-10-0278.

47. LK Sprod et al., "Three versus six months of exercise training in breast cancer survivors," *Breast Cancer Research and Treatment*, 2010 Jun, 121(2):413–9, https://doi. org/10.1007/s10549-010-0913-0.

48. J Hamer and E Warner, "Lifestyle modifications for patients with breast cancer to improve prognosis and optimize overall health," *Canadian Medical Association Journal*, 2017 Feb 21, 189(7), https://doi.org/10.1503/cmaj.160464.

49. Hamer and Warner, "Lifestyle modifications for patients with breast cancer."

50. Hamer and Warner, "Lifestyle modifications for patients with breast cancer."

51. SA Kenfield et al, "Physical activity and survival after prostate cancer diagnosis in the health professionals follow-up study," *Journal of Clinical Oncology*, 2011 Feb, 29(6): 726–732, https://doi.org/10.1200/JCO.2010.31.5226.

52. EL Richman et al, "Physical activity after diagnosis and risk of prostate cancer progression: Data from the Cancer of the Prostate Strategic Urologic Research Endeavor," *Cancer Research*, 2011 June, 71(11): 3889–3895, https://doi. org/10.1158/0008-5472.CAN-10-3932.

53. K Chandrasekhar et al., "A prospective, randomized double-blind, placebo-controlled study of safety and efficacy of a high-concentration full-spectrum extract of ashwagandha root in reducing stress in adults," *Indian Journal of Psychological Medicine*, 2012 Jul, 34(3):255–62, https://doi.org/10.4103/0253-7176.106022.

54. DL Barton et al., "Wisconsin Ginseng (Panax quinquefolius) to improve cancer-related fatigue: a randomized, double-blind trial, N07C2," *Journal of the National Cancer Institute*, 2013, 105(16):1230–1238, https://doi.org/10.1093/jnci/djt181.

55. JP Medema, "Targeting the colorectal cancer stem cell," *New England Journal of Medicine*, 2017, 377(9):888–890, https://doi.org/10.1056/NEJMcibr1706541.

CHAPTER 4

1. DeVita, Lawrence, and Rosenberg, *Cancer: Principles & Practice*, 142.

2. DeVita, Lawrence, and Rosenberg, *Cancer: Principles & Practice*, 142.

3. "Radiation Therapy," National Cancer Institute, accessed July 2, 2017, https://www.cancer.gov/about-cancer/treatment/types/radiation-therapy.

4. K Eda et al., "The effects of enteral glutamine on radiotherapy induced dermatitis in breast cancer," *Clinical Nutrition*, 2016 Apr, 35(2):436–9, https://doi.org/10.1016/j.clnu.2015.03.009.

5. V DeVita, Jr., and E Chu, "A history of cancer chemotherapy," *Cancer Research*, 2008 Nov 1, 68:21, https://doi.org/10.1158/0008-5472.CAN-07-6611.

6. DeVita and Chu, "A history of cancer chemotherapy."

7. DeVita and Chu, "A history of cancer chemotherapy."

8. DeVita and Chu, "A history of cancer chemotherapy."

9. DeVita and Chu, "A history of cancer chemotherapy."

10. "Chemotherapy," National Cancer Institute, accessed July 2, 2017, https://www.cancer.gov/about-cancer/treatment/types/chemotherapy.

11. DeVita, Lawrence, and Rosenberg, *Cancer: Principles & Practice*, 189.

12. "Chemotherapy: How Chemotherapy Drugs Work," American Cancer Society, accessed July 2, 2017, https://www.cancer.org/treatment/treatments-and-side-effects/treatment-types/chemotherapy/how-chemotherapy-drugs-work.html.

13. "Alkylating agents," Drugs.com, accessed July 2, 2017, https://www.drugs.com/drug-class/alkylating-agents.html.

14. "Chemotherapy: How Chemotherapy Drugs Work," American Cancer Society.

15. DeVita, Lawrence, and Rosenberg, *Cancer: Principles & Practice*, 195.

16. "Types of Chemotherapy," Chemocare, accessed October 29, 2017, http://chemocare.com/chemotherapy/what-is-chemotherapy/types-of-chemotherapy.aspx.

17. DeVita, Lawrence, and Rosenberg, *Cancer: Principles & Practice*, 189–193.

18. TC Johnstone et al., "Understanding and improving platinum anticancer drugs–phenanthriplatin." *Anticancer Research*, 2014, 34(1):471–476, PMID: 24403503, PMCID: PMC3937549.

19. JE Buckley et al., "Hypomagnesemia after cisplatin combination chemotherapy," *Archives of Internal Medicine*, 1984 Dec, 144(12):2347–8, https://doi.org/10.1001/archinte.1984.00350220063013.

20. E Hodgkinson et al., "Magnesium depletion in patients receiving cisplatin-based chemotherapy," *Clinical Oncology (Royal College of Radiologists (Great Britain))*, 2006 Nov, 18(9):710–8, PMID: 17100159.

21. RA Murphy et al., "Supplementation with fish oil increases first-line chemotherapy efficacy in patients with advanced nonsmall cell lung cancer," *Cancer*, 2011 Aug 15, 117(16):3774–80, https://doi.org/10.1002/cncr.25933.

22. "Chemotherapy: How Chemotherapy Drugs Work," American Cancer Society.

23. "Methotrexate Side Effects," Drugs.com, accessed July 2, 2017, https://www.drugs.com/sfx/methotrexate-side-effects.html.

24. "Types of Chemotherapy," Chemocare.

25. Y Panahi et al., "Adjuvant therapy with bioavailability-boosted curcuminoids suppresses systemic inflammation and improves quality of life in patients with solid tumors: a randomized double-blind placebo-controlled trial," *Phytotherapy Research*, 2014 Oct, 28(10):1461–7, https://doi.org/10.1002/ptr.5149.

26. DeVita, Lawrence, and Rosenberg, *Cancer: Principles & Practice*, 223.

27. DeVita, Lawrence, and Rosenberg, *Cancer: Principles & Practice*, 226.

28. "Mitomycin," Drugs.com, accessed July 2, 2017, https://www.drugs.com/sfx/mitomycin-side-effects.html.

29. "Chemotherapy: How Chemotherapy Drugs Work," American Cancer Society.

30. "Chemotherapy: How Chemotherapy Drugs Work," American Cancer Society.

31. DeVita, Lawrence, and Rosenberg, *Cancer: Principles & Practice*, 218.

32. "Chemotherapy: How Chemotherapy Drugs Work," American Cancer Society.

33. "Irinotecan," Drugs.com, accessed July 2, 2017, https://www.drugs.com/mtm/irinotecan.html.

34. "Etopside," Drugs.com, accessed July 2, 2017, https://www.drugs.com/mtm/etoposide.html.

35. "Mitoxantrone," Drugs.com, accessed July 2, 2017, https://www.drugs.com/mtm/mitoxantrone.html.

36. "Types of Chemotherapy," Chemocare.

37. "Chemotherapy: How Chemotherapy Drugs Work," American Cancer Society.

38. YM Wang et al., "The efficacy and safety of melatonin in concurrent chemotherapy or radiotherapy for solid tumors."

39. DeVita, Lawrence, and Rosenberg, *Cancer: Principles & Practice*, 228.

40. DeVita, Lawrence, and Rosenberg, *Cancer: Principles & Practice*, 228.

41. DeVita, Lawrence, and Rosenberg, *Cancer: Principles & Practice*, 230.

42. DeVita, Lawrence, and Rosenberg, *Cancer: Principles & Practice*, 232.

43. DeVita, Lawrence, and Rosenberg, *Cancer: Principles & Practice*, 232.

44. DeVita, Lawrence, and Rosenberg, *Cancer: Principles & Practice*, 232.

45. DeVita, Lawrence, and Rosenberg, *Cancer: Principles & Practice*, 232.

46. DeVita, Lawrence, and Rosenberg, *Cancer: Principles & Practice*, 233.

47. DeVita, Lawrence, and Rosenberg, *Cancer: Principles & Practice*, 234.

48. Y Sun et al., "A prospective study to evaluate the efficacy and safety of oral acetyl-L-carnitine for the treatment of chemotherapy-induced peripheral neuropathy," *Experimental and Therapeutic Medicine*, 2016, 12(6):4017–4024, https://doi.org/10.3892/etm.2016.3871.

49. Kris Novak, "Conference Report-Protein Kinase Inhibitors in Cancer Treatment: Mixing and Matching?" Medscape.com, accessed July 6, 2017, https://www.medscape.com/viewarticle/471462_7.

50. "Kinase Inhibitors," CHemoth.com, accessed July 6, 2017, http://chemoth.com/types/kinaseinhibitors.

51. DeVita, Lawrence, and Rosenberg, *Cancer: Principles & Practice*, 237.

52. DeVita, Lawrence, and Rosenberg, *Cancer: Principles & Practice*, 237.

53. "Tyrosine Kinase Inhibitors (TKIs)," Michigan Medicine, University of Michigan, accessed July 6, 2017, http://www.uofmhealth.org/health-library/tv7950.

54. "Tyrosine Kinase Inhibitors (TKIs)," Michigan Medicine.

55. "Tyrosine Kinase Inhibitors (TKIs)," Michigan Medicine.

56. E Ceccacci and S Minucci, "Inhibition of histone deacetylases in cancer therapy: lessons from leukaemia," *British Journal of Cancer*, 2016 Mar 15, 114(6):605–611, https://doi.org/10.1038/bjc.2016.36.

57. Stephanie Liou, "Histones and HDAC Inhibitors," HOPES: Huntington's Outreach Project for Education, Stanford, accessed July 7, 2017, https://web.stanford.edu/group/hopes/cgi-bin/hopes_test/hdac-inhibitors/#histones-and-dna.

58. "Histone deacetylase inhibitors," Drugs.com, accessed July 7, 2017, https://www.drugs.com/drug-class/histone-deacetylase-inhibitors.html.

59. "Azacitidine," Drugs.com, accessed July 7, 2017, https://www.drugs.com/cdi/azacitidine.html.

60. "Decitabine," Drugs.com, accessed July 7, 2017, https://www.drugs.com/mtm/decitabine.html.

61. "Azacitidine," Drugs.com.

62. "Decitabine," Drugs.com.

63. "PARP Inhibitor," National Cancer Institute, accessed July 7, 2017, https://www.cancer.gov/publications/dictionaries/cancer-terms?cdrid=660869.

64. "What Is Targeted Cancer Therapy?" American Cancer Society, accessed July 7, 2017, https://www.cancer.org/treatment/treatments-and-side-effects/treatment-types/targeted-therapy/what-is.html.

65. "Olaparib," Drugs.com, accessed July 7, 2017, https://www.drugs.com/mtm/olaparib.html.

66. "Niraparib," Drugs.com, accessed July 7, 2017, https://www.drugs.com/mtm/niraparib.html.

67. "Olaparib," Drugs.com.

68. "Niraparib," Drugs.com.

69. DeVita, Lawrence, and Rosenberg, *Cancer: Principles & Practice*, 271–275.

70. Roxane Nelson, "Nurses Poorly Protected from 'Second-Hand Exposure' to Chemo," Medscape, accessed May 30, 2017, http://www.medscape.com/viewarticle/879449#vp_1.

71. CR Friese et al., "Structures and processes of care in ambulatory oncology settings and nurse-reported exposure to chemotherapy," *BMJ Quality & Safety*, 2012, 21(9):753–759, https://doi.org/10.1136/bmjqs-2011-000178.

72. "Hormone Therapy," Chemocare.com, accessed July 7, 2017, http://chemocare.com/chemotherapy/what-is-chemotherapy/hormone-therapy.aspx.

73. DeVita, Lawrence, and Rosenberg, *Cancer: Principles & Practice*, 278.

74. "Types of Hormone Therapy," Stanford Health Care, accessed July 7, 2017, https://stanfordhealthcare.org/medical-treatments/h/hormone-therapy/types.html.

75. L Santacroce et al., "Paraneoplastic Syndromes," Medscape.com, accessed July 7, 2017, http://emedicine.medscape.com/article/280744-overview.

76. DeVita, Lawrence, and Rosenberg, *Cancer: Principles & Practice*, 278.

77. "Selective Estrogen Receptor Modulators (SERMs)," BreastCancer.org, accessed July 7, 2017, http://www.breastcancer.org/treatment/hormonal/serms.

78. DeVita, Lawrence, and Rosenberg, *Cancer: Principles & Practice*, 278.

79. DeVita, Lawrence, and Rosenberg, *Cancer: Principles & Practice*, 278.

80. "Selective Estrogen Receptor Modulators (SERMs)," BreastCancer.org.

81. "Aromatase Inhibitors," BreastCancer.org, accessed July 7, 2017, http://www.breastcancer.org/treatment/hormonal/aromatase_inhibitors.

82. Carolyn Vachani, "Hormone Therapy: The Basics," OncoLink, accessed July 7, 2017, https://www.oncolink.org/cancer-treatment/hormone-therapy/hormone-therapy-the-basics.

83. DeVita, Lawrence, and Rosenberg, *Cancer: Principles & Practice*, 283.

84. DeVita, Lawrence, and Rosenberg, *Cancer: Principles & Practice*, 283.

85. DeVita, Lawrence, and Rosenberg, *Cancer: Principles & Practice*, 282.

86. DeVita, Lawrence, and Rosenberg, *Cancer: Principles & Practice*, 282.

87. "Fulvestrant," National Cancer Institute, accessed July 7, 2017, https://www.cancer.gov/about-cancer/treatment/drugs/fulvestrant.

88. "Faslodex, BreastCancer.org, accessed July 7, 2017, http://www.breastcancer.org/treatment/hormonal/erds/faslodex.

89. Vachani, "Hormone Therapy: The Basics."

90. "Zoladex," Zoldex.com, accessed July 7, 2017, https://www.zoladex.com/prostate-cancer.html.

91. "Zoladex," Zoldex.com.

92. "Goserelin Acetate for Men," OncoLink, accessed July 8, 2017, https://www.oncolink.org/cancer-treatment/chemotherapy/oncolink-rx/goserelin-acetate-zoladex-r-for-men.

93. "Leuprolide Acetate for Men," OncoLink, accessed July 8, 2017, https://www.oncolink.org/cancer-treatment/chemotherapy/oncolink-rx/leuprolide-acetate-lupron-r-lupron-depot-r-eligard-r-prostap-r-viadur-r-for-men.

94. "Goserelin Acetate for Women," OncoLink, accessed July 8, 2017, https://www.oncolink.org/cancer-treatment/chemotherapy/oncolink-rx/goserelin-acetate-zoladex-r-for-women.

95. "Leuprolide Acetate for Women," OncoLink, accessed July 8, 2017, https://www.oncolink.org/cancer-treatment/chemotherapy/oncolink-rx/leuprolide-acetate-lupron-r-lupron-depot-r-eligard-r-prostap-r-viadur-r-for-women.

96. "Degarelix," OncoLink, accessed July 8, 2017, https://www.oncolink.org/cancer-treatment/chemotherapy/oncolink-rx/degarelix-firmagon-r.

97. "Hormone Therapy for Prostate Cancer," American Cancer Society, accessed July 8, 2017, https://www.cancer.org/cancer/prostate-cancer/treating/hormone-therapy.html.

98. "Degarelix," OncoLink.

99. Vachani, "Hormone Therapy: The Basics."

100. Vachani, "Hormone Therapy: The Basics."

101. "Hormone Therapy for Prostate Cancer," American Cancer Society.

102. "Casodex Side Effects," Drugs.com, accessed July 9, 2017, https://www.drugs.com/sfx/casodex-side-effects.html.

103. "Eulexin Side Effects," Drugs.com, accessed July 9, 2017, https://www.drugs.com/sfx/eulexin-side-effects.html.

104. DeVita, Lawrence, and Rosenberg, *Cancer: Principles & Practice*, 286.

105. "Hormone Therapy for Prostate Cancer," American Cancer Society.

106. "Hormone Therapy for Prostate Cancer," American Cancer Society.

107. "Zytiga Side Effects," Drugs.com, accessed July 9, 2017, https://www.drugs.com/sfx/zytiga-side-effects.html.

108. "Mechanism of Action," Xtandihcp.com, accessed July 9, 2017, https://www.xtandihcp.com/mechanism-of-action.

109. "Xtandi," Drugs.com, accessed July 9, 2017, https://www.drugs.com/xtandi.html.

110. DeVita, Lawrence, and Rosenberg, *Cancer: Principles & Practice*, 286.

111. RM Griffin, "Hormone Treatment Fights Prostate Cancer," WebMD, accessed July 8, 2017, http://www.webmd.com/prostate-cancer/features/hormone-therapy-for-prostate-cancer#2.

112. DeVita, Lawrence, and Rosenberg, *Cancer: Principles & Practice*, 286–287.

113. DeVita, Lawrence, and Rosenberg, *Cancer: Principles & Practice*, 287.

114. DeVita, Lawrence, and Rosenberg, *Cancer: Principles & Practice*, 287.

115. DeVita, Lawrence, and Rosenberg, *Cancer: Principles & Practice*, 287.

116. "Megestrol," Drugs.com, accessed July 9, 2017, https://www.drugs.com/mtm/megestrol.html.

117. "Hormone Therapy for Prostate Cancer," American Cancer Society.

118. "Nizoral," Rxlist.com, accessed July 9, 2017, http://www.rxlist.com/nizoral-side-effects-drug-center.htm.

119. "Octreotide," Chemocare.com, accessed July 9, 2017, http://chemocare.com/chemotherapy/drug-info/Octreotide.aspx.

120. DeVita, Lawrence, and Rosenberg, *Cancer: Principles & Practice*, 288.

121. "Evolution of Cancer Treatments: Targeted Therapy," American Cancer Society, accessed July 9, 2017, https://www.cancer.org/cancer/cancer-basics/history-of-cancer/cancer-treatment-targeted-therapy.html.

122. "Angiogenesis inhibitors," National Cancer Institute, accessed July 9, 2017, https://www.cancer.gov/about-cancer/treatment/types/immunotherapy/angiogenesis-inhibitors-fact-sheet.

123. "Angiogenesis inhibitors," National Cancer Institute.

124. "Angiogenesis and Angiogenesis Inhibitors to Treat Cancer," Cancer.net, accessed July 9, 2017, http://www.cancer.net/navigating-cancer-care/how-cancer-treated/personalized-and-targeted-therapies/angiogenesis-and-angiogenesis-inhibitors-treat-cancer.

125. "Immunotherapy," National Cancer Institute, accessed July 9, 2017, https://www.cancer.gov/about-cancer/treatment/types/immunotherapy.

126. "Immunotherapy," National Cancer Institute.

127. DeVita, Lawrence, and Rosenberg, *Cancer: Principles & Practice*, 300.

128. "Monoclonal antibody drugs for cancer: How they work," Mayo Clinic, accessed July 9, 2017, http://www.mayoclinic.org/diseases-conditions/cancer/in-depth/monoclonal-antibody/art-20047808.

129. "Monoclonal antibodies to treat cancer," American Cancer Society, accessed July 9, 2017, https://www.cancer.org/treatment/treatments-and-side-effects/treatment-types/immunotherapy/monoclonal-antibodies.html.

130. "Monoclonal antibodies to treat cancer," American Cancer Society.

131. "Monoclonal antibodies to treat cancer," American Cancer Society.

132. "Monoclonal antibodies to treat cancer," American Cancer Society.

133. "Immunotherapy," National Cancer Institute.

134. "Immunotherapy," National Cancer Institute.

135. SA Rosenberg and NP Restifo, "Adoptive cell transfer as personalized immunotherapy for human cancer," *Science*, 2015 Apr 3, 348(6230):62–68, http://science.sciencemag.org/content/348/6230/62.full.

136. "Immunotherapy," National Cancer Institute.

137. S-K Tey, "Adoptive T-cell therapy: adverse events and safety switches," *Clinical & Translational Immunology*, 2014 Jun, 3(6): e17, https://doi.org/10.1038/cti.2014.11.

138. "Immunotherapy," National Cancer Institute.

139. "Immunotherapy," National Cancer Institute.

140. J Weber, "Cytokines and Cancer Therapy," Meds.com, accessed July 9, 2017, http://www.meds.com/immunotherapy/cytokines.html.

141. "Immunotherapy for Kidney Cancer," American Cancer Society, accessed July 9, 2017, https://www.cancer.org/cancer/kidney-cancer/treating/immunotherapy.html.

142. "Immunotherapy for Kidney Cancer," American Cancer Society.

143. "Biological Therapies for Cancer," National Cancer Institute, accessed July 9, 2017, https://www.cancer.gov/about-cancer/treatment/types/immunotherapy/bio-therapies-fact-sheet.

144. "Biological Therapies for Cancer," National Cancer Institute.

145. "Biological Therapies for Cancer," National Cancer Institute.

146. "Sipuleucel-T," Drugs.com, accessed July 9, 2017, https://www.drugs.com/mtm/sipuleucel-t.html.

147. "Sipuleucel-T," Drugs.com.

148. "Sipuleucel-T," Drugs.com.

149. "Bacillus Calmette-Guerin (BCG) Vaccine," MedlinePlus, accessed July 10, 2017, https://medlineplus.gov/druginfo/meds/a682809.html.

150. GD Steinberg et al., "Bacillus Calmette-Guérin Immunotherapy for Bladder Cancer Overview of BCG Immunotherapy," Medscape.com, accessed July 10, 2017, http://emedicine.medscape.com/article/1950803-overview?.

151. GD Steinberg et al., "Bacillus Calmette-Guérin Immunotherapy for Bladder Cancer."

152. GD Steinberg et al., "Bacillus Calmette-Guérin Immunotherapy for Bladder Cancer."

153. GD Steinberg et al., "Bacillus Calmette-Guérin Immunotherapy for Bladder Cancer."

154. "Non-specific cancer immunotherapies and adjuvants," American Cancer Society, accessed July 10, 2017, https://www.cancer.org/treatment/treatments-and-side-effects/treatment-types/immunotherapy/nonspecific-immunotherapies.html.

155. "Imiquimod," Medscape.com, accessed July 10, 2017, http://reference.medscape.com/drug/aldara-zyclara-imiquimod-343508.

156. "Imiquimod," Medscape.com.

157. "Aldara," Drugs.com, accessed July 10, 2017, https://www.drugs.com/aldara.html.

158. "Photodynamic Therapy," American Cancer Society, accessed July 14, 2017, https://www.cancer.org/treatment/treatments-and-side-effects/treatment-types/photodynamic-therapy.html.

159. "Photodynamic Therapy," American Cancer Society.

160. "Photodynamic Therapy," American Cancer Society.

161. GW Cole, "Photodynamic Therapy," Medicinenet.com, accessed July 14, 2017, http://www.medicinenet.com/photodynamic_therapy/article.htm.

162. "Photodynamic Therapy," American Cancer Society.

163. "Photodynamic Therapy," American Cancer Society.

164. GW Cole, "Photodynamic Therapy."

165. GW Cole, "Photodynamic Therapy."

166. "Photodynamic Therapy," American Cancer Society.

167. GW Cole, "Photodynamic Therapy."

168. "Lasers in Cancer Treatment," American Cancer Society, accessed July 14, 2017, https://www.cancer.org/treatment/treatments-and-side-effects/treatment-types/lasers-in-cancer-treatment.html.

169. "Lasers in Cancer Treatment," American Cancer Society.

170. "Lasers in Cancer Treatment," National Cancer Institute, accessed July 14, 2017, https://www.cancer.gov/about-cancer/treatment/types/surgery/lasers-fact-sheet.

171. "Lasers in Cancer Treatment," American Cancer Society.

172. "Lasers in Cancer Treatment," National Cancer Institute.

173. "Lasers in Cancer Treatment," National Cancer Institute.

174. "Lasers in Cancer Treatment," National Cancer Institute.

175. "Lasers in Cancer Treatment," American Cancer Society.

176. "Lasers in Cancer Treatment," American Cancer Society.

177. "Lasers in Cancer Treatment," American Cancer Society.

178. "Lasers in Cancer Treatment," National Cancer Institute.

179. "Stem Cell Transplant," National Cancer Institute, accessed July 14, 2017, https://www.cancer.gov/about-cancer/treatment/types/stem-cell-transplant.

180. "Why Are Stem Cell Transplants Used as Cancer Treatment?" American Cancer Society, accessed July 14, 2017, https://www.cancer.org/treatment/treatments-and-side-effects/treatment-types/stem-cell-transplant/why-stem-cell-transplants-are-used.html.

181. "Why Are Stem Cell Transplants Used as Cancer Treatment?" American Cancer Society.

182. "Why Are Stem Cell Transplants Used as Cancer Treatment?" American Cancer Society.

183. "Why Are Stem Cell Transplants Used as Cancer Treatment?" American Cancer Society.

184. "Why Are Stem Cell Transplants Used as Cancer Treatment?" American Cancer Society.

185. "Why Are Stem Cell Transplants Used as Cancer Treatment?" American Cancer Society.

186. "Why Are Stem Cell Transplants Used as Cancer Treatment?" American Cancer Society.

187. "Why Are Stem Cell Transplants Used as Cancer Treatment?" American Cancer Society.

188. "Why Are Stem Cell Transplants Used as Cancer Treatment?" American Cancer Society.

CHAPTER 5

1. M Maurizio et al, "Prevalence of malnutrition in patients at first medical oncology visit: the PreMiO study,"*Oncotarget*, 2017, 8(45): 79884–79896, https://doi.org/10.18632/oncotarget.20168.

2. Patrick Quillin, *Beating Cancer with Nutrition* (Nutrition Times Press, Inc., 2005), 95.

3. G Supic et al., "Epigenetics: a new link between nutrition and cancer," *Nutrition and Cancer*, 2013, 65(6):781–92, https://doi.org/10.1080/01635581.2013.805794.

4. TO Tollefsbol, "Dietary epigenetics in cancer and aging," *Cancer Treatment and Research*, 2014; 159:257–67, https://doi.org/10.1007/978-3-642-38007-5_15.

5. TO Tollefsbol, "Dietary epigenetics in cancer and aging."

6. Dean Ornish et al., "Intensive lifestyle changes may affect the progression of prostate cancer," *The Journal of Urology*, 2005, 174(3):1065–1070, http://dx.doi.org/10.1097/01. ju.0000169487.49018.73.

7. John Pierce et al., "Greater Survival after breast cancer in physically active women with high vegetable-fruit intake regardless of obesity," *Journal of Clinical Oncology*, 2007, 25(17):2345–2351, https://doi.org/10.1200/JCO.2006.08.6819.

8. J LaMantia and N Berinstein, *The Essential Cancer Treatment Nutrition Guide & Cookbook* (Toronto: Robert Rose Inc, 2012), 11.

9. "The Expert Reports," American Institute for Cancer Research, accessed September 16, 2017, http://www.aicr.org/research/research_science_expert_report.html.

10. "Continuous Update Project: findings & reports," World Cancer Research Fund International, accessed September 16, 2017, http://www.wcrf.org/int/ research-we-fund/continuous-update-project-findings-reports.

11. "Cancer Prevention & Survival. Summary of global evidence on diet, weight, physical activity & what increases or decreases your risk of cancer. September 2017 edition," World Cancer Research Fund International, accessed September 16, 2017, http://www.wcrf.org/sites/default/files/CUP_Summary_Report_Sept17.pdf.

12. "Summary of global evidence on cancer prevention," World Cancer Research Fund International, accessed September 16, 2017, http://www. wcrf.org/int/research-we-fund/continuous-update-project-findings-reports/ summary-global-evidence-cancer.

13. "WCRF/AICR Systematic Literature Review Continuous Update Project Report: The Associations between Food, Nutrition, and Physical Activity and the Risk of Ovarian Cancer," World Cancer Research Fund International, accessed Decemeber 8, 2017, http://www.wcrf.org/sites/default/files/Ovarian-Cancer-SLR-2013.pdf.

14. E Riboli and T Norat, "Epidemiologic evidence of the protective effect of fruit and vegetables on cancer risk," *American Journal Clinical of Nutrition*, 2003, 78(3 suppl):559S–569S.

15. "Phytochemicals: The Cancer Fighters in Your Foods," American Institute for Cancer Research, accessed September 2017, http://www.aicr.org/reduce-your-cancer-risk/diet/ elements_phytochemicals.html.

16. D Boivin et al., "Antiproliferative and antioxidant activities of common vegetables: A comparative study," *Food Chemistry*, 2009 Jan 15, 112(2):374–380, https://doi. org/10.1016/j.foodchem.2008.05.084.

17. Boivin et al., "Antiproliferative and antioxidant activities of common vegetables."

18. Boivin et al., "Antiproliferative and antioxidant activities of common vegetables."

19. "Phytochemicals: The Cancer Fighters in Your Foods," American Institute for Cancer Research, accessed September 2017, http://www.aicr.org/reduce-your-cancer-risk/diet/elements_phytochemicals.html.

20. I Robey, "Examining the relationship between diet-induced acidosis and cancer," *Nutrition & Metabolism*, 2012, 9:72. https://doi.org/10.1186/1743-7075-9-72.

21. Robey, "Examining the relationship between diet-induced acidosis and cancer."

22. Robey, "Examining the relationship between diet-induced acidosis and cancer."

23. "Chronic Inflammation," National Cancer Institute, accessed September 22, 2017, https://www.cancer.gov/about-cancer/causes-prevention/risk/chronic-inflammation.

24. "Foods that Fight Inflammation," Harvard Health Publishing, accessed September 22, 2017, https://www.health.harvard.edu/staying-healthy/foods-that-fight-inflammation.

25. "Foods that Fight Inflammation," Harvard Health Publishing.

26. "Overview of Inflammation," Linus Pauling Institute, accessed September 22, 2017, http://lpi.oregonstate.edu/mic/health-disease/inflammation#reference19.

27. D Giugliano et al., "The effects of diet on inflammation: emphasis on the metabolic syndrome," *Journal of the American College of Cardiology*, 2006 Aug 15, 48(4):677–85, https://doi.org/10.1016/j.jacc.2006.03.052.

28. D Giugliano et al., "The effects of diet on inflammation."

29. Katherine Esposito et al., "Inflammatory cytokine concentrations are acutely increased by hyperglycemia in humans," *Circulation*, 2002, 106:2067–2072, https://doi.org/10.1161/01.CIR.0000034509.14906.AE.

30. A Menke et al., "Prevalence of and trends in diabetes among adults in the United States, 1988–2012," *JAMA*, 2015, 314(10):1021–1029, https://doi.org/10.1001/jama.2015.10029.

31. A Menke et al., "Prevalence of and trends in diabetes."

32. A Menke et al., "Prevalence of and trends in diabetes."

33. A Menke et al., "Prevalence of and trends in diabetes."

34. IF Godsland, "Insulin resistance and hyperinsulinaemia in the development and progression of cancer," *Clinical Science* (London, England: 1979), 2009, 118(Pt 5):315–332, https://doi.org/10.1042/CS20090399.

35. IF Godsland, "Insulin resistance and hyperinsulinaemia in the development and progression of cancer."

36. IF Godsland, "Insulin resistance and hyperinsulinaemia in the development and progression of cancer."

37. "WHO calls on countries to reduce sugars intake among adults and children," World Health Organization, accessed September 23, 2017, http://www.who.int/mediacentre/news/releases/2015/sugar-guideline/en.

38. "How Much Is Too Much? The growing concern over too much added sugar in our diets," Sugar Science: The Unsweetened Truth, University of California–San Francisco, http://sugarscience.ucsf.edu/the-growing-concern-of-overconsumption.

39. "Glycemic index and glycemic load for 100+ foods," Harvard Health Publishing, accessed September 23, 2017, https://www.health.harvard.edu/diseases-and-conditions/glycemic-index-and-glycemic-load-for-100-foods.

40. "Glycemic index and glycemic load for 100+ foods," Harvard Health Publishing.

41. T Brown, "'Caution' Warranted if Consuming Artificial Sweeteners," Medscape.com, accessed September 30, 2017, http://www.medscape.com/viewarticle/807615.

42. ES Schernhammer et al., "Consumption of artificial sweetener- and sugar-containing soda and risk of lymphoma and leukemia in men and women," *American Journal of Clinical Nutrition*, 2012 Dec, 96(6):1419–28, https://doi.org/10.3945/ajcn.111.030833.

43. T Seyfried et al., "Cancer as a metabolic disease: implications for novel therapeutics." *Carcinogenesis*, 2014, 35(3):515–527, https://doi.org/10.1093/carcin/bgt480.

44. M Liberti and J Locasale, "The Warburg effect: how does it benefit cancer cells?" *Trends in Biochemical Sciences*, 2016 Mar, 41(3):211–218, https://doi.org/10.1016/j.tibs.2015.12.001.

45. Seyfried et al., "Cancer as a metabolic disease."

46. Travis Christofferson, *Tripping Over the Truth: How the Metabolic Theory of Cancer Is Overturning One of Medicine's Most Entrenched Paradigms* (White River Junction: Chelsea Green Publishing, 2017), 145.

47. Seyfried et al., "Cancer as a metabolic disease."

48. Christofferson, *Tripping Over the Truth*, 64.

49. Christofferson, *Tripping Over the Truth*, 64.

50. Christofferson, *Tripping Over the Truth*, 64.

51. NA Graham et al., "Glucose deprivation activates a metabolic and signaling amplification loop leading to cell death," *Molecular Systems Biology*, 2012 Jun 26, 8:589, https://doi.org/10.1038/msb.2012.20.

52. PN Mitrou et al., "Mediterranean dietary pattern and prediction of all-cause mortality in a US population: results from the NIH-AARP Diet and Health Study," *Archives of Internal Medicine*, 2007, 167(22):2461–2468, https://doi.org/10.1001/archinte.167.22.2461.

53. C Bamia et al., "Mediterranean diet and colorectal cancer risk: results from a European cohort," *European Journal of Epidemiology*, 2013, 28(4):317–328, https://doi.org/10.1007/s10654-013-9795-x.

54. C Agnoli et al., "Italian mediterranean index and risk of colorectal cancer in the Italian section of the EPIC cohort," *International Journal of Cancer*, 132:1404–1411, https://doi.org/10.1002/ijc.27740.

55. L Schwingshackl et al., "Does a Mediterranean-type diet reduce cancer risk?" *Current Nutrition Reports*, 2016, 5:9–17, https://doi.org/10.1007/s13668-015-0141-7.

56. E Toledo et al., "Mediterranean diet and invasive breast cancer risk among women at high cardiovascular risk in the PREDIMED trial: a randomized clinical trial," *JAMA Internal Medicine*, 2015, 175(11):1752–1760, https://doi.org/10.1001/jamainternmed.2015.4838.

57. A Castelló et al., "Spanish Mediterranean diet and other dietary patterns and breast cancer risk: case–control EpiGEICAM study," *British Journal of Cancer*, 2014, 111(7):1454–1462, https://doi.org/10.1038/bjc.2014.434.

58. L Schwingshackl and G Hoffmann, "Adherence to Mediterranean diet and risk of cancer: A systematic review and meta-analysis of observational studies," *International Journal of Cancer*, 2014, 135:1884–1897, https://doi.org/10.1002/ijc.28824.

59. Schwingshackl and Hoffmann, "Adherence to Mediterranean diet and risk of cancer."

60. Schwingshackl and Hoffmann, "Adherence to Mediterranean diet and risk of cancer."

61. SA Kenfield et al., "Mediterranean diet and prostate cancer risk and mortality in the health professionals follow-up study," *European Urology*, 2014, 65(5):887–894, https://doi.org/10.1016/j.eururo.2013.08.009.

62. C Bosetti et al., "Influence of the Mediterranean diet on the risk of cancers of the upper aerodigestive tract," *Cancer Epidemiology, Biomarkers & Prevention*, 2003 Oct, 12(10):1091–4, PMID: 14578148.

63. Toledo et al., "Mediterranean Diet and Invasive Breast Cancer."

64. R Etzel, "Mycotoxins," JAMA, 2002, 287(4):425–427, https://doi.org/10.1001/jama.287.4.425.

65. D Kaufmann, "One Man's Hypothesis On An Unknown Cause of Cancer," Knowthecause.com, accessed October 1, 2017, http://www.knowthecause.com/index.php/cancer.

66. "The Genetics of Cancer," Cancer.Net, accessed October 1, 2017, http://www.cancer.net/navigating-cancer-care/cancer-basics/genetics/genetics-cancer.

67. "The Genetics of Cancer," Cancer.Net.

68. F Aguilar et al., "Aflatoxin B1 induces the transversion of G-->T in codon 249 of the p53 tumor suppressor gene in human hepatocytes," *Proceedings of the National Academy of Sciences of the United States of America*, 1993, 90(18):8586–8590.

69. D Kaufmann, "Integrative 2016 Oncology Presentation."

70. KW Barañano and AL Hartman, "The ketogenic diet: uses in epilepsy and other neurologic illnesses," *Current Treatment Options In Neurology*, 2008, 10(6):410–419.

71. A Paoli, "Ketogenic diet for obesity: friend or foe?" *International Journal of Environmental Research and Public Health*, 2014, 11(2):2092–2107, https://doi.org/10.3390/ijerph110202092.

72. TN Seyfried et al., "Cancer as a metabolic disease: implications for novel therapeutics," *Carcinogenesis*. 2014;35(3):515–527. doi:10.1093/carcin/bgt480.

73. Seyfried et al., "Cancer as a metabolic disease."

74. Seyfried et al., "Cancer as a metabolic disease."

75. BG Allen et al., "Ketogenic diets as an adjuvant cancer therapy: History and potential mechanism," *Redox Biology*, 2014; 2:963–970, https://doi.org/10.1016/j.redox.2014.08.002.

76. Seyfried et al., "Cancer as a metabolic disease."

77. JC Newman and E Verdin, "Ketone bodies as signaling metabolites," *Trends in Endocrinology and Metabolism*, 2014, 25(1):42–52, https://doi.org/10.1016/j.tem.2013.09.002.

78. IF Godsland, "Insulin resistance and hyperinsulinaemia in the development and progression of cancer."

79. S Braun, K Bitton-Worms, D LeRoith, "The link between the metabolic syndrome and cancer," *International Journal of Biological Sciences*, 2011, 7(7):1003–1015.

80. MJ Tisdale et al., "Reduction of weight loss and tumour size in a cachexia model by a high fat diet," *British Journal of Cancer*, 1987, 56(1):39–43.

81. Allen et al., "Ketogenic diets as an adjuvant cancer therapy."

82. MG Abdelwahab et al., "The ketogenic diet is an effective adjuvant to radiation therapy for the treatment of malignant glioma," *PLoS ONE*, 2012, 7(5):e36197, https://doi.org/ 10.1371/journal.pone.0036197.

83. L C Nebeling et al., "Effects of a ketogenic diet on tumor metabolism and nutritional status in pediatric oncology patients: two case reports," *Journal of the American College of Nutrition*, 1995, 14(2):202–208.

84. M Schmidt et al., "Effects of a ketogenic diet on the quality of life in 16 patients with advanced cancer: A pilot trial," *Nutrition & Metabolism*, 2011, 8:54, https://doi.org/10.1186/1743-7075-8-54.

85. EJ Fine et al., "Targeting insulin inhibition as a metabolic therapy in advanced cancer: A pilot safety and feasibility dietary trial in 10 patients," *Nutrition*, 2012 Oct, 28(10):1028–35, https://doi.org/10.1016/j.nut.2012.05.001.

86. N Jansen and H Walach, "The development of tumours under a ketogenic diet in association with the novel tumour marker TKTL1: A case series in general practice," *Oncology Letters*, 2016, 11(1):584–592, https://doi.org/10.3892/ol.2015.3923.

87. Allen et al., "Ketogenic diets as an adjuvant cancer therapy."

88. Allen et al., "Ketogenic diets as an adjuvant cancer therapy."

89. Allen et al., "Ketogenic diets as an adjuvant cancer therapy."

90. E Davis, *Fight Cancer with a Ketogenic Diet*, 3rd ed. (Cheyenne: Gutsy Badger Publishing, 2017), 29–33.

91. Allen et al., "Ketogenic diets as an adjuvant cancer therapy."

92. Allen et al., "Ketogenic diets as an adjuvant cancer therapy."

93. Davis, *Fight Cancer with a Ketogenic Diet*, 23.

94. A Hayashi et al., "[Changes in serum levels of selenium, zinc and copper in patients on a ketogenic diet using Ketonformula]," *No To Hattastu*, 2013 Jul, 45(4):288–93.

95. N Winters and J Higgins Kelley, *The Metabolic Approach to Cancer* (White River Junction: Chelsea Green Publishing, 2017), 73.

96. Allen et al., "Ketogenic diets as an adjuvant cancer therapy."

97. Allen et al., "Ketogenic diets as an adjuvant cancer therapy."

98. Davis, *Fight Cancer with A Ketogenic Diet*, 41.

99. J Meidenbauer et al., "The glucose ketone index calculator: a simple tool to monitor therapeutic efficacy for metabolic management of brain cancer," *Nutrition & Metabolism*, 2015, 12:12, https://doi.org/10.1186/s12986-015-0009-2.

100. J Meidenbauer et al., "The glucose ketone index calculator."

101. J Meidenbauer et al., "The glucose ketone index calculator."

102. S Brandhorst and VD Longo, "Fasting and Caloric Restriction in Cancer Prevention and Treatment," *Recent Results in Cancer Research*, 2016, 207:241–66, https://doi.org/10.1007/978-3-319-42118-6_12.

103. Brandhorst and Longo, "Fasting and Caloric Restriction in Cancer Prevention and Treatment."

104. RJ Colman et al., "Caloric restriction delays disease onset and mortality in rhesus monkeys," *Science* (New York, NY), 2009, 325(5937):201–204, https://doi.org/10.1126/science.1173635.

105. Brandhorst and Longo, "Fasting and Caloric Restriction in Cancer Prevention and Treatment."

106. S Brandhorst et al., "A periodic diet that mimics fasting promotes multi-system regeneration, enhanced cognitive performance and healthspan," *Cell Metabolism*, 2015,22(1):86–99, https://doi.org/10.1016/j.cmet.2015.05.012.

107. Brandhorst et al., "A periodic diet that mimics fasting."

108. FM Safdie et al., "Fasting and cancer treatment in humans: A case series report," *Aging* (Albany NY), 2009, 1(12):988–1007, https://doi.org/10.18632/aging.100114.

109. S De Groot et al., "The effects of short-term fasting on tolerance to (neo) adjuvant chemotherapy in HER2-negative breast cancer patients: a randomized pilot study," BMC Cancer, 2015, 15:652, https://doi.org/10.1186/s12885-015-1663-5.

110. "Tackling the Conundrum of Cachexia in Cancer," National Cancer Institute, accessed September 15, 2017, https://www.cancer.gov/about-cancer/treatment/research/cachexia.

111. NP Gullett et al., "Nutritional interventions for cancer-induced cachexia," *Current Problems in Cancer*, 2011, 35(2):58–90, https://doi.org/10.1016/j.currproblcancer.2011.01.001.

112. A Utech et al., "Predicting survival in cancer patients: the role of cachexia and hormonal, nutritional and inflammatory markers," *Journal of Cachexia, Sarcopenia and Muscle*, 2012 Dec, 3(4): 245–251, https://doi.org/10.1007/s13539-012-0075-5.

113. A Nicolini et al., "Malnutrition, anorexia and cachexia in cancer patients: A mini-review on pathogenesis and treatment," *Biomedicine & Pharmacotherapy*, 2013, 67(8):807–817, https://doi.org/10.1016/j.biopha.2013.08.005.

114. E Bruera et al., "Effect of fish oil on appetite and other symptoms in patients with advanced cancer and anorexia/cachexia: a double-blind, placebo-controlled study," *Journal of Clinical Oncology*, 2003 Jan 1, 21(1):129–34, https://doi.org/10.1200/JCO.2003.01.101.

115. MD Barber et al., "The effect of an oral nutritional supplement enriched with fish oil on weight-loss in patients with pancreatic cancer," *British Journal of Cancer*, 1999 Sep, 81(1):80–6, https://doi.org/10.1038/sj.bjc.6690654.

116. R Colomer et al., "N-3 fatty acids, cancer and cachexia: a systematic review of the literature," *British Journal of Nutrition*, 2007 May, 97(5):823–31, https://doi.org/10.1017/S000711450765795X.

117. MD Barber et al., "Fish oil-enriched nutritional supplement attenuates progression of the acute-phase response in weight-losing patients with advanced pancreatic cancer," *The Journal of Nutrition*, 1999 June, 129(6):1120–5.

CHAPTER 6

1. Y Gao et al., "Active hexose correlated compound enhances tumor surveillance through regulating both innate and adaptive immune responses," *Cancer Immunology, Immunotherapy*, 2006, 55(10):1258–1266, https://doi.org/10.1007/s00262-005-0111-9.

2. Z Yin et al., "Effects of active hexose correlated compound on frequency of CD4+ and CD8+ T cells producing interferon-γ and/or tumor necrosis factor-α in healthy adults," *Human Immunology*, 2010 Dec, 71(12):1187–90, https://doi.org/10.1016/j.humimm.2010.08.006.

3. K Uno et al., "Active hexose correlated compound (AHCC) improves immunological parameters and performance status of patients with solid tumors," *Biotherapy* (Tokyo), 2000, 14(3):303–309.

4. Y Matsui et al., "Improved prognosis of postoperative hepatocellular carcinoma patients when treated with functional foods: a prospective cohort study," *Journal of Hepatology*, 2002, 37(1):78–86, http://dx.doi.org/10.1016/S0168-8278(02)00091-0.

5. S Cowawintaweewat et al., "Prognostic improvement of patients with advanced liver cancer after active hexose correlated compound (AHCC) treatment," *Asian Pacific Journal of Allergy and Immunology*, 2006, 24(1):33–45.

6. Y Matsui et al., "Improved prognosis of postoperative hepatocellular carcinoma patients when treated with functional foods: a prospective cohort study," *Journal of Hepatology*, 2002, 37(1):78–86, http://dx.doi.org/10.1016/S0168-8278(02)00091-0.

7. Cowawintaweewat et al., "Prognostic improvement of patients with advanced liver cancer."

8. T Ito et al., "Reduction of adverse effects by a mushroom product, active hexose correlated compound (AHCC) in patients with advanced cancer during chemotherapy—the significance of the levels of HHV-6 DNA in saliva as a surrogate biomarker during chemotherapy," *Nutrition and Cancer*, 2014, 66(3):377–82, https://doi.org/10.1080/01635581.2014.884232.

9. H Yanagimoto et al., "Alleviating effect of active hexose correlated compound (AHCC) on chemotherapy-related adverse events in patients with unresectable pancreatic ductal adenocarcinoma," *Nutrition and Cancer*, 2016, 68(2):234–40, https://doi.org/10.1080/01635581.2016.1134597.

10. CM Mach et al., "Evaluation of active hexose correlated compound hepatic metabolism and potential for drug interactions with chemotherapy agents," *Journal of the Society for Integrative Oncology*, 2008, 6:105–109.

11. T Kaczor, "The therapeutic effects of acetyl-l-carnitine on peripheral neuropathy: a review of the literature," *Natural Medicine Journal*, 2010 Aug, 2(8).

12. Kaczor, "The Therapeutic Effects of Acetyl-L-Carnitine on Peripheral Neuropathy."

13. G Bianchi et al., "Symptomatic and neurophysiological responses of paclitaxel- or cisplatin-induced neuropathy to oral acetyl-l-carnitine," *European Journal of Cancer*, 41(12):1746–1750, http://dx.doi.org/10.1016/j.ejca.2005.04.028.

14. A Maestri et al., "A pilot study on the effect of acetyl-L-carnitine in paclitaxel- and cisplatin-induced peripheral neuropathy," *Tumori*, 2005, 91(2):135–138.

15. M Malaguarnera et al., "Effects of L-Carnitine in Patients with Hepatic Encephalopathy," *World Journal of Gastroenterology*, 2005, 11(45): 7197–7202, https://doi.org/10.3748/wjg.v11.i45.7197.

16. "Artemisia annua," Memorial Sloan Kettering Cancer Center, accessed August 2, 2017, https://www.mskcc.org/cancer-care/integrative-medicine/herbs/artemisia-annua.

17. S Zhu et al., "Artemisinin reduces cell proliferation and induces apoptosis in neuroblastoma," *Oncology Reports*, 2014 Sep, 32(3):1094–100, https://doi.org/10.3892/or.2014.3323.

18. M Lu et al., "Dihydroartemisinin induces apoptosis in colorectal cancer cells through the mitochondria-dependent pathway," *Tumour Biology,* 2014 Jun, 35(6):5307–14, https://doi.org/10.1007/s13277-014-1691-9.

19. LH Stockwin et. al., "Artemisinin dimer anti-cancer activity correlates with heme catalyzed ROS generation and ER stress induction," *International Journal of Cancer,* 2009 Sep\ 15, 125(6):1266–1275, https://doi.org/10.1002/ijc.24496.

20. T Efferth, "Molecular pharmacology and pharmacogenomics of artemisinin and its derivatives in cancer cells," *Current Drug Targets,* 2006, 7:407–21.

21. IH Paik et al., "Second generation, orally active, antimalarial, artemisinin-derived trioxane dimers with high stability, efficacy, and anticancer activity," *Journal of Medicinal Chemistry,* 2006, 49(9):2731–4, https://doi.org/10.1021/jm058288w.

22. W Nam et al., "Effects of artemisinin and its derivatives on growth inhibition and apoptosis of oral cancer cells," *Head & Neck,* 2007, 29(4):335–40, https://doi.org/10.1002/hed.20524.

23. H Lai et al., "Targeted treatment of cancer with artemisinin and artemisinin-tagged iron-carrying compounds," *Expert Opinions on Therapeutic Targets,* 2005 Oct, 9(5):995–1007, https://doi.org/10.1517/14728222.9.5.995.

24. S Zhu et al., "Artemisinin reduces cell proliferation and induces apoptosis in neuroblastoma," *Oncology Reports,* 2014 Sep, 32(3):1094–100, https://doi.org/10.3892/or.2014.3323.

25. Lu et al., "Dihydroartemisinin induces apoptosis in colorectal cancer cells."

26. JA Willoughby et al., "Artemisinin blocks prostate cancer growth and cell cycle progression by disrupting Sp1 interactions with the cyclin-dependent kinase-4 (CDK4) promoter and inhibiting CDK4 gene expression," *The Journal of Biological Chemistry,* 2009, 284:2203–2213, https://doi.org/10.1074/jbc.M804491200.

27. AS Tin et al., "Antiproliferative effects of artemisinin on human breast cancer cells requires the downregulated expression of the E2F1 transcription factor and loss of E2F1-target cell cycle genes," *Anticancer Drugs,* 2012, 23(4):370–379, https://doi.org/10.1097/CAD.0b013e32834f6ea8.

28. T Weifeng et al., "Artemisinin inhibits in vitro and in vivo invasion and metastasis of human hepatocellular carcinoma cells," *Phytomedicine,* 2011, 18(2–3):158–162, https://doi.org/10.1016/j.phymed.2010.07.003.

29. P Reungpatthanaphong and S Mankhetkorn, "Modulation of multidrug resistance by artemisinin, artesunate and dihydroartemisinin in K562/adr and GLC4/adr resistant cell lines," *Biological & Pharmaceutical Bulletin,* 2002, 25(12):1555–1561, http://doi.org/10.1248/bpb.25.1555.

30. E Yamachika et al., "Artemisinin: an alternative treatment for oral squamous cell carcinoma," *Anticancer Research,* 2004, 24:2153–2160.

31. "Artemisia annua," Memorial Sloan Kettering Cancer Center, accessed August 2, 2017, https://www.mskcc.org/cancer-care/integrative-medicine/herbs/artemisia-annua.

32. "Sweet Wormwood," Drugs.com, accessed August 2, 2017, https://www.drugs.com/npp/sweet-wormwood.html.

33. KK Auyeung et al., "Astragalus membranaceus: A Review of its Protection Against Inflammation and Gastrointestinal Cancers," *The American Journal of Chinese Medicine*, 2016,44(1):1-22, https://doi.org/10.1142/S0192415X16500014.

34. T Fleischer et al., "Improved Survival With Integration of Chinese Herbal Medicine Therapy in Patients With Acute Myeloid Leukemia: A Nationwide Population-Based Cohort Study," *Integrative Cancer Therapies*, 2016 Aug 16, 16(2):156–164, https://doi.org/10.1177/1534735416664171.

35. T Wu et al., "Chinese medical herbs for chemotherapy side effects in colorectal cancer patients," *Cochrane Database of Systematic Reviews*, 2005 Jan 25, 1:CD004540, https://doi.org/10.1002/14651858.CD004540.pub2.

36. DT Chu et al., "Immunotherapy with Chinese medicinal herbs. II. Reversal of cyclophosphamide-induced immune suppression by administration of fractionated *Astragalus membranaceus* in vivo," *Journal of Clinical & Laboratory Immunology*, 1988, 25(3):125–9.

37. J Zhu et al., "Effects and mechanism of flavonoids from Astragalus complanatus on breast cancer growth," *Naunyn-Schmiedeberg's Archives of Pharmacology*, 2015, 388(9):965–972, https://doi.org/10.1007/s00210-015-1127-0.

38. KK Auyeung et al., "*Astragalus* saponins modulate cell invasiveness and angiogenesis in human gastric adenocarcinoma cells," *Journal of Ethnopharmacology*, 2012 Jun 1, 141(2):635–641, https://doi.org/10.1016/j.jep.2011.08.010.

39. MM Tin et al., "*Astragalus* saponins induce growth inhibition and apoptosis in human colon cancer cells and tumor xenograft," *Carcinogenesis*, 2007 Jun, 28(6):1347–1355, https://doi.org/10.1093/carcin/bgl238.

40. KK Auyeung et al., "Combined therapeutic effects of vinblastine and Astragalus saponins in human colon cancer cells and tumor xenograft via inhibition of tumor growth and proangiogenic factors," *Nutrition and Cancer*, 2014, 66(4):662–674, http://dx.doi.org/10.1080/01635581.2014.894093.

41. Y Wang et al., "Astragalus saponins modulates colon cancer development by regulating calpain-mediated glucose-regulated protein expression," *BMC Complementary and Alternative Medicine*, 2014, 14:401, https://doi.org/10.1186/1472-6882-14-401.

42. WH Huang et al., "Astragalus polysaccharide induces the apoptosis of human hepatocellular carcinoma cells by decreasing the expression of Notch1," *International Journal of Molecular Medicine*, 2016 Aug, 38(2):551–557, https://doi.org/10.3892/ijmm.2016.2632.

43. B Cham, "Solasodine rhamnosyl glycosides in a cream formulation is effective for treating large and troublesome skin cancers," *Research Journal Biological Science*, 2007, 2(7):749–761.

44. Cham, "Solasodine rhamnosyl glycosides in a cream formulation."

45. LY Shiu et al., "Solamargine induces apoptosis and sensitizes breast cancer cells to cisplatin," *Food and Chemical Toxicology*, 2007, 45(11):2155–2164, https://doi.org/10.1016/j.fct.2007.05.009.

46. CH Liang et al., "Solamargine upregulation of fas, downregulation of HER 2, and enhancement of cytotoxicity using epirubicin in NSCLC cells," *Molecular Nutrition Food Research*, 2007, 51:999–1005, https://doi.org/10.1002/mnfr.200700044.

47. Cham, "Solasodine rhamnosyl glycosides in a cream formulation."

48. B Daunter and BE Cham, "Solasodine glycosides, in vitro preferential cytotoxicity for human cancer cells," *Cancer Letters*, 1990, 55(3:209–220, http://dx.doi.org/10.1016/0304-3835(90)90121-D.

49. Cham, "Solasodine rhamnosyl glycosides in a cream formulation."

50. B Cham, "Solasodine glycosides: a topical therapy for actinic keratosis. A single-blind, randomized, placebo-controlled, parallel group study with CuradermBEC5." *Journal of Cancer Therapy*, 2013, 4(2), https://doi.org/10.4236/jct.2013.42076.

51. S Punjabi et al., "Solasodine glycoalkaloids: a novel topical therapy for basal cell carcinoma. A double-blind, randomized, placebo-controlled, parallel group, multicenter study," *International Journal of Dermatology*, 47(1): 78–82, https://doi.org/10.1111/j.1365-4632.2007.03363.x.

52. K Cham et al., "Treatment of non melanoma skin cancers: an intra-comparison study of CuradermBEC5 and various established modalities," *Journal of Cancer Therapy*, 6(12): 1045–1053, https://doi.org/10.4236/jct.2015.612114.

53. S Punjabi et al., "Solasodine glycoalkaloids: a novel topical therapy for basal cell carcinoma. A double-blind, randomized, placebo-controlled, parallel group, multicenter study," *International Journal of Dermatology*, 47(1): 78–82, https://doi.org/10.1111/j.1365-4632.2007.03363.x.

54. B Cham, "Topical Curaderm BEC5 therapy for periocular nonmelanoma skin cancers: a review of clinical outcomes," *International Journal of Clinical Medicine*, 2013, 4(5):233–238, https://doi.org/10.4236/ijcm.2013.45041.

55. H Safayhi et al., "Concentration-dependent potentiating and inhibitory effects of Boswellia extracts on 5-lipoxygenase product formation in stimulated PMNL," *Planta Medica*, 2000 Mar, 66(2):110–113, https://doi.org/10.1055/s-2000-11136.

56. T Glaser et al., "Boswellic acids and malignant glioma: induction of apoptosis but no modulation of drug sensitivity," *British Journal of Cancer*, 1999 May, 80(5–6):756–765, https://doi.org/10.1038/sj.bjc.6690419.

57. H Wang et al., "Targeting NF-KB with a natural triterpenoid alleviates skin inflammation in a mouse model of psoriasis," *The Journal of Immunology*, 2009 Oct, 183(7):4755–63, https://doi.org/10.4049/jimmunol.0900521.

58. Glaser et al., "Boswellic acids and malignant glioma."

59. Y Jing et al "Boswellic acid acetate induces differentiation and apoptosis in leukemia cell lines," *Leukemia Research*, 1999 Jan, 23(1):43–50, http://dx.doi.org/10.1016/S0145-2126(98)00096-4.

60. M Winking et al "Boswellic acids inhibit glioma growth: a new treatment option?" *Journal of Neuro-oncology*, 2000, 46(2):97–103.

61. T Syrovets et al., "Acetyl-boswellic acids are novel catalytic inhibitors of human topoisomerases I and IIalpha," *Molecular Pharmacology*, 2000 Jul, 58(1):71–81.

62. S Kirste et al., "*Boswellia serrata* acts on cerebral edema in patients irradiated for brain tumors: A prospective, randomized, placebo-controlled, double-blind pilot trial," *Cancer*, 2011, 117(16):3788–95, https://doi.org/10.1002/cncr.25945.

63. S Togni et al., "Clinical evaluation of safety and efficacy of Boswellia-based cream for prevention of adjuvant radiotherapy skin damage in mammary carcinoma: a randomized placebo controlled trial," *European Review for Medical and Pharmacological Sciences*, 2015 Apr, 19(8):1338–44.

64. PK Kokkiripati et al., "Gum resin of Boswellia serrata inhibited human monocytic (THP-1) cell activation and platelet aggregation," *Journal of Ethnopharmacology*, 2011 Sep 1, 137(1):893–901, https://doi.org/10.1016/j.jep.2011.07.004.

65. P Pacher et al., "The endocannabinoid system as an emerging target of pharmacotherapy," *Pharmacological Reviews*, 2006, 58(3):389–462, https://doi.org/10.1124/pr.58.3.2.

66. LM Borgelt et al., "The pharmacologic and clinical effects of medical cannabis," *Pharmacotherapy*, 2013, 33(2):195–209, https://doi.org/10.1002/phar.1187.

67. S Zhornitsky and S Potvin, "Cannabidiol in humans—the quest for therapeutic targets," *Pharmaceuticals (Basel)*, 2012, 5(5)–529–552, https://doi.org/10.3390/ph5050529.

68. E Martín-Sánchez et al., "Systematic review and meta-analysis of cannabis treatment for chronic pain," *Pain Medicine*, 2009; 10(8):1353–1368, https://doi.org/10.1111/j.1526-4637.2009.00703.x.

69. Donald Abrams et al., "Cannabinoid-opioid interaction in chronic pain." *Clinical Pharmacology & Therapeutics*, 2011 Dec, 90(6):844–851, https://doi.org/10.1038/clpt.2011.188.

70. KF Boehnke et al., "Medical cannabis use is associated with decreased opiate medication use in a retrospective cross-sectional survey of patients with chronic pain," *The Journal of Pain*, 2016 Jun, 17(6):739–44, https://doi.org/10.1016/j.jpain.2016.03.002.

71. B Chakravarti et al., "Cannabinoids as therapeutic agents in cancer: current status and future implications," *Oncotarget*, 2014, 5(15):5852–5872, https://doi.org/10.18632/oncotarget.2233.

72. KA Scott et al., "The combination of cannabidiol and δ9-tetrahydrocannabinol enhances the anticancer effects of radiation in an orthotopic murine glioma model," *Molecular Cancer Therapeutics*, 2014 Dec, 13(12):2955–67, https://doi.org/10.1158/1535 -7163.MCT-14-0402.

73. Y Singh et al., "Cannabis extract treatment for terminal acute lymphoblastic leukemia with a philadelphia chromosome mutation," *Case Reports in Oncology*, 2013, 6(3):585–592, https://doi.org/10.1159/000356446.

74. C Twelves et al., "A two-part safety and exploratory efficacy randomized double-blind, placebo-controlled study of a 1:1 ratio of the cannabinoids cannabidiol and delta-9-tetrahydrocannabinol (CBD: THC) plus dose-intense temozolomide in patients with recurrent glioblastoma multiforme (GBM)," *Journal of Clinical Oncology*, 2017, 35(15_suppl):2046–2046.

75. J Sachs, E McGlade , D Yurgelun-Todd," Safety and Toxicology of Cannabinoids," *Neurotherapeutics*. 2015;12(4):735-746. doi:10.1007/s13311-015-0380-8.

76. Marijuana, Drug Facts. National Institute on Drug Abuse, accessed November 23, 2017, https://www.drugabuse.gov/publications/drugfacts/marijuana.

77. BC He et al., "Ginsenoside Rg3 inhibits colorectal tumor growth through the down-regulation of Wnt/ß-catenin signaling." *International Journal of Oncology*, 2011 Feb, 38(2):437–45, https://doi.org/10.3892/ijo.2010.858.

78. JH Kang et al., "Ginsenoside Rp1 from panax ginseng exhibits anti-cancer activity by down-regulation of the IGF-1R/Akt pathway in breast cancer cells," *Plant Foods for Human Nutrition*, 2011 Jul 12, 66(3):298–305, https://doi.org/10.1007/ s11130-011-0242-4.

79. HR Shin et al., "The cancer-preventive potential of panax ginseng: a review of human and experimental evidence," *Cancer Causes Control*, 2000 Jul, 11(6):565–76.

80. TK Yun and SY Choi, "Non-organ specific cancer prevention of ginseng: a prospective study in Korea," *International Journal of Epidemiology*, 1998, 27:359–64.

81. B Li et al., "Antioxidants potentiate American ginseng-induced killing of colorectal cancer cells," *Cancer Letters*, 2010, 289(1):62–70, https://doi.org/10.1016/j. canlet.2009.08.002.

82. XL Li et al., "American ginseng berry enhances chemopreventive effect of 5-FU on human colorectal cancer cells," *Oncology Reports*, 2009 Oct, 22(4):943–52. https://doi. org/10.3892/or_00000521.

83. Y Cui et al., "Association of ginseng use with survival and quality of life among breast cancer patients," *American Journal of Epidemiology*, 2006, 163(7):645–53, https:// doi.org/10.1093/aje/kwj087.

84. DL Barton et al., "Wisconsin Ginseng (Panax quinquefolius) to improve cancer-related fatigue: a randomized, double-blind trial, N07C2," *Journal of the National Cancer Institute,* 2013 Aug 21, 105(16):1230–8, https://doi.org/10.1093/jnci/djt181.

85. HR Shin et al., "The cancer-preventive potential of Panax ginseng: a review of human and experimental evidence," *Cancer Causes Control*, 2000,11(6):565–76.

86. CZ Wang et al., "Ginsenoside compound K, not Rb1, possesses potential chemopreventive activities in human colorectal cancer," *International Journal of Oncology*, 2012 Jun, 40(6):1970–6, https://doi.org/10.3892/ijo.2012.1399.

87. He et al., "Ginsenoside Rg3 inhibits colorectal tumor growth."

88. Kang et al., "Ginsenoside Rp1 from panax ginseng exhibits anti-cancer activity."

89. Cui et al., "Association of ginseng use with survival and quality of life."

90. WL Hsu et al., "The prescription pattern of chinese herbal products containing ginseng among tamoxifen-treated female breast cancer survivors in taiwan: a population-based study," *Evidence Based Complementary and Alternative Medicine*, 2015, 385204, http://dx.doi.org/10.1155/2015/385204.

91. DL Barton et al., "Wisconsin Ginseng (Panax quinquefolius) to improve cancer-related fatigue: a randomized, double-blind trial, N07C2," *Journal of the National Cancer Institute*, 2013 Aug 21, 105(16):1230–8, https://doi.org/10.1093/jnci/djt181.

92. JZ Luo, L Luo L, "Ginseng on hyperglycemia: Effects and mechanisms," *Evidence-Based Complementary and Alternative Medicine*, 2009, 6(4):423–427, https://doi.org/10.1093/ecam/nem178.

93. MK Ang-Lee, J Moss, and CS Yuan, "Herbal medicines and perioperative care," *Journal of the American Medical Association*, 2001 Jul 11, 286(2):208–16, https://doi.org/10.1001/jama.286.2.208.

94. Joseph Pizzorno, "Glutathione!" *Integrative Medicine*, 2014, 13(1):8–12.

95. DP Jones, "The health dividend of glutathione," *Natural Medicine Journal*, 2011 Feb, 3(2).

96. S Cascinu et al., "Neuroprotective effect of reduced glutathione on cisplatin-based chemotherapy in advanced gastric cancer: a randomized double-blind placebo-controlled trial," *Journal of Clinical Oncology*, 1995 Jan, 13(1):26–32, https://doi.org/10.1200/JCO.1995.13.1.26.

97. Cascinu et al., " Neuroprotective Effect of Reduced Glutathione on Oxaliplatin-Based Chemotherapy."

98. JF Smyth et al., "Glutathione reduces the toxicity and improves quality of life of women diagnosed with ovarian cancer treated with cisplatin: results of a double-blind, randomized trial," *Annals of Oncology*, 1997 Jun, 8(6):569–73, https://doi.org/10.1023/A:1008211226339.

99. JP Richie, Jr, et al., "Randomized controlled trial of oral glutathione supplementation on body stores of glutathione," *European Journal of Nutrition*, 2015 Mar, 54(2):251–63, https://doi.org/10.1007/s00394-014-0706-z.

100. "Germanium," Memorial Sloan Kettering Cancer Center, accessed August 13, 2017, https://www.mskcc.org/cancer-care/integrative-medicine/herbs/germanium.

101. BJ Kaplan et al., "Germane facts about germanium sesquioxide: I. Chemistry and anticancer properties," *The Journal of Alternative and Complementary Medicine*, 2004 Jul, 10(2):337–44, https://doi.org/10.1089/107555304323062329.

102. N Tanaka et al., "[Augmentation of NK activity in peripheral blood lymphocytes of cancer patients by intermittent GE-132 administration]," *Gan To Kagaku Ryoho*, 1984 Jun, 11(6):1303–6.

103. Tanaka et al., "[Augmentation of NK activity in peripheral blood lymphocyte]."

104. Kaplan et al., "Germane facts about germanium sesquioxide."

105. Kaplan et al., "Germane facts about germanium sesquioxide."

106. Y Chen et al., "Resveratrol-induced cellular apoptosis and cell cycle arrest in neuroblastoma cells and antitumor effects on neuroblastoma in mice," *Surgery*, Jul 2004, 136(1):57–66, https://doi.org/10.1016/j.surg.2004.01.017.

107. R Lu and G Serrero, "Resveratrol, a natural product derived from grape, exhibits antiestrogenic activity and inhibits the growth of human breast cancer cells," *Journal of Cellular Physiology*, Jun 1999, 179(3):297–304, https://doi.org/10.1002/(SICI)1097-4652(199906)179:3<297::AID-JCP7>3.0.CO;2-P.

108. YJ Surh et al., "Resveratrol, an antioxidant present in red wine, induces apoptosis in human promyelocytic leukemia (HL-60) cells," *Cancer Letters*, Jun 1 1999, 140(1–2):1–10, http://dx.doi.org/10.1016/S0304-3835(99)00039-7.

109. Chen et al., "Resveratrol-induced cellular apoptosis and cell cycle arrest in neuroblastoma cells and antitumor effects."

110. R Lu and G Serrero, "Resveratrol, a natural product derived from grape, exhibits antiestrogenic activity."

111. Surh et al., "Resveratrol, an antioxidant present in red wine, induces apoptosis in human promyelocytic leukemia (HL-60) cells."

112. TT Wang et al., "Differential effects of resveratrol on androgen-responsive LNCaP human prostate cancer cells in vitro and in vivo," *Carcinogenesis*, Oct 2008, 29(10):2001–2010, https://doi.org/10.1093/carcin/bgn131.

113. Wang et al., "Differential effects of resveratrol on androgen-responsive LNCaP human prostate cancer cells."

114. H Cai et al., "Cancer chemoprevention: Evidence of a nonlinear dose response for the protective effects of resveratrol in humans and mice," *Science Translational Medicine*, 2015 Jul 29, 7(298):298ra117, https://doi.org/10.1126/scitranslmed.aaa7619.

115. C la Porte et al., "Steady-State pharmacokinetics and tolerability of trans-resveratrol 2000 mg twice daily with food, quercetin and alcohol (ethanol) in healthy human subjects," *Clinical Pharmacokinetics*, Jul 2010, 49(7):449-454, https://doi.org/10.2165/11531820-000000000-00000.

116. BD Gehm et al., "Resveratrol, a polyphenolic compound found in grapes and wine, is an agonist for the estrogen receptor," *Proceedings of the National Academy of Sciences U S A,* 1997 Dec 9, 94(25):14138–14143.

117. Mark Stengler, *Maitake Gold 404,* (North Bergen: Basic Health Publications, 2002), 4.

118. M Mayell, "Maitake Extracts and Their Therapeutic Potential-A Review," *Alternative Medicine Review,* 2001, 6(1):51.

119. K Adachi et al., "Potentiation of host-mediated antitumor activity in mice by beta glucan obtained from *Grifola frondosa* (maitake)," *Chemical and Pharmaceutical Bulletin* (Tokyo), 1987 Jan, 35(1):262–70.

120. Y Masuda et al., "Inhibitory effect of MD-Fraction on tumor metastasis: involvement of NK cell activation and suppression of intercellular adhesion molecule (ICAM)-1 expression in lung vascular endothelial cells," *Biological and Pharmaceutical Bulletin,* 2008 Jun, 31(6):1104–8, http://doi.org/10.1248/bpb.31.1104.

121. SP Wasser and A Weis, "Medicinal Properties of Substances Occurring in Higher Basidiomycetes Mushrooms: Current Perspectives (Review)," *International Journal of Medicinal Mushrooms,* 1999, 1:31–62.

122. B Louie et al., "Synergistic potentiation of interferon activity with maitake mushroom d-fraction on bladder cancer cells," *BJU International,* 2010 Apr, 105(7):1011–5, https://doi.org/10.1111/j.1464-410X.2009.08870.x.

123. "Maitake," Memorial Sloan Kettering Cancer Center, accessed August 13, 2017, https://www.mskcc.org/cancer-care/integrative-medicine/herbs/maitake.

124. R Soares et al., "Maitake (D fraction) mushroom extract induces apoptosis in breast cancer cells by BAK-1 gene activation," *Journal of Medicinal Food,* 2011 May, 14(6):563–72, https://doi.org/10.1089/jmf.2010.0095.

125. Stengler, *Maitake Gold 404,* 22.

126. G Deng et al., "A phase I/II trial of a polysaccharide extract from Grifola frondosa (Maitake mushroom) in breast cancer patients: immunological effects," *Journal of Cancer Research and Clinical Oncology,* 2009 Sep, 135(9):1215–21, https://doi.org/10.1007/s00432-009-0562-z.

127. H Nanba, "Maitake Glucan (MD-Fraction) can stop the cancer growth?" presented at the 3rd International Conference on Mushroom Biology and Mushroom Products in Sydney, Australia (October 1999).

128. H Nanba, *Maitake Challenges Cancer* (Kobe, Japan: Socio Health Group, 1998).

129. EN Alonso et al., "Antitumoral Effects of D-Fraction from Grifola Frondosa (Maitake) Mushroom in Breast Cancer," *Nutrition and Cancer,* 2017 Jan, 69(1):29–43, https://doi.org/10.1080/01635581.2017.1247891.

130. S Konno et al., "A possible hypoglycaemic effect of maitake mushroom on Type 2 diabetic patients." *Diabetic Medicine,* 2001 Dec, 18(12):1010, https://doi.org/10.1046/j.1464-5491.2001.00532-5.x.

131. MR Hanselin et al., "INR elevation with maitake extract in combination with warfarin," *The Annals of Pharmacotherapy,* 2010 Jan, 44(1):223–4, https://doi.org/10.1345/aph.1M510.

132. "Wheat germ extract," Memorial Sloan Kettering Cancer Center, accessed August 13, 2017, https://www.mskcc.org/cancer-care/integrative-medicine/herbs/wheat-germ-extract.

133. T Mueller and W Voigt, "Fermented wheat germ extract - nutritional supplement or anticancer drug?" *Nutrition Journal,* 2011, 10: 89, https://doi.org/10.1186/1475-2891-10-89.

134. B Comin-Anduix et al., "Fermented wheat-germ extract inhibits glycolysis/pentose cycle enzymes and induces apoptosis through poly(ADP-ribose) polymerase activation in Jurkat T-cell leukemia tumor cells," *Journal of Biological Chemistry,* 2002 Nov 29, 277(48):46408–14.

135. A Telekes et al., "Avemar (wheat germ extract) in cancer prevention and treatment," *Nutrition and Cancer,* 2009, 61(6):891–899, https://doi.org/10.1080/01635580903285114.

136. R Fajka-Boja et al., "Fermented wheat germ extract induces apoptosis and downregulation of major histocompatibility complex class I proteins in tumor T and B cell lines," *International Journal of Oncology,* 2002 Mar, 20(3):563–570, https://doi.org/10.3892/ijo.20.3.563.

137. F Jakab et al., "A medical nutriment has supportive value in the treatment of colorectal cancer," *British Journal of Cancer,* 2003 Aug 4, 89(3):465–469, https://doi.org/10.1038/sj.bjc.6601153.

138. LV Demidov et al., "Adjuvant fermented wheat germ extract (Avemar) nutraceutical improves survival of high-risk skin melanoma patients: a randomized, pilot, phase II clinical study with a 7-year follow-up," *Cancer Biotherapy & Radiopharmaceuticals,* 2008 Aug, 23(4):477–482, https://doi.org/10.1089/cbr.2008.0486.

139. J Barabás and Z Németh, "[Recommendation of the Hungarian Society for Face, Mandible and Oral Surgery in the indication of supportive therapy with Avemar]," *Orvosi Hetilap,* 2006, 147(35):1709–11.

140. LG Boros et al., "Fermented wheat germ extract (Avemar) in the treatment of cancer and autoimmune diseases," *Annals of the NY Academy of Sciences,* 2005 Jun, 1051:529–42, https://doi.org/10.1196/annals.1361.097.

141. Z Marcsek et al., "The efficacy of tamoxifen in estrogen receptor–positive breast cancer cells is enhanced by a medical nutriment," *Cancer Biotherapy & Radiopharmaceuticals,* 2005 Jan, 19(6):746–53, https://doi.org/10.1089/cbr.2004.19.746.

142. M Garami et al., "Fermented wheat germ extract reduces chemotherapy-induced febrile neutropenia in pediatric cancer patients," *Journal of Pediatric Hematology/Oncology,* 2004, 26(10):631–5.

143. "Wheat germ extract," Memorial Sloan Kettering Cancer Center, accessed August 13, 2017, https://www.mskcc.org/cancer-care/integrative-medicine/herbs/ wheat-germ-extract.

144. "Wheat Germ Extract," Medscape.com, accessed August 13, 2017, http://reference. medscape.com/drug/avemar-wheat-germ-extract-344559.

145. SM Henning et al., "Bioavailability and antioxidant activity of tea flavanols after consumption of green tea, black tea, or a green tea extract supplement," *American Journal of Clinical Nutrition*, 2004, 80(6):1558–1564.

146. NT Zaveri, "Green tea and its polyphenolic catechins: Medicinal uses in cancer and noncancer applications," *Life Sciences*, 2006, 78(18):2073–2080.

147. CA Elmets et al., "Cutaneous photoprotection from ultraviolet injury by green tea polyphenols," *Journal of the American Academy of Dermatology*, 2001, 44(3):425–432.

148. VE Steele et al., "Comparative chemopreventive mechanisms of green tea, black tea and selected polyphenol extracts measured by in vitro bioassays," *Carcinogenesis*, 2000, 21(1):63–67.

149. Steele et al., "Comparative chemopreventive mechanisms of green tea, black tea and selected polyphenol extracts."

150. S Nechuta et al., "Prospective cohort study of tea consumption and risk of digestive system cancers: results from the Shanghai Women's Health Study," *American Journal of Clinical Nutrition*, 2012 Nov, 96(5):1056–63, https://doi.org/10.3945/ ajcn.111.031419.

151. J Liu et al., "Green tea (Camellia sinensis) and cancer prevention: a systematic review of randomized trials and epidemiological studies," *Chinese Medicine*, 2008 Oct 22, 3:12, https://doi.org/10.1186/1749-8546-3-12.

152. TD Shanafelt et al., "Phase I trial of daily oral Polyphenon E in patients with asymptomatic Rai stage 0 to II chronic lymphocytic leukemia," *Journal of Clinical Oncology*, 2009 Aug 10, 27(23):3808–14, https://doi.org/10.1200/JCO.2008.21.1284.

153. S Bettuzzi et al., "Chemoprevention of human prostate cancer by oral administration of green tea catechins in volunteers with high-grade prostate intraepithelial neoplasia: A preliminary report from a one-year proof-of-principle study," *Cancer Research*, 2006, 66(2):1234–1240.

154. ME Stearns and M Wang, "Synergistic effects of the green tea extract epigallocatechin-3-gallate and taxane in eradication of malignant human prostate tumors," *Translational Oncology*, 2011, 4(3):147–156.

155. M Shimizu et al., "Green tea extracts for the prevention of metachronous colorectal adenomas: a pilot study," *Cancer Epidemiology*, Biomarkers & Prevention, 2008, 17(11):3020–3025, https://doi.org/10.1158/1055-9965.EPI-08-0528.

156. Memorial Sloan Kettering Cancer Center, "Green Tea," accessed August 13, 2017, https://www.mskcc.org/cancer-care/integrative-medicine/herbs/green-tea.

157. HH Chow et al., "Pharmacokinetics and safety of green tea polyphenols after multiple-dose administration of epigallocatechin gallate and polyphenon E in healthy individuals," *Clinical Cancer Research*, 2003, 9(9):3312–3319.

158. Z Yu et al., "Effect of green tea supplements on liver enzyme elevation: results from a randomized intervention study in the united states," *Cancer Prevention Research (Phila)*, 2017 Aug 1, https://doi.org/10.1158/1940-6207.CAPR-17-0160.

159. SC Shin and JS Choi, "Effects of epigallocatechin gallate on the oral bioavailability and pharmacokinetics of tamoxifen and its main metabolite, 4-hydroxytamoxifen, in rats," *Anticancer Drugs*, 2009 Aug, 20(7):584–8, https://doi.org/10.1097/CAD.0b013e32832d6834.

160. Mark Stengler, *The Natural Physician's Healing Therapies*. (New York, NY: Penguin Group: 2010), 451.

161. JM Yun et al., "Epigenetic regulation of high glucose-induced proinflammatory cytokine production in monocytes by curcumin," *The Journal of Nutritional Biochemistry*, May 2011, 22(5):450–458, https://doi.org/10.1016/j.jnutbio.2010.03.014.

162. "Curcumin," Linus Pauling Institute, accessed August 15, 2017, http://lpi.oregonstate.edu/mic/dietary-factors/phytochemicals/curcumin#biological-activities.

163. AB Kunnumakkara et al., "Curcumin inhibits proliferation, invasion, angiogenesis and metastasis of different cancers through interaction with multiple cell signaling proteins," *Cancer Letters*, 2008, 269(2):199–225, https://doi.org/10.1016/j.canlet.2008.03.009.

164. G Kuttan et al., "Antitumor, anti-invasion, and antimetastatic effects of curcumin," In Aggarwal B.B., Surh YJ., Shishodia S. (eds) *The Molecular Targets and Therapeutic Uses of Curcumin in Health and Disease. Advances in Experimental Medicine and Biology*, vol 595. (Boston: Springer).

165. "Curcumin," Linus Pauling Institute.

166. "Curcumin," Linus Pauling Institute.

167. A Goel et al., "Multi-targeted therapy by curcumin: how spicy is it?" *Molecular Nutrition & Food Research*, 2008 Sep, 52(9):1010–1030, https://doi.org/10.1002/mnfr.200700354.

168. ZY He et al., "Upregulation of p53 expression in patients with colorectal cancer by administration of curcumin," *Cancer Investigation*, Mar 2011, 29(3):208–213, https://doi.org/10.3109/07357907.2010.550592.

169. S Gupta et al., "Therapeutic roles of curcumin: lessons learned from clinical trials," *The APPS Journal*, 2013 Jan, 15(1):195–218, https://doi.org/10.1208/s12248-012-9432-8.

170. Timothy J. Moynihan, "Can curcumin slow cancer growth?" Mayo Clinic, accessed August 16, 2017, http://www.mayoclinic.org/diseases-conditions/cancer/expert-answers/curcumin/faq-20057858.

171. MC Fadus et al., "Curcumin: An age-old anti-inflammatory and anti-neoplastic agent," *Journal of Traditional and Complementary Medicine*, 2016 Sep 9, 7(3):339–346, https://doi.org/10.1016/j.jtcme.2016.08.002.

172. I Jantan et al., "Inhibitory effect of compounds from Zingiberaceae species on human platelet aggregation," *Phytomedicine*, 2008 Apr, 15(4):306–309.

173. VV Glinsky and A Raz, "A Modified citrus pectin anti-metastatic property: one bullet, multiple targets," *Carbohydrate Research*, 2009 Sep 28, 344(14):1788–91.

174. P Nangia-Makker et al., "Galectin-3 binding and metastasis," *Methods in Molecular Biology*, 2012, 878:251–66, https://doi.org/10.1007/978-1-61779-854-2_17.

175. N Tehranian et al., "Combination effect of PectaSol and Doxorubicin on viability, cell cycle arrest and apoptosis in DU-145 and LNCaP prostate cancer cell lines," *Cell Biology International*, 2012 Jul, 36(7):601–10, https://doi.org/10.1042/CBI20110309.

176. C Ramachandran et al., "Activation of human T-helper/inducer cell, T-cytotoxic cell, B-cell, and natural killer (NK)-cells and induction of natural killer cell activity against K562 chronic myeloid leukemia cells with modified citrus pectin," *BMC Complementary and Alternative Medicine*, 2011 Aug 4, 11:59, http://www.biomedcentral.com/1472-6882/11/59.

177. Tehranian et al., "Combination effect of PectaSol and Doxorubicin on viability, cell cycle arrest and apoptosis."

178. Nangia-Makker et al., "Inhibition of human cancer cell growth and metastasis."

179. BW Guess et al., "Modified citrus pectin (MCP) increases the prostate-specific antigen doubling time in men with prostate cancer: a phase II pilot study," *Prostate Cancer and Prostatic Disease*, 2003, 6(4):301–304.

180. J Yan and A Katz, "Pectasol-C modified citrus pectin induces apoptosis and inhibition of proliferation in human and mouse androgen-dependent and-independent prostate cancer cells," *Integrative Cancer Therapies*, 2010 Jun,9(2):197–203, https://doi.org/10.1177/1534735410369672.

181. Marc Azémar et al., "Clinical benefit in patients with advanced solid tumors treated with modified citrus pectin: a prospective pilot study," *Clinical Medicine Insights: Oncology*, 2007,1:73–80, https://doi.org/10.4137/CMO.S285.

182. "Milk Thistle," University of Maryland Medical Center, accessed August 27, 2017, http://www.umm.edu/health/medical/altmed/herb/milk-thistle.

183. "Milk Thistle," University of Maryland Medical Center.

184. M Kaur and R Agarwal, "Silymarin and Epithelial Cancer Chemoprevention: How close we are to bedside?" *Toxicology and Applied Pharmacology*, 2007 November 1, 224(3): 350–359, https://doi.org/10.1016 /j.taap.2006.11.011.

185. Kaur and Agarwal, "Silymarin and Epithelial Cancer Chemoprevention."

186. Brittany Cordeiro, "Probiotics: Healthy bacteria for your gut." MD Anderson Cancer Center, accessed August 27, 2017, https://www.mdanderson.org/publications/focused-on-health/may-2015/FOH-probiotics.html.

187. Erika Isolauri et al., "Probiotics: effects on immunity," *The American Journal of Clinical Nutrition*, 2001 Feb, 73(2):444s–450s.

188. I Wollowski et al., "Protective role of probiotics and prebiotics in colon cancer," *The American Journal of Clinical Nutrition*. 2001 Feb, 73(2):451s–455s.

189. JY Lee et al., "Effects of 12 weeks of probiotic supplementation on quality of life in colorectal cancer survivors: a double-blind, randomized, placebo-controlled trial," *Digestive and Liver Disease*, 2014 Dec, 46(12):1126–32, https://doi.org/10.1016/j.dld.2014.09.004.

190. MG Redman et al., "The efficacy and safety of probiotics in people with cancer: a systematic review," *Annals of Oncology*, 2014 Oct, 25(10):1919–29, https://doi.org/10.1093/annonc/mdu106.

191. N Aisu et al., "Impact of perioperative probiotic treatment for surgical site infections in patients with colorectal cancer," *Experimental and Therapeutic Medicine*, 2015 Sep, 10(3):966–972, https://doi.org/10.3892/etm.2015.2640.

192. Y Yang et al., "The effect of perioperative probiotics treatment for colorectal cancer: short-term outcomes of a randomized controlled trial," *Oncotarget*, 2016, 7(7):8432–8440, https://doi.org/10.18632/oncotarget.7045.

193. Redman et al., "The efficacy and safety of probiotics in people with cancer."

194. EH Jo et al., "Modulations of the Bcl-2/Bax family were involved in the chemopreventive effects of licorice root (Glycyrrhiza uralensis Fisch) in MCF-7 human breast cancer cell," *Journal of Agricultural and Food Chemistry*, 2004 Mar 24, 52(6):1715–1719.

195. T Takahashi et al., "Isoliquiritigenin, a flavonoid from licorice, reduces prostaglandin E2 and nitric oxide, causes apoptosis, and suppresses aberrant crypt foci development," *Cancer Science*, 2004 May, 95(5):448–453.

196. SY Park et al., "Hexane-ethanol extract of Glycyrrhiza uralensis containing licoricidin inhibits the metastatic capacity of DU145 human prostate cancer cells," *British Journal of Nutrition*, 2010 Nov, 104(9):1272–82, https://doi.org/10.1017/S0007114510002114.

197. Ao Guo et al., "Promotion of regulatory T cell induction by immunomodulatory herbal medicine licorice and its two constituents," *Scientific Reports*, 2015, 5:14046, https://doi.org/10.1038/srep14046.

198. ZY Wang and DW Nixon, Licorice and cancer," *Nutrition and Cancer*, 2001, 39(1):1–11.

199. Jo et al., "Modulations of the Bcl-2/Bax family were involved in the chemopreventive effects of licorice root."

200. SM Nourazarian et al., "Effect of Root Extracts of Medicinal Herb Glycyrrhiza glabra on HSP90 Gene Expression and Apoptosis in the HT-29 Colon Cancer Cell Line," *Asian Pacific Journal of Cancer Prevention*, 2015, 16(18):8563–6.

201. "Licorice," Memorial Sloan Kettering Cancer Center, accessed August 27, 2017, https://www.mskcc.org/cancer-care/integrative-medicine/herbs/licorice.

202. G Weiss et al., "Immunomodulation by perioperative administration of n-3 fatty acids," *British Journal of Nutrition*, 2002, 87(Suppl 1):S89–S94.

203. Y Zhao et al., "Eicosapentaenoic acid prevents LPS-induced TNF-alpha expression by preventing NF-kappaB activation," *Journal of the American College of Nutrition*, 2004 Feb, 23(1):71–8.

204. TR Chagas et al., "Oral fish oil positively influences nutritional-inflammatory risk in patients with haematological malignancies during chemotherapy with an impact on long-term survival: a randomised clinical trial," *Journal of Human Nutrition and Dietetics*, 2017 Apr 4, https://doi.org/10.1111/jhn.12471.

205. N Merendino et al., "Dietary ω-3 polyunsaturated fatty acid DHA: a potential adjuvant in the treatment of cancer," *BioMed Research International*, 2013, 2013:310186, 11 pages, https://doi.org/10.1155/2013/310186.

206. CJ Fabian et al., "Omega-3 fatty acids for breast cancer prevention and survivorship," *Breast Cancer Research*, 2015, 17:62, https://doi.org/10.1186/s13058-015-0571-6.

207. TR Chagas et al., "Oral fish oil positively influences nutritional-inflammatory risk in patients with haematological malignancies during chemotherapy with an impact on long-term survival: a randomised clinical trial," *Journal of Human Nutrition and Dietetics*, 2017 Apr 4, https://doi.org/10.1111/jhn.12471.

208. Y Shirai et al., "Fish oil-enriched nutrition combined with systemic chemotherapy for gastrointestinal cancer patients with cancer cachexia," *Scientific Reports*, 2017; 7:4826, https://doi.org/10.1038/s41598-017-05278-0.

209. TM Brasky et al., "Specialty supplements and breast cancer risk in the VITamins And Lifestyle (VITAL) cohort," *Cancer Epidemiology, Biomarkers & Prevention*, 2010, 19(7); 1696–708, https://doi.org/10.1158/1055-9965.EPI-10-0318.

210. JY Lee et al., "Chemopreventive and chemotherapeutic effects of fish oil derived omega-3 polyunsaturated fatty acids on colon carcinogenesis," *Clinical Nutrition Research*, 2017, 6(3):147–160, https://doi.org/10.7762/cnr.2017.6.3.147.

211. RA Murphy et al., "Supplementation with fish oil increases first-line chemotherapy efficacy in patients with advanced nonsmall cell lung cancer," *Cancer*, 2011 Aug 15, 117(16):3774–80, https://doi.org/10.1002/cncr.25933.

212. "Quercetin," University of Maryland Medical Center, accessed September 1, 2017, http://www.umm.edu/health/medical/altmed/supplement/Quercetin.

213. J-H Jeong, "Effects of low dose quercetin: Cancer cell-specific inhibition of cell cycle progression," *Journal of Cellular Biochemistry*, 2009,106(1):73–82, https://doi.org/10.1002/jcb.21977.

214. Jeong, "Effects of low dose quercetin."

215. C Chen and AN Kong, "Dietary cancer-chemopreventive compounds: from signaling and gene expression to pharmacological effects," *Trends in Pharmacological Sciences*, 2005, 26(6):318–326.

216. J Jeong, "Effects of low dose quercetin."

217. E Angst et al., "The flavonoid quercetin inhibits pancreatic cancer growth in vitro and in vivo," *Pancreas*, 2013, 42(2):223–229, https://doi.org/10.1097/MPA.0b013e318264ccae.

218. "Quercetin," Memorial Sloan Kettering Cancer Center, accessed September 1, 2017, https://www.mskcc.org/cancer-care/integrative-medicine/herbs/quercetin.

219. "Quercetin," Memorial Sloan Kettering Cancer Center.

220. "Iodine", Linus Pauling Institute, accessed September 2, 2017, http://lpi.oregonstate.edu/mic/minerals/iodine.

221. David Brownstein, *Iodine: Why You Need It, Why You Can't Live Without It*. 4th ed. (Michigan: Medical Alternatives Press, 2009), 21.

222. Brownstein, *Iodine*, 21.

223. Brownstein, *Iodine*, 65.

224. FR Stoddard et al., "Iodine alters gene expression in the MCF7 breast cancer cell line: evidence for an anti-estrogen effect of iodine," *International Journal of Medical Sciences*, 2008, 5(4):189–196, https://doi.org/10.7150/ijms.5.189.

225. Brownstein, *Iodine*, 21.

226. Brownstein, *Iodine*, 21.

227. C Aceves et al., "Is iodine a gatekeeper of the integrity of the mammary gland?" *Journal of Mammary Gland Biology and Neoplasia*, 2005 Apr, 10(2):189–96.

228. Brownstein, *Iodine*, 21.

229. Brownstein, *Iodine*, 65.

230. Aceves et al., "Is iodine a gatekeeper of the integrity of the mammary gland?"

231. T Kawamura and T Sobue, "Comparison of breast cancer mortality in five countries: France, Italy, Japan, the UK and the USA from the WHO mortality database (1960–2000)," *Japanese Journal of Clinical Oncology*, 2005 Dec, 35(12):758–759, https://doi.org/10.1093/jjco/hyi201.

232. Aceves et al., "Is iodine a gatekeeper of the integrity of the mammary gland?"

233. Aceves et al., "Is iodine a gatekeeper of the integrity of the mammary gland?"

234. T Kaczor, "Iodine and Cancer," *Natural Medicine Journal*, 2014 Jun, 6(6).

235. SA Hoption Cann et al., "A prospective study of iodine status, thyroid function, and prostate cancer risk: follow-up of the First National Health and Nutrition Examination Survey," *Nutrition and Cancer,* 2007, 58(1):28–34.

236. R Rahn et al., "Povidone-iodine to prevent mucositis in patients during antineoplastic radiochemotherapy," *Dermatology,* 1997, 195(Suppl 2):57–61.

237. "Iodine," WebMD, accessed September 2, 2017, http://www.webmd.com/vitamins -supplements/ingredientmono-35-iodine.aspx?activeingredientid=35.

238. "Iodine," Linus Pauling Institute.

239. "Proteolytic enzymes," Memorial Sloan Kettering Cancer Center, accessed September 1, 2017, https://www.mskcc.org/cancer-care/integrative-medicine/herbs/ proteolytic-enzymes.

240. NJ Gonzalez and LL Isaacs, "Evaluation of pancreatic proteolytic enzyme treatment of adenocarcinoma of the pancreas, with nutrition and detoxification support," *Nutrition and Cancer,* 1999 33(2), 117–124.

241. NJ Gonzalez and LL Isaacs, "The Gonzalez therapy and cancer: a collection of case reports," *Alternative Therapies in Health and Medicine,* 2007, 13(1), 46–55.

242. MS Gujral et al., "Efficacy of hydrolytic enzymes in preventing radiation therapy-induced side effects in patients with head and neck cancers," *Cancer Chemotherapy and Pharmacology,* 2001 Jul, 47(Suppl):S23–28.

243. A Sakalová et al., "Retrolective cohort study of an additive therapy with an oral enzyme preparation in patients with multiple myeloma," *Cancer Chemotherapy and Pharmacology,* 2001 Jul, 47(Suppl):S38–44.

244. J Beuth et al., "Impact of complementary oral enzyme application on the postoperative treatment results of breast cancer patients—results of an epidemiological multicentre retrolective cohort study," *Cancer Chemotherapy and Pharmacology,* 2001 Jul, 47(Suppl):S45–54.

245. PS Dale et al., "Co-medication with hydrolytic enzymes in radiation therapy of uterine cervix: evidence of the reduction of acute side effects," *Cancer Chemotherapy and Pharmacology,* 2001 Jul, 47(Suppl):S29–34.

246. T Popiela et al., "Influence of a complementary treatment with oral enzymes on patients with colorectal cancers—an epidemiological retrolective cohort study," *Cancer Chemotherapy and Pharmacology,* 2001 Jul, 47(Suppl):S55–63.

247. JK Roberts et al., "Pancreas exocrine replacement therapy is associated with increased survival following pancreatoduodenectomy for periampullary malignancy," *HPB* (Oxford), 2017 Oct, 19(10):859–867, http://dx.doi.org/10.1016/j.hpb.2017.05.009.

248. Popiela et al., "Influence of a complementary treatment with oral enzymes on patients with colorectal cancers."

249. BE Licznerska et al., "Modulation of CYP19 expression by cabbage juices and their active components: indole-3-carbinol and 3,3'-diindolylmethene in human breast epithelial cell lines," *European Journal of Nutrition*, 2013, 52(5):1483–1492, https://doi.org/10.1007/s00394-012-0455-9.

250. HL Bradlow et al., "Long-term responses of women to indole-3-carbinol or a high fiber diet," *Cancer Epidemiology and Biomarkers Prevention*, 1994, 3(7):591–5.

251. "Indole-3-Carbinol," Linus Pauling Institute, accessed September 3, 2017, http://lpi.oregonstate.edu/mic/dietary-factors/phytochemicals/indole-3-carbinol.

252. CN Marconett et al., "Indole-3-carbinol disrupts estrogen receptor-alpha dependent expression of insulin-like growth factor-1 receptor and insulin receptor substrate-1 and proliferation of human breast cancer cells," *Molecular and Cellular Endocrinology*, 2012, 363(1–2):74–84, https://doi.org/10.1016/j.mce.2012.07.008.

253. CN Marconett et al., "Indole-3-carbinol triggers aryl hydrocarbon receptor-dependent estrogen receptor (ER)alpha protein degradation in breast cancer cells disrupting an ERalpha-GATA3 transcriptional cross-regulatory loop," *Molecular Biology of the Cell*, 2010, 21(7):1166–1177, https://doi.org/10.1091/mbc.E09-08-0689.

254. ML Wang et al., "Antiangiogenic activity of indole-3-carbinol in endothelial cells stimulated with activated macrophages," *Food Chemistry*, 2012, 134(2):811–820, https://doi.org/10.1016/j.foodchem.2012.02.185.

255. HT Wu et al., "Inhibition of cell proliferation and in vitro markers of angiogenesis by indole-3-carbinol, a major indole metabolite present in cruciferous vegetables," *Journal of Agricultural and Food Chemistry*, 2005, 53(13):5164–5169.

256. K Kunimasa et al., "Antiangiogenic effects of indole-3-carbinol and 3,3'-diindolylmethane are associated with their differential regulation of ERK1/2 and Akt in tube-forming HUVEC," *Journal of Nutrition*, 2010, 140(1):1–6, https://doi.org/10.3945/jn.109.112359.

257. EJ Kim et al., "3,3'-diindolylmethane suppresses 12-O-tetradecanoylphorbol-13-acetate-induced inflammation and tumor promotion in mouse skin via the downregulation of inflammatory mediators," *Molecular Carcinogenesis*, 2010, 49(7):672–683, https://doi.org/10.1002/mc.20640.

258. ZJ D'Costa et al., "Screening of drugs to counteract human papillomavirus 16 E6 repression of E-cadherin expression," *Investigational New Drugs*, 2012 Dec, 30(6):2236–2251, https://doi.org/10.1007/s10637-012-9803-0.

259. SM Kim, "Cellular and Molecular Mechanisms of 3,3'-Diindolylmethane in Gastrointestinal Cancer," *International Journal of Molecular Sciences*, 2016, 17(7):1155, https://doi.org/10.3390/ijms17071155.

260. L Chen et al., "Indole-3-carbinol (I3C) increases apoptosis, represses growth of cancer cells, and enhances adenovirus-mediated oncolysis," *Cancer Biology & Therapy*, 2014 Sep, 15(9):1256–1267, https://doi.org/10.4161/cbt.29690.

261. MC Bellet al., "Placebo-controlled trial of indole-3-carbinol in the treatment of CIN," *Gynecologic Oncology*, 2000, 78(2):123–129.

262. L Ashrafian et al., "Double-blind randomized placebo-controlled multicenter clinical trial (phase IIa) on diindolylmethane's efficacy and safety in the treatment of CIN: implications for cervical cancer prevention," *EPMA Journal*, 2015 Dec 21, 6:25, https://doi.org/10.1186/s13167-015-0048-9.

263. R Naik, "A randomized phase II trial of indole-3-carbinol in the treatment of vulvar intraepithelial neoplasia," *International Journal of Gynecological Cancer*, 2006, 16(2):786–790.

264. CA Thomson et al., "A randomized, placebo-controlled trial of diindolylmethane for breast cancer biomarker modulation in patients taking tamoxifen," *Breast Cancer Research Treatment*, 2017 Aug, 165(1):97–107, https://doi.org/10.1007/s10549-017-4292-7.

265. Marconett et al., "Indole-3-carbinol disrupts estrogen receptor-alpha dependent expression of insulin-like growth factor-1 receptor and insulin receptor substrate-1 and proliferation."

266. JA Caruso et al., "Indole-3-carbinol and its N-alkoxy derivatives preferentially target ER alpha-positive breast cancer cells," *Cell Cycle*. 2014;13(16):2587–2599. doi: 10.4161/15384101.2015.942210.

267. JN Ho et al., "I3C and ICZ inhibit migration by suppressing the EMT process and FAK expression in breast cancer cells," *Molecular Medicine Reports*. Feb 2013;7(2):384–388. doi: 10.3892/mmr.2012.119.

268. Licznerska et al., "Modulation of CYP19 expression by cabbage juices and their active components."

269. Licznerska et al., "Modulation of CYP19 expression by cabbage juices and their active components."

270. B Parajuli et al., "The synergistic apoptotic interaction of Indole-3-Carbinol and Genistein with TRAIL on endometrial cancer cells," *Journal of Korean Medical Science*, 2013 Apr, 28(4):527–533, https://doi.org/10.3346/jkms.2013.28.4.527.

271. V Krajka-Kuźniak et al., "The activation of the Nrf2/ARE pathway in HepG2 hepatoma cells by phytochemicals and subsequent modulation of phase II and antioxidant enzyme expression," *Journal of Physiology and Biochemistry*, 2015 Jun, 71(2):227–238, https://doi.org/10.1007/s13105-015-0401-4.

272. X Wang et al., "Indole-3-carbinol inhibits tumorigenicity of hepatocellular carcinoma cells via suppression of microRNA-21 and upregulation of phosphatase and tensin homolog," *Biochimica et Biophysica Acta*, 2015 Jan, 1853(1):244–253, https://doi.org/10.1016/j.bbamcr.2014.10.017.

273. I Aronchik et al., "The antiproliferative response of indole-3-carbinol in human melanoma cells is triggered by an interaction with NEDD4-1 and disruption of wild-type PTEN degradation," *Molecular Cancer Research*, 2014, 12(11):1621–1634, https://doi.org/10.1158/1541-7786.MCR-14-0018.

274. WH Paik et al., "Chemosensitivity induced by down-regulation of microRNA-21 in gemcitabine-resistant pancreatic cancer cells by indole-3-carbinol," *Anticancer Research*, 2013 Apr, 33(4):1473–1481.

275. Licznerska et al., "Modulation of CYP19 expression by cabbage juices and their active components."

276. HS Choi et al., "Indole-3-carbinol induces apoptosis through p53 and activation of caspase-8 pathway in lung cancer A549 cells," *Food and Chemical Toxicology,* 2010 Mar, 48(3):883–90, https://doi.org/10.1016/j.fct.2009.12.028.

277. YQ Wang et al., "Indole-3-carbinol inhibits cell proliferation and induces apoptosis in Hep-2 laryngeal cancer cells," *Oncology Reports*, 2013 Jul, 30(1):227–233, https://doi.org/10.3892/or.2013.2411.

278. Z Chen et al., "Indole-3-carbinol inhibits nasopharyngeal carcinoma growth through cell cycle arrest in vivo and in vitro," *PLoS One*, 2013, 8(12): e82288, https://doi.org/10.1371/journal.pone.0082288.

279. GA Reed et al., "Single-dose and multiple-dose administration of indole-3-carbinol to women: pharmacokinetics based on 3,3'-diindolylmethane," *Cancer Epidemiology Biomarkers & Prevention*, 2006, 15(12):2477–2481.

280. AM Shamsuddin, "Metabolism and cellular functions of IP6: a review," *Anticancer Research*, 1999, 19(5A):3733–6.

281. K Raina et al., "Inositol hexaphosphate inhibits tumor growth, vascularity, and metabolism in TRAMP mice: a multiparametric magnetic resonance study," *Cancer Prevention Research (Phila)*, 2013 Jan, 6(1):40–50, https://doi.org/10.1158/1940-6207.CAPR-12-0387.

282. I Bacić et al., "Efficacy of IP6 + inositol in the treatment of breast cancer patients receiving chemotherapy: prospective, randomized, pilot clinical study," *Journal of Experimental & Clinical Cancer Research*, 2010 Feb 12, 29:12, https://doi.org/10.1186/1756-9966-29-12.

283. RF Hurrell, "Influence of vegetable protein sources on trace element and mineral bioavailability," *Journal of Nutrition,* 2003 Sep, 133(9):2973S–7S.

284. I Vucenik et al., "Antiplatelet activity of inositol hexaphosphate (IP6)," *Anticancer Research*, 1999, 19(5A):3689–94.

285. SC Miller et al., "The role of melatonin in immuno-enhancement: potential application in cancer," *International Journal of Experimental Pathology*, 2006, 87(2):81–87, https://doi.org/10.1111/j.0959-9673.2006.00474.x.

286. RJ Reiter et al., "Biochemical reactivity of melatonin with reactive oxygen and nitrogen species: a review of the evidence," *Cell Biochemistry and Biophysics,* 2001, 34(2):237–256.

287. K Zwirska-Korczala et al., "Influence of melatonin on cell proliferation, antioxidative enzyme activities and lipid peroxidation in 3T3-L1 preadipocytes—an in vitro study," *Journal of Physiology and Pharmacology,* 2005 Dec, 56 (Suppl 6):91–99.

Endnotes

288. DX Tan et al., "Chemical and physical properties and potential mechanisms: melatonin as a broad spectrum antioxidant and free radical scavenger," *Current Topics in Medical Chemistry*, 2002, 2(2):181–197.

289. EJ Sánchez-Barceló et al., "Clinical uses of melatonin: evaluation of human trials," *Current Topics in Medical Chemistry*, 2010, 17(19):2070–95.

290. EJ Sánchez-Barceló et al., "Melatonin-estrogen interactions in breast cancer," *Journal of Pineal Research*, 2005, 38(4):217–222.

291. MD Mediavilla et a., "Melatonin increases p53 and p21WAF1 expression in MCF-7 human breast cancer cells in vitro." *Life Sciences*, 1999, 65(4):415–420.

292. S Cos et al., "Influence of melatonin on invasive and metastatic properties of MCF-7 human breast cancer cells," *Cancer Research*, 1998, 58(19):4383–4390.

293. P Lissoni et al., "Anti-angiogenic activity of melatonin in advanced cancer patients," *NeuroEndocrinology Letters*, 2001, 22(1):45–47.

294. A Gonzalez et al., "Selective estrogen enzyme modulator actions of melatonin in human breast cancer cells," *Journal of Pineal Research*, 2008, 45(1):86–92, https://doi.org/10.1111/j.1600-079X.2008.00559.x.

295. MD Mediavilla et al., "Effects of melatonin on mammary gland lesions in transgenic mice overexpressing N-ras proto-oncogene," *Journal of Pineal Research*, 1997, 22(2):86–94.

296. MM Leon-Blanco et al., "Melatonin inhibits telomerase activity in the MCF-7 tumor cell line both in vivo and in vitro," *Journal of Pineal Research*, 2004 Oct, 35(3):204–11.

297. YM Wang et al., "The efficacy and safety of melatonin in concurrent chemotherapy or radiotherapy for solid tumors: a meta-analysis of randomized controlled trials," *Cancer Chemotherapy and Pharmacology*, 2012 May, 69(5):1213–20, https://doi.org/10.1007/s00280-012-1828-8.

298. P Lissoni et al., "Modulation of cancer endocrine therapy by melatonin: a phase II study of tamoxifen plus melatonin in metastatic breast cancer patients progressing under tamoxifen alone," *British Journal of Cancer*, 1995, 71(4):854–856.

299. P Lissoni et al., "Chemoneuroendocrine therapy of metastatic breast cancer with persistent thrombocytopenia with weekly low-dose epirubicin plus melatonin: a phase II study," *Journal of Pineal Research*, 1999 Apr, 26(3):169–73.

300. G Messina et al., "Enhancement of the efficacy of cancer chemotherapy by the pineal hormone melatonin and its relation with the psychospiritual status of cancer patients," *Journal of Research in Medical Sciences*, 2010 Jul, 15(4):225–8.

301. P Lissoni et al., "Five years survival in metastatic non-small cell lung cancer patients treated with chemotherapy alone or chemotherapy and melatonin: a randomized trial," *Journal of Pineal Research*, 2003 Aug, 35(1):12–5.

302. P Lissoni, "Is there a role for melatonin in supportive care?" *Supportive Care in Cancer.* 2002 Mar;10(2):110–6.

303. Lissoni, "Is there a role for melatonin in supportive care?"

304. K Onseng et al., "Beneficial Effects of Adjuvant Melatonin in Minimizing Oral Mucositis Complications in Head and Neck Cancer Patients Receiving Concurrent Chemoradiation," *Journal of Alternative and Complementary Medicine*, 2017 Jun 28, https://doi.org/10.1089/acm.2017.0081.

305. MA Ben-David, "Melatonin for Prevention of Breast Radiation Dermatitis: A Phase II, Prospective, Double-Blind Randomized Trial," *The Israeli Medical Association*, 2016 Mar–Apr, 18(3–4):188–92.

306. EJ Sánchez-Barceló et al., "Clinical uses of melatonin: evaluation of human trial," *Current Medicinal Chemistry*, 2010, 17(19):2070–95.

307. K Hirsch et al., "Effect of purified allicin, the major ingredient in freshly crushed garlic, on cancer cell proliferation," *Nutrition and Cancer*, 2000, 38(2):245–54.

308. H Ishikawa et al., "Aged garlic extract prevents a decline of NK cell number and activity in patients with advanced cancer," *Journal of Nutrition*, Mar 2006, 136(3 Suppl):816S–820S.

309. SC Ho and MS Su, "Evaluating the anti-neuroinflammatory capacity of raw and steamed garlic as well as five organosulfur compounds," *Molecules*, 2014, 19(11):17697–17714, https://doi.org/10.3390/molecules191117697.

310. KL Liu, "DATS reduces LPS-induced iNOS expression, NO production, oxidative stress, and NF-κB activation in RAW 264.7 macrophages," *Journal of Agricultural and Food Chemistry*, 2006, 54(9):3472–3478.

311. S You et al., "Inhibitory effects and molecular mechanisms of garlic organosulfur compounds on the production of inflammatory mediators," *Molecular Nutrition and Food Research*, 2013, 57(11):2049–2060, https://doi.org/10.1002/mnfr.201200843.

312. R Munday and CM Munday, "Induction of phase II enzymes by aliphatic sulfides derived from garlic and onions: an overview," *Methods in Enzymology*, 2004, 382:449–456.

313. S Hatono et al., "Chemopreventive effect of S-allylcysteine and its relationship to the detoxification enzyme glutathione S-transferase," *Carcinogenesis*, 1996, 17(5):1041–1044.

314. R Munday and CM Munday, "Relative activities of organosulfur compounds derived from onions and garlic in increasing tissue activities of quinone reductase and glutathione transferase in rat tissues," *Nutrition and Cancer*, 2001, 40(2):205–210.

315. PP Tadi et al., "Organosulfur compounds of garlic modulate mutagenesis, metabolism, and DNA binding of aflatoxin B1," *Nutrition and Cancer*, 1991, 15(2):87–95.

316. PZ Trio et al., "Chemopreventive functions and molecular mechanisms of garlic organosulfur compounds," *Food & Function*, 2014, 5(5):833–844, https://doi.org/10.1039/c3fo60479a.

317. AA Powolny and SV Singh, "Multitargeted prevention and therapy of cancer by diallyl trisulfide and related Allium vegetable-derived organosulfur compounds," *Cancer Letters*, 2008, 269(2):305–314, https://doi.org/10.1016/j.canlet.2008.05.027.

318. S Balasenthil et al., "Apoptosis induction by S-allylcysteine, a garlic constituent, during 7,12-dimethylbenz[a]anthracene-induced hamster buccal pouch carcinogenesis," *Cell Biochemistry and Function*, 2002, 20(3):263–268.

319. Powolny and Singh, "Multitargeted prevention and therapy of cancer by diallyl trisulfide."

320. RB Walter et al., "Vitamin, mineral, and specialty supplements and risk of hematologic malignancies in the prospective VITamins And Lifestyle (VITAL) study," *Cancer Epidemiology, Biomarkers & Prevention*, 2011 Oct, 20(10):2298–308, https://doi.org/10.1158/1055-9965.EPI-11-0494.

321. S Tanaka et al., "Aged garlic extract has potential suppressive effect on colorectal adenomas in humans," *Journal of Nutrition*, 2006, 136(3 Suppl):821S–826S.

322. L Bayan et al., "Garlic: a review of potential therapeutic effects," *Avicenna Journal of Phytomedicine*, 2014, 4(1):1–14.

323. F Borrelli et al., "Garlic (Allium sativum L.): adverse effects and drug interactions in humans," *Molecular Nutrition & Food Research*, 2007, 51(11):1386–1397.

324. H Amagase, "Clarifying the real bioactive constituents of garlic," *Journal of Nutrition*, 2006, 136(3 Suppl):716S–725S.

325. L Ernster, G Dallner, "Biochemical, physiological and medical aspects of ubiquinone function," *Biochimica et Biophysica Acta*, 1995, 1271(1):195–204.

326. R Saini, "Coenzyme Q10: The essential nutrient," *Journal of Pharmacy & BioAllied Sciences*, 2011 Jul–Sep, 3(3): 466–467. https://doi.org/10.4103/0975-7406.84471.

327. Saini, "Coenzyme Q10."

328. K Lockwood et al., "Partial and complete regression of breast cancer in patients in relation to dosage of coenzyme Q10," *Biochemical and Biophysical Research Communications*, 1994, 199(3):1504–8.

329. K Lockwood et al., "Progress on therapy of breast cancer with vitamin Q10 and the regression of metastasis," *Biochemical and Biophysical Research Communications*, 1995, 212(1):172–7.

330. EP Cortes et al., "Adriamycin cardiotoxicity: early detection by systolic time interval and possible prevention by coenzyme Q10," *Cancer Treatment Reports*, 1978, 62(6):887–91.

331. D Iarussi et al., "Protective effect of coenzyme Q10 on anthracyclines cardiotoxicity: control study in children with acute lymphoblastic leukemia and non-Hodgkin lymphoma," *Molecular Aspects of Medicine*, 1994, 15 (Suppl):S207–12.

332. F Scasso et al., "Dietary supplementation of coenzyme Q10 plus multivitamins to hamper the ROS mediated cisplatin ototoxicity in humans: A pilot study," *Heliyon*, 2017, 3(2):e00251, https://doi.org/10.1016/j.heliyon.2017.e00251.

333. L Rusciani et al., "Recombinant interferon alpha-2b and coenzyme Q10 as a postsurgical adjuvant therapy for melanoma: a 3-year trial with recombinant interferon-alpha and 5-year follow-up," *Melanoma Research*, 2007 Jun, 17(3):177–83.

334. K Folkers et al., "Activities of vitamin Q10 in animal models and a serious deficiency in patients with cancer," *Biochemical and Biophysical Research Communications*, 1997, 234(2):296–299.

335. CW Shults et al., "Effects of coenzyme Q10 in early Parkinson disease: evidence of slowing of the functional decline," *Archives of Neurology*, 2002, 59(10):1541–1550.

336. AM Heck et al., "Potential interactions between alternative therapies and warfarin," *American Journal of Health System Pharmacy*, 2000, 57(13):1221–1227, quiz 1228–1230.

337. S Shalansky et al., "Risk of warfarin-related bleeding events and supratherapeutic international normalized ratios associated with complementary and alternative medicine: a longitudinal analysis," *Pharmacotherapy*, 2007, 27(9):1237–47.

338. D Lopez-Vaquero et al., "Double-blind randomized study of oral glutamine on the management of radio/chemotherapy-induced mucositis and dermatitis in head and neck cancer," *Molecular and Clinical Oncology*, 2017 Jun, 6(6):931–936, https://doi.org/10.3892/mco.2017.1238.

339. HW Leung and AL Chan, "Glutamine in Alleviation of Radiation-Induced Severe Oral Mucositis: A Meta-Analysis," *Nutrition and Cancer*, 2016 Jul, 68(5):734–42, https://doi.org/10.1080/01635581.2016.1159700.

340. K Gul et al., "Oral glutamine supplementation reduces radiotherapy- induced esophagitis in lung cancer patients," *Asian Pacific Journal of Cancer Prevention*, 2015, 16(1):53–8.

341. A Papanikolopoulou et al., "The role of glutamine supplementation in thoracic and upper aerodigestive malignancies," *Nutrition and Cancer*, 2015, 67(2):231–7, https://doi.org/10.1080/01635581.2015.990572.

342. K Eda et al., "The effects of enteral glutamine on radiotherapy induced dermatitis in breast cancer," *Clinical Nutrition*, 2016 Apr, 35(2):436–9, https://doi.org/10.1016/j.clnu.2015.03.009.

343. SJ Padayatty et al., "Vitamin C pharmacokinetics: implications for oral and intravenous use," *Annals of Internal Medicine*, 2004 Apr 6, 140(7):533–7.

344. "Vitamin C," Linus Pauling Institute, accessed September 5, 2017, http://lpi.oregonstate.edu/mic/vitamins/vitamin-C.

345. G Muralikrishnan et al., "Effect of vitamin C on lipidperoxidation and antioxidant status in tamoxifen-treated breast cancer patients," *Chemotherapy*, 2010, 56(4):298–302, https://doi.org/10.1159/000320030.

346. S Zhang et al., "Dietary carotenoids and vitamins A, C, and E and risk of breast cancer," *Journal of the National Cancer Institute*, 1999, 91(6):547–556.

347. KB Michels, "Dietary antioxidant vitamins, retinol, and breast cancer incidence in a cohort of Swedish women," *International Journal of Cancer*, 2001, 91(4):563–567.

348. S Tsugane and S Sasazuki, "Diet and the risk of gastric cancer: review of epidemiological evidence," *Gastric Cancer*, 2007, 10(2):75–83.

349. CA Thompson and JR Cerhan, "Fruit and vegetable intake and survival from non-Hodgkin lymphoma: does an apple a day keep the doctor away?" *Leukemia & Lymphoma*, 2010, 51(6):963–964, https://doi.org/10.3109/10428194.2010.483305.

350. Y Park et al., "Intakes of vitamins A, C, and E and use of multiple vitamin supplements and risk of colon cancer: a pooled analysis of prospective cohort studies," *Cancer Causes Control*, 2010, 21(11):1745–1757, https://doi.org/10.1007/s10552-010-9549-y.

351. GC Kabat et al., "Intake of antioxidant nutrients and risk of non-Hodgkin's Lymphoma in the Women's Health Initiative," *Nutrition and Cancer*, 2012, 64(2):245–254, https://doi.org/10.1080/01635581.2012.642454.

352. LD Thomas et al., "Ascorbic acid supplements and kidney stone incidence among men: a prospective study," *JAMA Internal Medicine*, 2013 Mar 11, 173(5):386–388, https://doi.org/10.1001/jamainternmed.2013.2296.

353. L Zhang and IR Tizard, "Activation of a mouse macrophage cell line by acemannan: the major carbohydrate fraction from Aloe vera gel," *Immunopharmacology*, 1996 Nov, 35(2):119–28.

354. JK Lee et al., "Acemannan purified from Aloe vera induces phenotypic and functional maturation of immature dendritic cells," *International Immunopharmacology*, 2001 Jul, 1(7):1275–84.

355. KH Lee et al., "Anti-leukaemic and anti-mutagenic effects of di(2-ethylhexyl) phthalate isolated from Aloe vera Linne," *Journal of Pharmacy and Pharmacology*, 2000 May, 52(5):593–8.

356. X Chang et al., "Aloe-emodin suppresses esophageal cancer cell TE1 proliferation by inhibiting AKT and ERK phosphorylation," *Oncology Letters*, 2016 Sep, 12(3):2232–2238, https://doi.org/10.3892/ol.2016.4910.

357. PL Kuo et al., "The antiproliferative activity of aloe-emodin is through p53-dependent and p21-dependent apoptotic pathway in human hepatoma cell lines," *Life Sciences*, 2002 Sep 6, 71(16):1879–92.

358. P Lissoni et al., "A randomized study of chemotherapy versus biochemotherapy with chemotherapy plus Aloe arborescens in patients with metastatic cancer," *In Vivo*, 2009 Jan–Feb, 23(1):171–5.

359. M Sahebjamee et al., "Comparative efficacy of Aloe vera and benzydamine mouthwashes on radiation-induced oral mucositis: a triple-blind, randomised, controlled clinical trial," *Oral Health & Preventive Dentistry*, 2015, 13(4):309–15, https://doi.org/10.3290/j.ohpd.a33091.

360. A Ruban et al., "Blood glutamate scavengers prolong the survival of rats and mice with brain-implanted gliomas," *Investigational New Drugs*, 2012, 30(6): 2226–2235, https://doi.org/10.1007/s10637-012-9794-x.

361. M Boyko et al. "Brain to blood glutamate scavenging as a novel therapeutic modality: a review," *Journal of Neural Transmission* (Vienna, Austria: 1996), 2014, 121(8):971–979, https://doi.org/10.1007/s00702-014-1181-7.

362. M Gottlieb et al., "Blood-mediated scavenging of cerebrospinal fluid glutamate," *Journal of Neurochemistry*, 2003 Oct, 87(1):119–26, https://doi.org/10.1046/j.1471-4159.2003.01972.x.

363. A Zlotnik et al., "The contribution of the blood glutamate scavenging activity of pyruvate to its neuroprotective properties in a rat model of closed head injury," *Neurochemical Research*, 2008 Jun, 33(6):1044–50, https://doi.org/10.1007/s11064-007-9548-x.

364. A Zlotnik et al., "The Neuroprotective Effects of Oxaloacetate in Closed Head Injury in Rats is Mediated by its Blood Glutamate Scavenging Activity: Evidence From the Use of Maleate," *Journal of Neurosurgical Anesthesiology*, 2009 Jul, 21(3):235–241, https://doi.org/10.1097/ANA.0b013e3181a2bf0b.

365. A Zlotnik et al., "Effect of glutamate and blood glutamate scavengers oxaloacetate and pyruvate on neurological outcome and pathohistology of the hippocampus after traumatic brain injury in rats," *Anesthesiology*, 2012 Jan, 116(1):73–83, https://doi.org/10.1097/ALN.0b013e31823d7731.

366. W Rzeski et al., "Glutamate antagonists limit tumor growth," *Proceedings of the National Academy of Sciences*, 2001, 98(11):6372–6377, https://doi.org/10.1073pnas.091113598.

367. A Stepulak et al., "Glutamate and its receptors in cancer," *Journal of Neural Transmission* (Vienna), 2014, 121(8):933–944, https://doi.org/10.1007/s00702-014-1182-6.

368. HM Wilkins et al., "Oxaloacetate activates brain mitochondrial biogenesis, enhances the insulin pathway, reduces inflammation and stimulates neurogenesis," *Human Molecular Genetics*, 2014, 23(24) 6528–6541, https://doi.org/10.1093/hmg/ddu371.

369. RH Swerdlow et al., "Tolerability and pharmacokinetics of oxaloacetate 100 mg capsules in Alzheimer's subjects." *BBA Clinical*, 2016, 10(5):120–123, https://doi.org/10.1016/j.bbacli.2016.03.005.

370. FJ Antonawich et al., "Regulation of ischemic cell death by the lipoic acid-palladium complex, Poly MVA, in gerbils," *Experimental Neurology*, 2004 Sep, 189(1):10–5. PMID: 15296831.

371. NP Sudheesh, "Palladium-α-lipoic acid complex attenuates alloxan-induced hyperglycemia and enhances the declined blood antioxidant status in diabetic rats," *Journal of Diabetes*, 2011 Dec, 3(4):293–300, https://doi.org/10.1111/j.1753-0407.2011.00142.x.

372. RK Veena et al., "Antitumor Effects of Palladium-α-Lipoic Acid Complex Formulation as an Adjunct in Radiotherapy," *Journal of Environmental Pathology, Toxicology, and Oncology,* 2016, 35(4):333–342, https://doi.org/10.1615/JEnvironPatholToxicolOncol.2016016640.

373. L Wark, "Poly-MVA: A New Cancer Breakthrough for Advanced Cancer Patients," accessed September 1, 2017, http://www.centurywellness.com/article-archives/233-poly-mva-new-cancer-breakthrough-for-advanced-cancer-patients.

374. Wark, "Poly-MVA."

375. J Forsythe, "Forsythe Protocol/Poly-MVA," accessed September 1, 2017, http://www.drforsythe.com/main-news/309-forsythe-protocol-poly-mva.

376. Forsythe, "Forsythe Protocol/Poly-MVA."

377. Forsythe, "Forsythe Protocol/Poly-MVA."

378. Veena et al., "Antitumor Effects of Palladium-α-Lipoic Acid Complex."

379. V Sridharan et al., "Late administration of a palladium lipoic acid complex (POLY-MVA) modifies cardiac mitochondria but not functional or structural manifestations of radiation-induced heart disease in a rat model," *Radiation Research,* 2017 Mar, 187(3):361–366, https://doi.org/10.1667/RR14643.1.

380. "Palladium's uses in health care," *The Pharmaceutical Journal* (blog), accessed September 1, 2017, http://www.pharmaceutical-journal.com/opinion/blogs/palladiums-uses-in-health-care/10993897.blog.

381. K Nesaretnam, " Multitargeted therapy of cancer by tocotrienols," *Cancer Letters,* 2008 Oct 8, ;269(2):388–95. Doi: http://dx.doi.org/10.1016/j.canlet.2008.03.063.

382. E Pierpaoli, E et al., "Gamma- and delta-tocotrienols exert a more potent anticancer effect than alpha-tocopheryl succinate on breast cancer cell lines irrespective of HER-2/neu expression," *Life Sciences,* 2010, 86(17–18): p. 668–75, https://doi.org/10.1016/j.lfs.2010.02.018.

383. PW Sylvester et al, "Potential role of tocotrienols in the treatment and prevention of breast cancer. Biofactors," 2014; 40(1):49-58. Epub 2013/06/28.

384. K Nesaretnam et al., "Tocotrienol levels in adipose tissue of benign and malignant breast lumps in patients in Malaysia," *Asia Pacific Journal of Clinical Nutrition,* 2007, 16(3):498–504.

385. K Nesaretnam et al., "Effectiveness of tocotrienol-rich fraction combined with tamoxifen in the management of women with early breast cancer: a pilot clinical trial," *Breast Cancer Research: BCR,* 2010, 12(5):R81, https://doi.org/10.1186/bcr2726.

386. K Husain et al., "δ-Tocotrienol, a natural form of vitamin E, inhibits pancreatic cancer stem-like cells and prevents pancreatic cancer metastasis," *Oncotarget,* 2017, 8(19):31554–31567, https://doi.org/doi:10.18632/oncotarget.15767.

387. K Husain et al., "Vitamin E δ-Tocotrienol Augments the Anti-tumor Activity of Gemcitabine and Suppresses Constitutive NF-κB Activation in Pancreatic Cancer," *Molecular Cancer Therapeutics*, 2011, 10(12):2363–2372, https://doi.org/10.1158/1535-7163.MCT-11-0424.

388. D O''Byrneet al., "Studies of LDL oxidation following alpha-, gamma-, or delta-tocotrienyl acetate supplementation of hypercholesterolemic humans," *Free Radical Biology and Medicine*, 2000, 29(9): p. 834–45, https://doi.org/10.1016/S0891-5849(00)00371-3.

389. KW Tsang et al., "Coriolus versicolor polysaccharide peptide slows progression of advanced non-small cell lung cancer," *Respiratory Medicine*, 2003, 97(6): 618–24.

390. X Yang et al., "The cell death process of the anticancer agent polysaccharide-peptide (PSP) in human promyelocytic leukemic HL-60 cells," *Oncology Reports*, 2005, 13(6): 1201–10.

391. CB Lau et al., "Cytotoxic activities of Coriolus versicolor (Yunzhi) extract on human leukemia and lymphoma cells by induction of apoptosis," *Life Sciences*, 2004, 75(7): 797–808.

392. JM Wan et al., "Polysaccharopeptides derived from Coriolus versicolor potentiate the S-phase specific cytotoxicity of Camptothecin (CPT) on human leukemia HL-60 cells," *Chinese Medicine*, 2010, 5:16, https://doi.org/10.1186/1749-8546-5-16.

393. J Jiang and D Sliva, "Novel medicinal mushroom blend suppresses growth and invasiveness of human breast cancer cells," *International Journal of Oncology*, 2010 Dec, 37(6):1529–36.

394. M Kato et al., "Induction of gene expression for immunomodulating cytokines in peripheral blood mononuclear cells in response to orally administered PSK, an immunomodulating protein-bound polysaccharide," *Cancer Immunology and Immunotherapy*, 1995, 40(3):152–6.

395. PM Kidd, "The use of mushroom glucans and proteoglycans in cancer treatment," *Alternative Medicine Review*, 2000 Feb, 5(1):4–27.

396. Mark Stengler, *The Health Benefits of Medicinal Mushrooms* (North Bergen: Basic Health Publications, 2005), 19.

397. K Hayakawa et al., "Effect of krestin (PSK) as adjuvant treatment on the prognosis after radical radiotherapy in patients with non-small cell lung cancer," *Anticancer Research*, 1993 Sep–Oct, 13(5C):1815–20.

398. M Torisu et al., "Significant prolongation of disease-free period gained by oral polysaccharide K (PSK) administration after curative surgical operation of colorectal cancer," *Cancer Immunology and Immunotherapy*, 1990, 31(5):261–8.

399. H Nakazato et al., "Efficacy of immunochemotherapy as adjuvant treatment after curative resection of gastric cancer. Study Group of Immunochemotherapy with PSK for Gastric Cancer," *The Lancet*. 1994 May 7, 343(8906):1122–6, https://doi.org/10.1016/S0140-6736(94)90233-X.

400. Mark Stengler, *The Health Benefits of Medicinal Mushrooms* (North Bergen: Basic Health Publications, 2005), 19.

401. K Ogoshi et al., "Possible predictive markers of immunotherapy in esophageal cancer: retrospective analysis of a randomized study. The Cooperative Study Group for Esophageal Cancer in Japan," *Cancer Investigation*, 1995, 13:363–369.

402. M Toi et al., "Randomized adjuvant trial to evaluate the addition of tamoxifen and PSK to chemotherapy in patients with primary breast cancer. 5-Year results from the Nishi-Nippon Group of the Adjuvant Chemoendocrine Therapy for Breast Cancer Organization," *Cancer*, 1992, 70(10):2475–2483.

403. T Morimoto et al., "Postoperative adjuvant randomised trial comparing chemoendocrine therapy, chemotherapy and immunotherapy for patients with stage II breast cancer: 5-year results from the Nishinihon Cooperative Study Group of Adjuvant Chemoendocrine Therapy for Breast Cancer (ACETBC) of Japan," *European Journal of Cancer*, 1996, 32A(2):235–242.

404. T Yokoe et al., "HLA antigen as predictive index for the outcome of breast cancer patients with adjuvant immunochemotherapy with PSK," *Anticancer Research*, 1997 Jul–Aug, 17(4A):2815–8.

405. LJ Standish et al., "Trametes versicolor mushroom immune therapy in breast cancer," *Journal of the Society for Integrative Oncology*, 2008 Summer, 6(3):122–8, https://www.researchgate.net/publication/23668727_Trametes_versicolor_Mushroom_Immune_Therapy_in_Breast_Cancer.

406. Z Sun et al., "The ameliorative effect of PSP on the toxic and side reaction of chemo and radiotherapy of cancers," in *Advanced Research in PSP*, QY Yang, ed. (Hong Kong: Hong Kong Association for Health Care Ltd, 1999).

407. Mark Stengler, 22.

408. S Samuel and MD Sitrin, "Vitamin D's role in cell proliferation and differentiation," *Nutrition Reviews*, 2008 Oct, 66(10 Suppl 2):S116–24 https://doi.org/10.1111/j.1753-4887.2008.00094.x.

409. JC Fleet et al., "Vitamin D and Cancer: A Review of Molecular Mechanisms," *The Biochemical Journal*, 2012, 441(1):61–76, https://doi.org/10.1042/BJ20110744.

410. D Hummel et al., "The vitamin D system is deregulated in pancreatic diseases," *The Journal of Steroid Biochemistry and Molecular Biology*, 2014 Oct, 144 Pt. B:402–9, https://doi.org/10.1016/j.jsbmb.2014.07.011.

411. JM Lappe et al., "Vitamin D and calcium supplementation reduces cancer risk: results of a randomized trial," *American Journal of Clinical Nutrition*, 2007 Jun, 85(6):1586–91.

412. SL McDonnell et al., "Serum 25-Hydroxyvitamin D Concentrations ≥40 ng/ml Are Associated with >65% Lower Cancer Risk: Pooled Analysis of Randomized Trial and Prospective Cohort Study," *PLOS ONE*, 2016, https://doi.org/10.1371/journal.pone.0152441.

413. ML Neuhouser et al., "Vitamin D insufficiency in a multiethnic cohort of breast cancer survivors," *American Journal of Clinical Nutrition,* 2008 Jul, 88(1):133–139.

414. SR Bauer et al., "Plasma vitamin D levels, menopause, and risk of breast cancer: dose-response meta-analysis of prospective studies," *Medicine (Baltimore),* 2013, 92(3):123–131, https://doi.org/10.1097/MD.0b013e3182943bc2.

415. Y Kim and Y Je , "Vitamin D intake, blood 25(OH)D levels, and breast cancer risk or mortality: a meta-analysis," *British Journal of Cancer,* 2014 May 27, 110(11):2772–84, https://doi.org/10.1038/bjc.2014.175.

416. ST Lim et al., "Association between alterations in the serum 25-hydroxyvitamin d status during follow-up and breast cancer patient prognosis," *Asian Pacific Journal of Cancer Prevention,* 2015, 16(6):2507–13.

417. Y Ma et al., "Association between vitamin D and risk of colorectal cancer: a systematic review of prospective studies," *Journal of Clinical Oncology.* 2011 Oct 1;29(28):3775–3782. doi: 10.1200/JCO.2011.35.7566.

418. C Buttigliero et al., "Prognostic role of vitamin D status and efficacy of vitamin D supplementation in cancer patients: a systematic review," *The Oncologist,* 2011, 16(9):1215–1227, https://doi.org/10.1634/theoncologist.2011-0098.

419. DT Marshall et al., "Vitamin D3 supplementation at 4000 International Units per day for one year results in a decrease of positive cores at repeat biopsy in subjects with low-risk prostate cancer under active surveillance," *The Journal of Clinical Endocrinology & Metabolism,* 2012;9(7):2315–24. doi: 10.1210/jc.2012-1451.

420. IM Shui et al., "Vitamin D-related genetic variation, plasma vitamin D, and risk of lethal prostate cancer: a prospective nested case-control study," *Journal of the National Cancer Institute,* 2012, 104(9):690–9, https://doi.org/10.1093/jnci/djs189.

421. S Tretli, "Association between serum 25(OH)D and death from prostate cancer," *British Journal of Cancer,* 2009, 100(3):450–4 https://doi.org/10.1038/sj.bjc.6604865.

422. "Vitamin D," Linus Pauling Institute, accessed August 25, 2017, http://lpi.oregonstate.edu/mic/vitamins/vitamin-D#safety.

423. "Vitamin D," Linus Pauling Institute.

424. L Davenport, "Vitamin D3, Not D2, Is Key to Tackling Vitamin D Deficiency," Medscape.com, accessed July 5, 2017, http://www.medscape.com/viewarticle/882482.

425. SL McDonnell et al., "Serum 25-hydroxyvitamin D concentrations ≥40 ng/ml are associated with >65% lower cancer risk: pooled analysis of randomized trial and prospective cohort study," 2016 Apr 6, 11(4):e0152441, https://doi.org/10.1371/journal.pone.0152441.

CHAPTER 7

1. SJ Padayattyet al., "Vitamin C pharmacokinetics: implications for oral and intravenous use," *Annals of Internal Medicine*, 2004, 140(7):533–537, https://doi.org/10.7326/0003-4819-140-7-200404060-00010.

2. A Oppenheimer, "Turmeric (Curcumin) in Biliary Diseases," *The Lancet*, 1937 Mar 13, 229(5924):619–621, https://doi.org/10.1016/S0140-6736(00)98193-5.

3. F Klenner, "Virus Pneumonia and its Treatment with Vitamin C", *Southern Medicine & Surgery*, 1948 Feb, 110(2):36–38, 46.

4. F Klenner, "Encephalitis as a Sequela of the Pneumonias," *Tri-State Medical Journal*, 1960 Feb.

5. F Klenner, "An Insidious Virus", *Tri-State Medical Journal*, 1957 Jun.

6. Linus Pauling, *Vitamin C and the Common Cold*, San Francisco: W. F. Freeman & Co., 1970.

7. *Vitamin C as a Fundamental Medicine: Abstracts of Dr. Frederick R. Klenner, M.D.'s Published and Unpublished Work*, ISBN 0-943685-13-3, first printing 1988.

8. L Smith, "Clinical Guide to the Use of Vitamin C: The Clinical Experiences of Frederick R. Klenner, M.D.," https://www.seanet.com/~alexs/ascorbate/198x/smith-lh-clinical_guide_1988.htm.

9. Q Chen et al., "Ascorbate in pharmacologic concentrations selectively generates ascorbate radical and hydrogen peroxide in extracellular fluid in vivo", *Proceedings of the Natlional Academy of Sciences of the United States of America*, 2007, 104(21):8749–54, https://doi.org/10.1073/pnas.0702854104.

10. SJ Padayatty et al. "Vitamin C: Intravenous Use by Complementary and Alternative Medicine Practitioners and Adverse Effects", *PLoS ONE*, 2010, 5(7):e11414:1-8, https://doi.org/10.1371/journal.pone.0011414.

11. J Verrax and PB Calderon. "The controversial place of vitamin C in cancer treatment," *Biochemical Pharmacology*, 2008, 76(12):1644–1652, https://doi.org/10.1016/j.bcp.2008.09.024.

12. Q Chen et al. "Ascorbate in pharmacologic concentrations selectively generates ascorbate radical and hydrogen peroxide in extracellular fluid in vivo," *Proceedings of the Natlional Academy of Sciences of the United States of America*, 2007, 104(21):8749–54, https://doi.org/10.1073/pnas.0702854104.

13. Verrax and Calderon, "The controversial place of vitamin C in cancer treatment."

14. R Hunninghake, "Adjunctive IVC Therapy Help Cancer Patients Update." 3rd Annual Conference and Expo IV Therapies 2014 Integrative Oncology, January 25, 2014.

15. Hunninghake, "Adjunctive IVC Therapy."

16. NA Mikirova et al. "Intravenous ascorbic acid protocol for cancer patients: scientific rationale, pharmacology, and clinical experience," *Functional Foods in Health and Disease*, 2013, 3(8):344–366, http://functionalfoodscenter.net/files/73514619.pdf.

17. SJ Padayatty et al. "Vitamin C: intravenous use by complementary and alternative medicine practitioners and adverse effects."

18. Paul S Anderson, "Ascorbate and Oncologic Therapies: Research Review," 2013, https://www.academia.edu/10024397/Ascorbate_and_Oncologic_Therapies_Research_Review.

19. M Levine, et.al. "Vitamin C: a concentration-function approach yields pharmacology and therapeutic discoveries," *Advances in Nutrition*, 2011, 2:78–88, https://doi.org/10.3945/an.110.000109.

20. Verrax and Calderon, "The controversial place of vitamin C in cancer treatment."

21. JR Berensonet al., "Bortezomib, ascorbic acid and melphalan (BAM) therapy for patients with newly diagnosed multiple myeloma: an effective and well-tolerated frontline regimen" *European Journal of Haematology*, 2009, 82(6):433–9, https://doi.org/10.1111/j.1600-0609.2009.01244.x.

22. H Takahashi et al., "A High-dose intravenous vitamin C improves quality of life in cancer patients," *Personalized Medicine Universe*, 2012 Jul, 1(1):49–53, https://doi.org/10.1016/j.pmu.2012.05.008.

23. CH Yeom et al., "Changes of terminal cancer patients' health-related quality of life after high dose vitamin C administration," *Journal of Korean Medical Science*, 22(1):7–11, https://doi.org/10.3346/jkms.2007.22.1.7.

24. P Anderson, "Intravenous Vitamin C in Naturopathic Oncology," scientific presentation, Oncology Association of Naturopathic Physicians, Scottsdale, Arizona, 2012.

25. AC Carr et al., "The Effect of Intravenous Vitamin C on Cancer- and Chemotherapy-Related Fatigue and Quality of Life," *Frontiers in Oncology*, 2014, 4:283, https://doi.org/10.3389/fonc.2014.00283.

26. Roxanne Nelson, "Can Integrative Oncology Extend Life in Advanced Disease?" Medscape.com, accessed September 17, 2017, http://www.medscape.com/viewarticle/813217.

27. Paul S Anderson, "Updated Data Review and Policies for concurrent use at Anderson Medical Specialty Associates, Southwest College of Naturopathic Medicine Research Institute and Medical Center and Bastyr University Clinical Research Center." 3rd Annual Conference and Expo IV Therapies 2014 Integrative Oncology, January 25, 2014.

28. T Efferth and B Kaina, "Toxicity of the antimalarial artemisinin and its derivatives," *Critical Reviews in Toxicology*, 2010, 40(5):405–421, https://doi.org/10.3109/10408441003610571.

29. TME Davis et al., "Pharmacokinetics and Pharmacodynamics of Intravenous Artesunate in Severe Falciparum Malaria," *Antimicrobial Agents and Chemotherapy,* 2001 Jan, 45(1):181–186, https://doi.org/10.1128/AAC.45.1.181-186.2001.

30. T Gordi and EI Lepist, "Artemisinin derivatives: toxic for laboratory animals, safe for humans?" *Toxicology Letters,* 2004, 147(2):99–107.

31. B Medhi et al., "Pharmacokinetic and toxicological profile of artemisinin compounds: an update," *Pharmacology,* 2009; 84(6):323–332, https://doi.org/10.1159/000252658.

32. KL Jones, S Donegan, DG Lalloo, "Treating severe malaria: Artesunate versus quinine?" *Indian Pediatrics,* 2008 Jan 17, 45(41).

33. AM Dondorp et al., "Artesunate versus quinine in the treatment of severe falciparum malaria in African children (AQUAMAT): an open-label, randomised trial," *The Lancet,* 2010 Nov 13, 376(9753)1647–1657, https://doi.org/10.1016/S0140-6736(10)61924-1.

34. PJ Rosenthal, "Artesunate for the Treatment of Severe Falciparum Malaria," *The New England Journal of Medicine,* 2008, 358:1829–36, https://doi.org/ 10.1056/NEJMct0709050.

35. JH Du et al., "Artesunate induces oncosis-like cell death in vitro and has antitumor activity against pancreatic cancer xenografts in vivo," *Cancer Chemotherapy and Pharmacology,* 2010, 65(5):895–902, https://doi.org/10.1007/s00280-009-1095-5.

36. LH Stockwin, et. al. "Artemisinin dimer anticancer activity correlates with heme-catalyzed reactive oxygen species generation and endoplasmic reticulum stress induction," *International Journal of Cancer,* 2009 September 15, 125(6): 1266–1275, https://doi.org/10.1002/ijc.24496.

37. T Efferth, "Molecular pharmacology and pharmacogenomics of artemisinin and its derivatives in cancer cells," *Current Drug Targets,* 2006, 7:407–21.

38. IH Paik et al., "Second generation, orally active, antimalarial, artemisinin-derived trioxane dimers with high stability, efficacy, and anticancer activity," *Journal of Medicinal Chemistry,* 2006, 49(9):2731–4.

39. W Nam et al., "Effects of artemisinin and its derivatives on growth inhibition and apoptosis of oral cancer cells," *Head & Neck,* 2007, 29(4):335–40.

40. HH Chen et al., "Antimalarial dihydroartemisinin also inhibits angiogenesis," *Cancer Chemotherapy Pharmacology,* 2004, 53(5):423–432, https://doi.org/10.1007/s00280-003-0751-4.

41. G Kelter et al., "Role of Transferrin Receptor and the ABC Transporters ABCB6 and ABCB7 for Resistance and Differentiation of Tumor Cells towards Artesunate," *PLoS ONE,* 2007, 2(8):e798, https://doi.org/10.1371/journal.pone.0000798.

42. MP Crespo-Ortiz and MQ Wei, "Antitumor Activity of Artemisinin and Its Derivatives: From a Well-Known Antimalarial Agent to a Potential Anticancer Drug," *Journal of Biomedicine and Biotechnology,* 2012:247597, https://doi.org/10.1155/2012/247597.

43. C Shi et al., "Anti-Inflammatory and Immunoregulatory Functions of Artemisinin and Its Derivatives," *Mediators of Inflammation*, 2015:435713, http://dx.doi.org/10.1155/2015/435713.

44. Ouyang Jin et al., "A Pilot Study of the Therapeutic Efficacy and Mechanism of Artesunate in the MRL/lpr Murine Model of Systemic Lupus Erythematosus," *Cellular & Molecular Immunology*, 2009, 6:461-467, https://doi.org/10.1038/cmi.2009.58.

45. Z Wang et.al., "Anti-Inflammatory Properties and Regulatory Mechanism of a Novel Derivative of Artemisinin in Experimental Autoimmune Encephalomyelitis," *The Journal of Immunology*, 2007, 179(9):5958–5965.

46. L Hou et al., "Artesunate Abolishes Germinal Center B Cells and Inhibits Autoimmune Arthritis," *PLoS ONE*, 9(8): e104762, https://doi.org/10.1371/journal.pone.0104762.

47. Roxanne Nelson, "Can Integrative Oncology Extend Life in Advanced Disease?" 10th International Conference of the Society for Integrative Oncology (SIO): Abstract 79, presented October 21, 2013. http://www.medscape.com/viewarticle/813217.

48. Q Chen et. al., "Ascorbate in pharmacologic concentrations selectively generates ascorbate radical and hydrogen peroxide in extracellular fluid in vivo," *Proceedings of the National Academy of Sciences of the United States of America*, 2007, 104(21):8749–54, https://doi.org/10.1073/pnas.0702854104.

49. RC Siwaleet al., "The effect of intracellular antioxidant delivery (catalase) on hydrogen peroxide and proinflammatory cytokine synthesis: a new therapeutic horizon," *Journal of Drug Targeting*, 17(9):710–718, https://doi.org/10.3109/10611860903161328.

50. MS Zadeh et al. "Regulation of ICAM/CD54 expression on human endothelial cells by hydrogen peroxide involves inducible NO synthase," *Journal of Leukocyte Biology*, 2000, 67:327–334.

51. B Clavo et al., "Ozone Therapy in the Management of Persistent Radiation-Induced Rectal Bleeding in Prostate Cancer Patients," *Evidence-based Complementary and Alternative Medicine*, 2015:480369, https://doi.org/10.1155/2015/480369.

52. A Kucukgul et al., "Beneficial effects of nontoxic ozone on H2O2-induced stress and inflammation," *Biochemistry and Cell Biology*, 2016 Dec, 94(6):577–583.

53. M Luongo et al., "Possible Therapeutic Effects of Ozone Mixture on Hypoxia in Tumor Development," *Anticancer Research*, 2017 Feb, 37(2):425–435.

54. HS Kızıltan et al., "Medical ozone and radiotherapy in a peritoneal, Erlich-ascites, tumor-cell model," *Alternative Therapies in Health and Medicine*, 2015 Mar–Apr,21(2):24–9.

55. V Bocci et al., "The ozone paradox: ozone is a strong oxidant as well as a medical drug," *Medicinal Research Reviews*, 2009 Jul, 29(4):646–82, https://doi.org/10.1002/med.20150.

56. VV Velikaya et al., "[Ozone therapy for radiation reactions and skin lesions after neutron therapy in patients with malignant tumors]," *Voprosy Onkologii*, 2015, 61(4):571–4. PMID: 26571824.

57. V Travagli et al., "Effects of ozone blood treatment on the metabolite profile of human blood," *International Journal of Toxicology*, 2010 Mar–Apr, 29(2):165–74, https://doi.org/10.1177/1091581809360069.

58. IE Ganelina et al., "[Therapy of severe stenocardia with ultraviolet blood irradiation (UVB) and various action mechanisms of this therapy]," *Folia Haematologica (Leipzig)*, 1982 Jan 1, 109(3):470–482. PMID:6182067.

59. As Mazepin et al., "[Experience with the use of UV irradiation of autologous blood in oral surgery]," *Stomatologiia (Mosk)*, 1990 May–Jun, 69(3):49–50. PMID: 2389276.

60. VI Karandashov et al., "[The mechanism of the action of UV-irradiated autotransfusions in treating patients with suppurative-inflammatory diseases of the face and neck]," *Vestnik Khirurgii Imini I. I. Grekova*, 1989 Oct, 143(10):92–4. PMID: 2631372.

61. TG van Rossum et al., "Intravenous glycyrrhizin for the treatment of chronic hepatitis C: a double-blind, randomized, placebo-controlled phase I/II trial," *Journal of Gastroenterology and Hepatology*, 1999 Nov, 14(11):1093–9.

62. TG van Rossum et al., "Pharmacokinetics of intravenous glycyrrhizin after single and multiple doses in patients with chronic hepatitis C infection," *Clinical Therapeutics*, 1999 Dec, 21(12):2080–90.

63. Paul S Anderson and Brenden Cochran, "Personal experiences with the clinical use of intravenous substances," AMSA, BIORC and private clinic data, Seattle, Washington, 2014.

64. S Thirugnanam et al. "Glycyrrhizin induces apoptosis in prostate cancer cell lines DU-145 and LNCaP," *Oncology Reports*, 2008 Dec, 20(6):1387–92. PMID: 19020719.

65. TG van Rossum et al., "'Pseudo-aldosteronism' induced by intravenous glycyrrhizin treatment of chronic hepatitis C patients," *Journal of Gastroenterology and Hepatology*, 2001 Jul, 16(7):789–95.

66. CR Jonas et al., "Plasma antioxidant status after high-dose chemotherapy: a randomized trial of parenteral nutrition in bone marrow transplantation patients," *The American Journal of Clinical Nutrition*, 2000, 72(1):181–9.

67. J Midander et al., "Reduced repair of potentially lethal radiation damage in glutathione synthetase-deficient human fibroblasts after X-irradiation," *International Journal of Radiation Biology and Related Studies in Physics, Chemistry, and Medicine*, 1986 Mar, 49(3):403–13. PMID: 3485589.

68. G Pujari et al., "Influence of glutathione levels on radiation-induced chromosomal DNA damage and repair in human peripheral lymphocytes," *Mutation Research*, 2009 Apr, 675(1–2):23–8. PMID: 19386243.

OUTSIDE THE BOX CANCER THERAPIES

69. G De Mattia et al., "Influence of reduced glutathione infusion on glucose metabolism in patients with non-insulin-dependent diabetes mellitus," *Metabolism*, 1998 Aug, 47(8):993–7. PMID: 9711998.

70. S Cascinu et al., "Neuroprotective Effect of Reduced Glutathione on Oxaliplatin-Based Chemotherapy in Advanced Colorectal Cancer: A Randomized, Double-Blind, Placebo-Controlled Trial," *Journal of Clinical Oncology*, 2002 Aug 15, 20(16):3478–3483, https://doi.org/10.1200/JCO.2002.07.061.

71. P Milla et al., "Administration of reduced glutathione in FOLFOX4 adjuvant treatment for colorectal cancer: effect on oxaliplatin pharmacokinetics, Pt-DNA adduct formation, and neurotoxicity," *Anticancer Drugs*, 2009 Jun, 20(5):396–402, https://doi.org/10.1097/CAD.0b013e32832a2dc1 PMID: 19287306.

72. Paul S Anderson, "IV Therapy Use and Compatibility Chart," https://www.academia.edu/21926047/IV_Therapy_Use_and_Compatibility_Chart_-Prepared_for_Anderson_Medical_Group_BCRC_and_SCRI_All_rights_reserved.

73. I Elisia et al., "DMSO Represses Inflammatory Cytokine Production from Human Blood Cells and Reduces Autoimmune Arthritis," *PLoS ONE*, 2016;11(3):e0152538, https://doi.org/10.1371/journal.pone.0152538.

74. BX Hoang et al., "Dimethyl Sulfoxide–Sodium Bicarbonate Infusion for Palliative Care and Pain Relief in Patients With Metastatic Prostate Cancer," *Journal of Pain & Palliative Care Pharmacotherapy*, 2011, 25(4):350–355, https://doi.org/10.3109/15360288.2011.606294.

75. BX Hoang et al., "Dimethyl sulfoxide and sodium bicarbonate in the treatment of refractory cancer pain," *Journal of Pain & Palliative Care Pharmacotherapy*, 2011, 25(1):19–24, https://doi.org/10.3109/15360288.2010.536306.

76. ML Blanke and AMJ VanDongen, "Chapter 13: Activation Mechanisms of the NMDA Receptor," in *Biology of the NMDA Receptor*, AM Van Dongen, ed. (Boca Raton (FL): CRC Press/Taylor & Francis; 2009), http://www.ncbi.nlm.nih.gov/books/NBK5274.

77. Tuba Berra Saritas et al., "Is intra-articular magnesium effective for postoperative analgesia in arthroscopic shoulder surgery?" *Pain Research & Management*, 2015 Jan–Feb, 20(1): 35–38, PMCID: PMC4325888.

78. BJ Kaplan et al., "Germane facts about germanium sesquioxide: I. Chemistry and anticancer properties," *Journal of Alternative and Complementary Medicine*, 2004 Apr, 10(2):337–44, https://doi.org/10.1089/107555304323062329.

79. NTanaka et al., "[Augmentation of NK activity in peripheral blood lymphocytes of cancer patients by intermittent GE-132 administration]," *Gan To Kagaku Ryoho*, 1984 Jun, 11(6):1303–6. PMID: 6732257.

80. GT Bolger et al., "Distribution and Metabolism of Lipocurc™ (Liposomal Curcumin) in Dog and Human Blood Cells: Species Selectivity and Pharmacokinetic Relevance," *Anticancer Research*, 2017 Jul, 37(7):3483–3492, https://doi.org/10.21873/anticanres.11716.

81. S Chiu et al., "Liposomal-formulated curcumin [Lipocurc™] targeting HDAC (histone deacetylase) prevents apoptosis and improves motor deficits in Park 7 (DJ-1)-knockout rat model of Parkinson's disease: implications for epigenetics-based nanotechnology-driven drug platform," *Journal of Complementary & Integrative Medicine*, 2013 Nov 7, 10, https://doi.org/10.1515/jcim-2013-0020.

82. N Ghalandarlaki et al., "Nanotechnology-Applied Curcumin for Different Diseases Therapy," *BioMed Research International*, 2014, 2014:394264, https://doi.org/10.1155/2014/394264.

83. Y Rivera-Espinoza and P Muriel, "Pharmacological actions of curcumin in liver diseases or damage," *Liver International*, 2009 Nov, 29(10):1457–66, https://doi.org/10.1111/j.1478-3231.2009.02086.x.

84. SC Gupta et al., "Therapeutic roles of curcumin: lessons learned from clinical trials," *The AAPS Journal*, 2013, 15(1):195–218, http://doi.org/10.1208/s12248-012-9432-8.

85. Gupta et al., "Therapeutic roles of curcumin."

86. NM Rogers et al., "Amelioration of renal ischaemia–reperfusion injury by liposomal delivery of curcumin to renal tubular epithelial and antigen-presenting cells," *British Journal of Pharmacology*, 2012, 166(1):194–209, https://doi.org/10.1111/j.1476-5381.2011.01590.x.

87. SS Ghosh et al. "Curcumin and enalapril ameliorate renal failure by antagonizing inflammation in 5⁄6 nephrectomized rats: role of phospholipase and cyclooxygenase," *American Journal of Physiology. Renal Physiology*, 2012, 302:F439–F454, https://doi.org/10.1152/ajprenal.00356.2010.

88. J Trujillo et al., "Renoprotective effect of the antioxidant curcumin: Recent findings," *Redox Biology*, 2013, 1:448–456, https://doi.org/10.1016/j.redox.2013.09.003.

89. F Zhong et al., "Curcumin Attenuates Lipopolysaccharide-Induced Renal Inflammation," *Biol. Pharm. Bull.*, 2011, 34(2):226–232, PMID: 21415532.

90. P Singh et al., "Unexpected effect of angiotensin AT1 receptor blockade on tubuloglomerular feedback in early subtotal nephrectomy," *American Journal of Physiology. Renal Physiology*, 2009, 296(5): F1158–F1165.

91. V Soetikno et al., "Curcumin alleviates oxidative stress, inflammation, and renal fibrosis in remnant kidney through the Nrf2-keap1 pathway," *Molecular Nutrition & Food Research*, 2013 Sep, 57(9):1649–59, https://doi.org/10.1002/mnfr.201200540.

92. SC Gupta et al., "Multitargeting by curcumin as revealed by molecular interaction studies," *Natural Products Reports*, 2011, 28(12):1937–55, https://doi.org/10.1039/c1np00051a.

93. S Reuter et al., "Epigenetic changes induced by curcumin and other natural compounds," *Genes & Nutrition*, 2011, 6(2):93–108, https://doi.org/10.1007/s12263-011-0222-1.

94. P Anand et al., "Curcumin and cancer: An 'old-age' disease with an 'age-old' solution," *Cancer Letters*, 2008, 267(1):133–164, https://doi.org/10.1016/j.canlet.2008.03.025.

95. L Li et al., "Liposome encapsulated curcumin: in vitro and in vivo effects on proliferation, apoptosis, signaling, and angiogenesis," *Cancer*, 2005, 104(6):1322–1331, https://doi.org/10.1002/cncr.21300.

96. N Dhillon et al., "Curcumin and pancreatic cancer: phase II clinical trial experience," *Journal of Clinical Oncology*, 2007, 25(18 supplement):4599, https://doi.org/10.1200/jco.2007.25.18_suppl.4599.

97. C Chen et al., "An in vitro study of liposomal curcumin: Stability, toxicity and biological activity in human lymphocytes and Epstein-Barr virus-transformed human B-cells," *International Journal of Pharmaceutics*, 2009 Jan., 366(1–2): 133–139, DOI: 10.1016/j.ijpharm.2008.09.009.

98. R Wilken et al. "Curcumin: A review of anti-cancer properties and therapeutic activity in head and neck squamous cell carcinoma," *Molecular Cancer*, 2011, 10:12, https://doi.org/10.1186/1476-4598-10-12.

99. R Kurzrock and L Li, "Liposome-encapsulated curcumin: in vitro and in vivo effects on proliferation, apoptosis, signaling, and angiogenesis," *Journal of Clinical Oncology*, 2005 June, 23(16S): 4091, DOI: 10.1200/jco.2005.23.16_suppl.4091.

100. MC Comelli et al. "Toward the definition of the mechanism of action of silymarin: activities related to cellular protection from toxic damage induced by chemotherapy," *Integrative Cancer Therapies*, 2007 Jun, 6(2):120–9, PMID: 17548791. DOI: 10.1177/1534735407302349.

101. K Ramasamy and R Agarwal, "Multitargeted therapy of cancer by silymarin," *Cancer Letters*, 2008 October 8, 269(2): 352–362. doi:10.1016/j.canlet.2008.03.053.

102. Kaur M and Agarwal R, "Silymarin and Epithelial Cancer Chemoprevention: How close we are to bedside?" *Toxicology and Applied Pharmacology*, 2007 November 1, 224(3): 350–359. doi:10.1016 /j.taap.2006.11.011.

103. M Vaid and SK Katiyar, "Molecular mechanisms of inhibition of photocarcinogenesis by silymarin, a phytochemical from milk thistle (Silybum marianum L. Gaertn)," *International Journal of Oncology*, 2010 May, 36(5): 1053–1060, PMID: 20372777.

104. C Sergides et al., "Bioavailability and safety study of resveratrol 500 mg tablets in healthy male and female volunteers." *Experimental and Therapeutic Medicine*, 2016, 11(1):164–170, doi:10.3892/etm.2015.2895.

105. LG Carter, JA D'Orazio and KJ Pearson, "Resveratrol and cancer: focus on in vivo evidence," *Endocrine-Related Cancer*, 2014, 21(3):R209–R225, doi:10.1530/ERC-13-0171.

106. S Gupta et al., "Chemosensitization of tumors by resveratrol," *Annals of the New York Academy of Sciences*, 1215 (2011) 150–160, doi: 10.1111/j.1749-6632.2010.05852.x.

107. M Athar et al., "Multiple molecular Targets of Resveratrol: Anti-carcinogenic Mechanisms," *Archives of Biochemistry and Biophysics*, 2009 June, 486(2): 95–102, doi:10.1016/j.abb.2009.01.018.

108. A Amri et al. "Administration of resveratrol: What formulation solutions to bioavailability limitations?" *Journal of Controlled Release*, 2012 Mar, 158(2): 182–193, doi: 10.1016/j.jconrel.2011.09.083.

109. JA Baur and DA Sinclair, "Therapeutic potential of resveratrol: the in vivo evidence," *Nature Reviews*. Drug Discovery, June 2006, 5(6):493–506, PMID: 16732220 DOI: 10.1038/nrd2060.

110. T Walle et al., "High Absorption But Very Low Bioavailability Of Oral Resveratrol In Humans," *Drug Metabolism and Disposition*, December 2004, 32(12): 1377–1382, doi: 10.1124/dmd.104.000885.

111. S Das, HS Lin, PC Ho and KY Ng, "The impact of aqueous solubility and dose on the pharmacokinetic profiles of resveratrol," *Pharmaceutical Research*, 2008 Nov, 25(11):2593–600, doi: 10.1007/s11095-008-9677-1, PMID: 18629618.

112. A Lodi et al., "Combinatorial treatment with natural compounds in prostate cancer inhibits prostate tumor growth and leads to key modulations of cancer cell metabolism," *Precision Oncology*, 2017, 1:18; doi:10.1038/s41698-017-0024-z.

113. R Gugler, M Leschik and HJ Dengler, "Disposition of quercetin in man after single oral and intravenous doses," *European Journal of Clinical Pharmacology*, 1975, 9(2–3): 229–234.

114. EU Graefe, H Derendorf and M Veit, "Pharmacokinetics and bioavailability of the flavonol quercetin in humans," *International Journal of Clinical Pharmacology and Therapeutics*, 1999 May, 37(5):219–33, PMID: 10363620.

115. DR Ferry, A Smith, J Malkhandi et al., "Phase I clinical trial of the flavonoid quercetin: pharmacokinetics and evidence for in vivo tyrosine kinase inhibition," *Clinical Cancer Research*, 1996, 2(4):659–668, PMID: 9816216.

116. Zhi-ping Yuan, Li-juan Chen, Lin-yu Fanet al., "Liposomal Quercetin Efficiently Suppresses Growth of Solid Tumors in Murine Models," *Clinical Cancer Research*, 2006, 12(10):3193–3199, PMID: 16707620, DOI: 10.1158/1078-0432.CCR-05-2365.

117. S Patel and S Panda, "Emerging roles of mistletoes in malignancy management," *3 Biotech*, 2014, 4(1):13–20, doi:10.1007/s13205-013-0124-6.

118. PR Bock et al., "Targeting inflammation in cancer-related-fatigue: a rationale for mistletoe therapy as supportive care in colorectal cancer patients," *Inflammation & Allergy Drug Targets*, 2014, 13(2):105–11, PMID 24766319.

119. S Braedel-Ruoff, "Immunomodulatory effects of Viscum album extracts on natural killer cells: review of clinical trials," *Forschende Komplementarmedizin*, 2010 Apr, 17(2):63–73, doi: 10.1159/000288702, PMID 20484913.

120. R Attar et al., "Natural products are the future of anticancer therapy: Preclinical and clinical advancements of Viscum album phytometabolites," *Cellular and Molecular Biology (Noisy-le-grand)*, 2015 Oct 30, 61(6):62–8, PMID 26518897.

121. U Weissenstein et al., "Interaction of standardized mistletoe (Viscum album) extracts with chemotherapeutic drugs regarding cytostatic and cytotoxic effects in vitro," *BMC Complementary and Alternative Medicine*, 2014 Jan 8, 14:6, doi: 10.1186/1472-6882-14-6, PMID 24397864.

122. SB Sunjic et al., "Adjuvant Cancer Biotherapy by Viscum Album Extract Isorel: Overview of Evidence Based Medicine Findings," *Collegium Antropologicum*, 2015, 39(3):701–8, PMID 26898069.

123. T Ostermann et al., "Retrospective studies on the survival of cancer patients treated with mistletoe extracts: a meta-analysis," *Explore (NY)*, 2012 Sep–Oct, 8(5):277–81, doi: 10.1016/j.explore.2012.06.005, PMID 22938746.

124. S Wrotek et al., "[Immunostimulatory properties of mistletoe extracts and their application in oncology]," *Postepy Higieny i Medycyny Doswiadczalnej* (Online), 2014 Oct 23, 68:1216–24, doi: 10.5604/17322693.1126850, PMID 25380204.

125. N Yamamoto, H Suyama and N Yamamoto, "Immunotherapy for Prostate Cancer with Gc Protein-Derived Macrophage-Activating Factor, GcMAF," *Translational Oncology*, 2008, 1(2):65–72, PMID: 18633461.

126. HM Arafa, "Possible contribution of beta-glucosidase and caspases in the cytotoxicity of glufosfamide in colon cancer cells," *European Journal of Pharmacology*, 2009 Aug 15, 616(1–3):58–63, doi: 10.1016/j.ejphar.2009.06.024, PMID: 19545561.

127. KN Syrigos, G Rowlinson-Busza and AA Epenetos, "In vitro cytotoxicity following specific activation of amygdalin by β-glucosidase conjugated to a bladder cancer-associated monoclonal antibody," *International Journal of Cancer*, 78(6):712–719, 1998, PMID: 9833764.

128. L Thyer, E Ward, R Smith et al., "GC protein-derived macrophage-activating factor decreases α-N-acetylgalactosaminidase levels in advanced cancer patients," *Oncoimmunology*, 2013, 2(8):e25769, doi:10.4161/onci.25769.

129. N Yamamoto, H Suyama and N Yamamoto, "Immunotherapy for Prostate Cancer with Gc Protein-Derived Macrophage-Activating Factor, GcMAF," *Translational Oncology*, 2008, 1(2):65–72, PMID: 18633461.

130. KN Syrigos, G Rowlinson-Busza and AA Epenetos, "In vitro cytotoxicity following specific activation of amygdalin by β-glucosidase conjugated to a bladder cancer-associated monoclonal antibody," *International Journal of Cancer*, 78(6):712–719, 1998, PMID: 9833764.

131. CG Moertel et al., "A clinical trial of amygdalin (Laetrile) in the treatment of human cancer," *New England Journal of Medicine*, 1982 Jan 28, 306(4):201–6, PMID: 7033783.

132. Z Song and X Xu, "Advanced research on anti-tumor effects of amygdalin," *Journal of Cancer Research and Therapeutics*, 2014 Aug, 10 Suppl 1:3–7, doi: 10.4103/0973-1482.139743, PMID: 25207888.

133. NP Sudheesh, TA Ajith, KK Janardhanan and CV Krishnan, "Palladium alpha-lipoic acid complex formulation enhances activities of Krebs cycle dehydrogenases and respiratory complexes I-IV in the heart of aged rats," *Food and Chemical Toxicology*, 2009 Aug, 47(8):2124–8, doi: 10.1016/j.fct.2009.05.032, PMID: 19500641.

134. TA Ajith, N Nima, RK Veena, KK Janardhanan, F Antonawich, "Effect of palladium α-lipoic acid complex on energy in the brain mitochondria of aged rats," *Alternative Therapies in Health and Medicine*, 2014 May–Jun, 20(3):27–35, PMID:24755568.

135. A Menon and CKK Nair, "Poly MVA–a dietary supplement containing α-lipoic acid palladium complex, enhances cellular DNA repair," *International Journal of Low Radiation*, 8(1): (2011) 42–54.

136. NP Sudheesh et al., "Effect of POLY-MVA, a palladium alpha-lipoic acid complex formulation against declined mitochondrial antioxidant status in the myocardium of aged rats," *Food and Chemical Toxicology*, 2010 Jul, 48(7):1858–62, doi: 10.1016/j.fct.2010.04.022, PMID: 20412826.

137. FJ Antonawich, SM Fiore and LM Welicky, "Regulation of ischemic cell death by the lipoic acid-palladium complex, Poly MVA, in gerbils," *Experimental Neurology*, 2004 Sep, 189(1):10–5, PMID: 15296831.

138. NP Sudheesh et al., "Palladium-α-lipoic acid complex attenuates alloxan-induced hyperglycemia and enhances the declined blood antioxidant status in diabetic rats," *Journal of Diabetes*, 2011 Dec, 3(4):293–300, doi: 10.1111/j.1753-0407.2011.00142.x, PMID: 21679354.

139. A Menon and CKK Nair, "POLY MVA, a dietary supplement containing α-lipoic acid palladium complex, enhances cellular DNA repair," *International Journal of Low Radiation*, 2011, 8(1): 42–54, DOI: 10.1504/IJLR.2011.040648.

140. L Ramachandran et al., "Radioprotection by α-Lipoic Acid Mineral Complex formulation, (POLY-MVA) in mice," *Cancer Biotherapy and Radiopharmaceuticals*, 2010, 25(4): 395–399, https://doi.org/10.1089/cbr.2009.0744.

141. A Menon, CV Krishnan, and CKK Nair, "Protection from gamma-radiation insult to antioxidant defense and cellular DNA by POLY-MVA, a dietary supplement containing palladium-lipoic acid formulation," *International Journal of Low Radiation*, 2009, 6(3): 248–262, DOI: 10.1504/IJLR.2009.028892.

142. A Menon, CV Krishnan, and CKK Nair, "Antioxidant and radioprotective activity of POLY-MVA against radiation induced damages," *Amala Cancer Bulletin*, 2008, 28: 167–173.

143. O Desouky et al., "Protection against Radiation-induced Genotoxic Damages in Cultured Human Fibroblast Cells by Treatment with Palladium-Lipoic Acid Complex," 2012, *Third International Conference on Radiation Sciences and Applications*, 897–907.

144. SM El-Marakby et al., "Prophylaxis And Mitigation Of Radiation-Induced Changes In The Electrical Properties Of Erythrocytes By Palladium Lipoic Acid Nano-Complex (Poly-MVA)," *Romanian Journal of Biophysics*, 2013, 23(3): 171–190.

145. NS Selim, "Radioprotective effect of palladium α-lipoic acid complex on the dielectric relaxation and AC conductivity of red blood cells," *Romanian Journal of Biophysics*, 2012, 22(3–4): 145–161.

146. NS Selim, "Influence Of Palladium α-Lipoic Acid Complex On The Mechanical Properties Of Blood Exposed To Gamma Radiation," *Romanian Journal of Biophysics*, 2012, 22(3–4): 163–179.

147. F Antonawich et al., "Preparatory Liquid Blend, Poly-MVA and Rejeneril-A Protect the Radiation-Induced DNA Damage and Lesions of Ileum," *Journal of Basic and Clinical Pharmacy*, 2017, 8:S054–S059.

148. V Sridharan et al., "Late Administration of a Palladium Lipoic Acid Complex (Poly-MVA) Modifies Cardiac Mitochondria Induced Heart Disease in a Rat Model," *Journal of Radiation Research*, 2017, 187(3): 361–366, doi: 10.1667/RR14643.1.

149. GK Ogilvie and AS Moore, *Managing the canine cancer patient: A practical guide to compassionate care*, Veterinary Learning Systems, Yardley, PA, 2006.

150. RK Veena et al., "Antitumor Effects of Palladium-Lipoic Acid Complex Formulation as an Adjunct in Radiotherapy," *Journal of Environmental Pathology, Toxicology and Oncology*, 2016, 35(4): 333–342, DOI: 10.1615/JEnvironPatholToxicolOncol.2016016640.

151. Frank Antonawich, "Cell death assay (U-87 glioblastoma cell line)" provided by Garnett McKeen Laboratory, Inc.

152. LH Stockwin et al., "Sodium dichloroacetate selectively targets cells with defects in the mitochondrial ETC," *International Journal of Cancer*, 2010 December, 127(11):2510–2519, DOI 10.1002/ijc.25499.

153. MG Vander Heiden et al., "Understanding the Warburg Effect: The Metabolic Requirements of Cell Proliferation," *Science*, 2009, 324(5930): 1029–1033, DOI: 10,1126/science.1160809.

154. M López-Lázaro, "A new view of carcinogenesis and an alternative approach to cancer therapy," *Molecular Medicine*, March–April 2010, 16(3–4): 144–153, doi: 10.2119/molmed.2009.00162.

155. ED Michelakis et al., "Metabolic Modulation of Glioblastoma with Dichloroacetate," *Science Translational Medicine*, 12 May 2010, 2(31):31ra34, DOI: 10.1126/scitranslmed.3000677.

156. B Yang and CP Reynolds, "Tirapazamine cytotoxicity for neuroblastoma is p53 dependent," *Clinical Cancer Research*, 2005 Apr 1, 11(7):2774–80, PMID: 15814660, DOI: 10.1158/1078-0432.CCR-04-2382.

157. JS Armstrong et al., "Role of glutathione depletion and reactive oxygen species generation in apoptotic signaling in human B lymphoma cell line," *Cell Death & Differentiation*, 2002, 9: 252–263, DOI: 10.1038/sj/cdd/4400959.

158. CV Ammini and PW Stacpool, "Biotransformation, Toxicology and Pharmacogenomics of Dichloroacetate," in G. Gribble (ed.), *Natural Production of Organohalogen Compounds*, The Handbook of Environmental Chemistry, 2003, 3, Part P: 215–234, https://doi.org/10.1007/b10453.

159. EA Hassoun and J Cearfoss, "Dichloroacetate- and trichloroacetate-induced modulation of superoxide dismutase, catalase, and glutathione peroxidase activities and glutathione level in the livers of mice after subacute and subchronic exposures," *Toxicological & Environmental Chemistry*, 2011, 93(2): 332–344, doi:10.1080/02772248.2010.509602.

160. R Cornett et al., "Inhibition of glutathione S-transferase zeta and tyrosine metabolism by dichloroacetate: a potential unifying mechanism for its altered biotransformation and toxicity," *Biochemical and Biophysical Research Communications*, 1999 Sep 7, 262(3):752–6, PMID: 10471397.

161. T Ohashi et al., "Dichloroacetate improves immune dysfunction caused by tumor-secreted lactic acid and increases antitumor immunoreactivity," *Interntional Journal of Cancer*, 2013, 133(5):1107–1118, doi: 10.1002/ijc.28114.

162. S Kankotia and PW Stacpoole "Dichloroacetate and cancer: new home for an orphan drug?" *Biochimica et Biophysica Acta*, 2014, 1846(2):617–629, doi: 10.1016/j.bbcan.2014.08.005.

163. D Heshe et al., "Dichloroacetate metabolically targeted therapy defeats cytotoxicity of standard anticancer drugs," *Cancer Chemotherapy and Pharmacology*, 2011, 67(3):647–655, doi: 10.1007/s00280-010-1361-6.

164. G Lin et al., "Dichloroacetate induces autophagy in colorectal cancer cells and tumours," *British Journal of Cancer*, 2014, 111(2):375–385, doi: 10.1038/bjc.2014.281.

165. S Shahrzad et al., "Sodium dichloroacetate (DCA) reduces apoptosis in colorectal tumor hypoxia," *Cancer Letters*, 2010, 297(1):75–83, doi: 10.1016/j.canlet.2010.04.027.

166. EM Dunbar et al., "Phase 1 trial of dichloroacetate (DCA) in adults with recurrent malignant brain tumors," *Investigational New Drugs*, 2014, 32(3):452–464, doi: 10.1007/s10637-013-0047-4.

167. A Khan et al., "A novel form of dichloroacetate therapy for patients with advanced cancer: a report of 3 cases," *Alternative Therapies in Health and Medicine*, 2014, 20(Suppl 2):21–28, PMID: 25362214.

168. SB Strum et al., "Case report: Sodium dichloroacetate (DCA) inhibition of the 'Warburg Effect' in a human cancer patient: complete response in non-Hodgkin's lymphoma after disease progression with rituximab-CHOP," *Journal of Bioenergetics and Biomembranes*, 2013, 45(3):307–315, doi: 10.1007/s10863-012-9496-2.

169. SB Strum et al., "Erratum to: Case Report: Sodium dichloroacetate (DCA) inhibition of the 'Warburg Effect' in a human cancer patient: response in non-Hodgkin's lymphoma after disease progression with rituximab-CHOP," *Journal of Bioenergetics and Biomembranes*, 2013, 45(3):317, https://doi.org/10.1007/s10863-013-9516-x.

170. QS Chu et al., "A phase I open-labeled, single arm, dose-escalation, study of dichloroacetate (DCA) in patients with advanced solid tumors," *Investigational New Drugs*, 2015, 33(3):603–610, doi: 10.1007/s10637-015-0221-y.

171. W Lemmo and G Tan, "Prolonged Survival After Dichloroacetate Treatment of Non-Small-Cell Lung Carcinoma-Related Leptomeningeal Carcinomatosis," *Journal of Medical Cases*, 2016, 7(4):136–142, http://dx.doi.org/10.14740/jmc2456w.

172. A Khan, "Case Report of Long Term Complete Remission of Metastatic Renal Squamous Cell Carcinoma after Palliative Radiotherapy and Adjuvant Dichloroacetate," *Advances in Cancer: Research & Treatment*, 2012, 2012, Article ID 441895, 7 pages, DOI: 10.5171/2012.441895, http://www.ibimapublishing.com/journals/ACRT/acrt.html.

173. A Khan, "Use of oral dichloroacetate for palliation of leg pain arising from metastatic poorly differentiated carcinoma: a case report," *Journal of Palliative Medicine*, 2011, 14(8):973–977, doi: 10.1089/jpm.2010.0472.

174. DF Flavin, "Non-Hodgkin's Lymphoma Reversal with Dichloroacetate," *Journal of Oncology*, 2010, Article ID 414726, 4 pages, 2010. doi:10.1155/2010/414726.

175. DF Flavin, "Medullary thyroid carcinoma relapse reversed with dichloroacetate: A case report," *Oncology Letters*, 2010, 1(5):889–891, doi: 10.3892/ol_00000158.

176. Sanford Health. "Study of DCA (Dichloroacetate) in Combination with Cisplatin and Definitive Radiation in Head and Neck Carcinoma," ClinicalTrials.gov, Identifier: NCT01386632, Downloaded from: https://clinicaltrials.gov/ct2/show/study/NCT01386632, August 28, 2017.

177. Frank Antonawich, "Cell death assay (U-87 glioblastoma cell line)" provided by Garnett McKeen Laboratory, Inc.

178. Leanna J Standish, Paul S Anderson et al., "Can Integrative Oncology Extend Life in Advanced Disease?" 10th International Conference of the Society for Integrative Oncology (SIO): Abstract 79, presented October 21, 2013.

179. TN Seyfried, RE Flores, AM Poff, DP D'Agostino, "Cancer as a metabolic disease: implications for novel therapeutics," *Carcinogenesis*, 2014, 35(3):515–527, doi:10.1093/carcin/bgt480.

180. V Gogvadze, S Orrenius, and B Zhivotovsky, "Mitochondria in cancer cells: what is so special about them?" *Trends in Cell Biology*, 2008, 18(4): 165173, doi: 10.1016/j.tcb.2008.01.006.

181. KA Miles and RE Williams, "Warburg revisited: imaging tumour blood flow and metabolism," *Cancer Imaging*, 2008, 8: 81–86, doi: 10.1102/1470-7330.2008.0011.

182. FS Collins, "Contemplating the end of the beginning," *Genome Research*, 2001, 11(5): 64–13, doi:10.1101/gr.1898.

183. D Escuin, JW Simons and P Giannakakou, "Exploitation of the HIF axis for cancer therapy," *Cancer Biology and Therapy*, 2004, 3(7):608–11, PMID: 15197342.

184. AL Bacon and AL Harris, "Hypoxia-inducible factors and hypoxic cell death in tumour physiology," *Annals of Medicine*, 2004, 36(7):530–9, http://dx.doi.org/10.1080/07853890410018231.

185. M Garnett, "Palladium Complexes and Methods for Using Same in the Treatment of Tumors and Psoriasis," U.S.Patent No. 5,463,093, Oct. 31. (1995).

186. I Hininger et al. "Acute prooxidant effects of vitamin C in EDTA chelation therapy and long-term antioxidant benefits of therapy," *Free Radical Biology & Medicine*, 2005, 38(12):1565–1570, https://doi.org/10.1016/j.freeradbiomed.2005.02.016.

187. AM Roussel et al. "EDTA Chelation Therapy, without Added Vitamin C, Decreases Oxidative DNA Damage and Lipid Peroxidation," *Alternative Medicine Review*, 2009, 14(1):56–61, PMID: 19364193.

188. A Mühlhöfer et al., "High-dose intravenous vitamin C is not associated with an increase of pro-oxidative biomarkers," *European Journal of Clinical Nutrition*, 2004 Aug, 58(8):1151–8, PMID: 15054428, DOI: 10.1038/sj.ejcn.1601943.

189. C Vollbracht et al., "Intravenous vitamin C administration improves quality of life in breast cancer patients during chemo-/radiotherapy and aftercare: results of a retrospective, multicentre, epidemiological cohort study in Germany," *In Vivo*, 2011 Nov–Dec, 25(6):983–90, PMID: 22021693.

190. CH Yeom, GC Jung, and KJ Song, "Changes of terminal cancer patients' health-related quality of life after high dose vitamin C administration," *Journal of Korean Medical Science*, 2007 Feb, 22(1):7–11, PMID: 17297243, DOI: 10.3346/jkms.2007.22.1.7.

191. E Klimant, H Wright, and H Hilewitz, "Guidelines for the Utilization of IV Vitamin C in the Supportive Care of Patients with Advanced Malignancies," SIO Poster Presentation, 2012.

192. EA Lutsenko et al., "Vitamin C Prevents DNA Mutation Induced by Oxidative Stress," *Journal of Biological Chemistry*, 2002 May 10, 277:16895–16899, DOI 10.1074/jbc.M201151200.

193. A Vojdani and G Namatella, "Enhancement of Human Natural Killer Cytotoxic Activity by Vitamin C in Pure and Augmented Formulations," *Journal of Nutritional and Environmental Medicine*, 1997, 7(3): 187–196, DOI: 10.1080/13590849762600.

194. J Tilton, "Benefits and risks of parenteral nutrition in patients with cancer," *Oncology Nurse Advisor*, July/August 2011, 28–34.

195. KA Kern and JA Norton, "Cancer cachexia," *Journal of Parenteral and Enteral Nutrition*, 1988, 12(3):286–298, PMID: 3292798, DOI: 10.1177/0148607188012003286.

196. F Bozzetti and L Mariani, "Defining and classifying cancer cachexia: a proposal by the SCRINIO Working Group," *Journal of Parenteral and Enteral Nutrition*, 2009, 33(4):361–367, doi: 10.1177/0148607108325076.

197. M Mirhosseini and R Faisinger, "Fast facts and concepts #190: Parenteral nutrition in advanced cancers patients," Palliative Care Network of Wisconsin, https://www.mypcnow.org/blank-cf128.

198. R Rabinovitch et al., "Impact of nutrition support on treatment outcome in patients with locally advanced head and neck squamous cell cancer treated with definitive radiotherapy: a secondary analysis of RTOG trial 90-03," *Head & Neck*, 2006, 28(4):287–296, PMID: 16287132, DOI: 10.1002/hed.20335.

199. DA August and MB Huhmann, "A.S.P.E.N. clinical guidelines: nutrition support therapy during adult anticancer treatment and in hematopoietic cell transplantation," *Journal of Parenteral and Enteral Nutrition*, 2009, 33(5):472–500, doi: 10.1177/0148607109341804.

200. F Bozzetti, "Total parenteral nutrition in cancer patients," *Current Opinion in Supportive and Palliative Care*, 2007, 1(4):281–286, doi: 10.1097/SPC.0b013e3282f1bf60.

201. BG Fan. Parenteral nutrition prolongs the survival of patients associated with malignant gastrointestinal obstruction. *Journal of Parenteral and Enteral Nutrition*, 2007, 31(6):508–510, PMID: 17947608, DOI: 10.1177/0148607107031006508.

202. G De Mattia et al., "Influence of reduced glutathione infusion on glucose metabolism in patients with non-insulin-dependent diabetes mellitus," *Metabolism*, 1998 Aug, 47(8):993–7, PMID: 9711998.

203. CR Jonas et al. "Plasma antioxidant status after high-dose chemotherapy: a randomized trial of parenteral nutrition in bone marrow transplantation patients," *The American Journal of Clinical Nutrition* 2000, 72(1):181–9, PMID: 10871578.

204. J Midander et al., "Reduced repair of potentially lethal radiation damage in glutathione synthetase-deficient human fibroblasts after X-irradiation," *International Journal of Radiation Biology and Related Studies in Physics, Chemistry, and Medicine*, 1986 Mar, 49(3):403–13, PMID: 3485589.

205. G Pujari, A Berni, F Palitti, and A Chatterjee, "Influence of glutathione levels on radiation-induced chromosomal DNA damage and repair in human peripheral lymphocytes," *Mutation Research*, 2009 Apr, 677(1–2):109–10, PMID: 19386243, doi: 10.1016/j.mrgentox.2009.02.001.

206. S Cascinu et al., "Neuroprotective Effect of Reduced Glutathione on Oxaliplatin-Based Chemotherapy in Advanced Colorectal Cancer: A Randomized, Double-Blind, Placebo-Controlled Trial," *Journal of Clinical Oncology*, 2002 Aug, 20(16):3478–3483, PMID: 12177109, DOI: 10.1200/JCO.2002.07.061.

207. P Milla et al., "Administration of reduced glutathione in FOLFOX4 adjuvant treatment for colorectal cancer: effect on oxaliplatin pharmacokinetics, Pt-DNA adduct formation, and neurotoxicity," *Anticancer Drugs*, 2009 Jun, 20(5):396–402, PMID: 19287306, doi: 10.1097/CAD.0b013e32832a2dc1.

CHAPTER 8

1. D MacKay and AL Miller. "Nutritional support for wound healing," *Alternative Medicine Review*, 2003 Nov, 8(4):359–77, PMID: 14653765.

2. JP McWhirter, CR Pennington, "The incidence and recognition of malnutrition in hospital," *BMJ*, 1994, 308(6934):945–8.

3. Ilksen Gurkan and James F Wenz, Sr., "Perioperative Infection Control: An Update for Patient Safety in Orthopedic Surgery," *Orthopedics*, 2006, 29(4):329, PMID: 16628993.

4. M Braga, L Gianotti, G Radaelli et al., "Perioperative immunonutrition in patients undergoing cancer surgery: results of a randomized double-blind phase 3 trial," *Archives of Surgery*, 1999, 134(4):428–433, PMID: 10199318.

5. L Gianotti, M Braga, L Nespoli, G Radaelli, A Beneduce, V Di Carlo, "A randomized controlled trial of preoperative oral supplementation with a specialized diet in patients with gastrointestinal cancer," *Gastroenterology*, 2002, 122(7):1763–1770, PMID: 12055582.

6. CH Snyderman, K Kachman, L Molseed et al., "Reduced postoperative infections with an immune-enhancing nutritional supplement," *Laryngoscope*, 1999, 109(6):915–921, PMID: 10369282.

7. National Cancer Institute, "Chemotherapy and You," https://www.cancer.gov/publications/patient-education/chemo-and-you, accessed September 20, 2017.

8. Paul S Anderson, "Ascorbate and Oncologic Therapies, a Review," 2013, https://www.academia.edu/10024397/Ascorbate_and_Oncologic_Therapies_-_Research_Review.

9. LJ Hoffer et al., "High-Dose Intravenous Vitamin C Combined with Cytotoxic Chemotherapy in Patients with Advanced Cancer: A Phase I-II Clinical Trial", *PLoS ONE*, 2015, 10(4), e0120228, doi:10.1371/journal.pone.0120228.

10. Y Ma et al., "High-dose parenteral ascorbate enhanced chemosensitivity of ovarian cancer and reduced toxicity of chemotherapy," *Science Translational Medicine*, 2014 Feb 5, 6(222):222ra18, doi: 10.1126/scitranslmed.3007154, PMID: 24500406.

11. C Vollbracht et al., "Intravenous vitamin C administration improves quality of life in breast cancer patients during chemo-/radiotherapy and aftercare: results of a retrospective, multicentre, epidemiological cohort study in Germany," *In Vivo*, 2011 Nov–Dec, 25(6):983–90, PMID: 22021693.

12. CH Yeom et al., "Changes of terminal cancer patients' health-related quality of life after high dose vitamin C administration" *Journal of Korean Medical Science*, 2007 Feb, 22(1):7–11, PMID: 17297243, PMCID: PMC2693571, DOI: 10.3346/jkms.2007.22.1.7.

13. Jan Axtner et al., "Health services research of integrative oncology in palliative care of patients with advanced pancreatic cancer," *BMC Cancer*, 2016, 16:579, DOI 10.1186/s12885-016-2594-5.

14. DM Seely et al., "A systematic review of integrative oncology programs," *Current Oncology*, 2012, 19(6): e436–461, doi: http://dx.doi.org/10.3747/co.19.1182.

15. BR Ferrell et al., "Integration of Palliative Care Into Standard Oncology Care: American Society of Clinical Oncology Clinical Practice Guideline Update," *Journal of Clinical Oncology*, 2017, 35(1):96–112.

16. G Lopez et al., "Integrative Oncology Outpatient Consultations: Long-Term Effects on Patient-Reported Symptoms and Quality of Life," *Journal of Cancer*, 2017, 8(9): 1640–1646, doi: 10.7150/jca.18875.

17. G Lopez et al., "Integrative Oncology Physician Consultations at a Comprehensive Cancer Center: Analysis of Demographic, Clinical and Patient Reported Outcomes," *Journal of Cancer*, 2017, 8(3): 395–402, doi: 10.7150/jca.17506.

18. G Lopez et al., "Integrative Oncology Physician Consultations at a Comprehensive Cancer Center: Analysis of Demographic, Clinical and Patient Reported Outcomes," *Journal of Cancer*, 2017, 8(3): 395–402, doi: 10.7150/jca.17506.

19. A Zbuchea, "Up-to-Date Use of Honey for Burns Treatment," *Annals of Burns and Fire Disasters*, 2014, 27(1): 22–30, PMCID: PMC4158441.

20. Rainer J Klement and Colin E Champ, "Calories, Carbohydrates, and Cancer Therapy with Radiation: Exploiting the Five R's through Dietary Manipulation," *Cancer Metastasis Reviews*, 2014, 33(1): 217–229, doi: 10.1007/s10555-014-9495-3.

21. Ayse Günes-Bayir & Huriye Senay Kiziltan, "Palliative Vitamin C Application in Patients with Radiotherapy-Resistant Bone Metastases: A Retrospective Study," *Nutrition and Cancer*, 2015, 67(6): 921–925, DOI: 10.1080/01635581.2015.1055366.

22. X Rong et al., "Radiation-induced cranial neuropathy in patients with nasopharyngeal carcinoma. A follow-up study," *Strahlentherapie und Onkologie*, 2012 Mar, 188(3):282–6, doi: 10.1007/s00066-011-0047-2.

23. Paul S Anderson, "Glutathione Augmentation in a Nerve Injury Model," published online, 2014, https://www.academia.edu/21925456/ Glutathione_Augmentation_in_a_nerve_injury_model.

24. K Irwin, "Radiation generates cancer stem cells from less aggressive breast cancer cells," *UCLA Newsroom*, 14 Feb 2012, http://newsroom.ucla.edu/releases/ radiation-treatments-generate-229002.

25. L Nurrual Abdullah and E Kai-Hua Chow, "Mechanisms of chemoresistance in cancer stem cells, "Mechanisms of chemoresistance in cancer stem cells," *Clinical and Translational Medicine,* 2013, 2(1):3, doi:10.1186/2001-1326-2-3.

26. Lagadec, Chann et al., "Radiation-Induced Reprograming of Breast Cancer Cells" *Stem Cells*, 2012, 30(5): 833–844, doi: 10.1002/stem.1058.

27. H Liu, L Lv, and K Yang, "Chemotherapy Targeting Cancer Stem Cells," *American Journal of Cancer Research*, 2015, 5(3): 880–893, PMCID: PMC4449424.

28. Robert S Kerbel and Yuval Shaked, "Therapy-activated stromal cells can dictate tumor fate," *Journal of Experimental Medicine*, Nov 2016, jem.20161845; DOI: 10.1084/ jem.20161845.

29. George S Karagiannis et al., "Neoadjuvant chemotherapy induces breast cancer metastasis through a TMEM-mediated mechanism," *Science Translational Medicine,*2017, 9(397):eaan0026, DOI: 10.1126/scitranslmed.aan0026.

30. Raffaghello, Lizzia et al., "Fasting and Differential Chemotherapy Protection in Patients," *Cell Cycle*, 2010, 9(22): 4474–4476, http://dx.doi.org/10.4161/cc.9.22.13954.

31. Naveed, Sidra, Muhammad Aslam, and Aftab Ahmad, "Starvation Based Differential Chemotherapy: A Novel Approach for Cancer Treatment," *Oman Medical Journal*, 2014, 29(6): 391–398, doi: 10.5001/omj.2014.107.

32. Mihaylova, Maria M, David M Sabatini, and Ömer H Yilmaz, "Dietary and Metabolic Control of Stem Cell Function in Physiology and Cancer," *Cell Stem Cell*, 2014, 14(3): 292–305, doi: 10.1016/j.stem.2014.02.008.

33. A Cangemi et al., "Dietary restriction: could it be considered as speed bump on tumor progression road?," *Tumour Biology*, 2016 Jun, 37(6):7109–18, doi: 10.1007/s13277-016-5044-8.

34. PP Sordillo and L Helson, "Curcumin and cancer stem cells: curcumin has asymmetrical effects on cancer and normal stem cells," *Anticancer Research*, 2015 Feb, 35(2):599–614, PMID: 25667437.

35. Y Li and T Zhang, "Targeting cancer stem cells by curcumin and clinical applications," *Cancer Letters*, 2014 May 1, 346(2):197–205, doi: 10.1016/j.canlet.2014.01.012. Epub 2014 Jan 23.

36. Gloria Bonuccelli et al., "NADH autofluorescence, a new metabolic biomarker for cancer stem cells: Identification of Vitamin C and CAPE as natural products targeting 'stemness'," *Oncotarget*, 2017; 8:20667-20678; DOI: 10.18632/oncotarget.15400.

CHAPTER 9

1. American Cancer Society, "Cancer Facts & Figures 2017," Atlanta, Ga, American Cancer Society, 2017, last accessed September 27, 2017, https://www.cancer.org/research/cancer-facts-statistics/all-cancer-facts-figures/cancer-facts-figures-2017.html.

2. Cancer Research UK, http://www.cancerresearchuk.org/sites/default/files/cstream-node/cs_surv_common.pdf, accessed September 27, 2017.

3. Cancer Research UK, http://www.cancerresearchuk.org/sites/default/files/cstream-node/cs_surv_common.pdf, accessed September 27, 2017.

4. American Cancer Society, https://www.cancer.org/cancer/breast-cancer/understanding-a-breast-cancer-diagnosis/breast-cancer-survival-rates.html.

5. American Cancer Society: Cancer Facts and Figures 2017, Atlanta, Ga, American Cancer Society, 2017, last accessed September 27, 2017, https://www.cancer.org/research/cancer-facts-statistics/all-cancer-facts-figures/cancer-facts-figures-2017.html.

6. Linda Sofie Lindström, E. Karlsson et al., "Clinically Used Breast Cancer Markers Such As Estrogen Receptor, Progesterone Receptor, and Human Epidermal Growth Factor Receptor 2 Are Unstable Throughout Tumor Progression," *Journal of Clinical Oncology*, 2012 July, 30(21): 2601–2608, DOI: 10.1200/JCO.2011.37.2482.

7. J Hamer and E Warner, "Lifestyle modifications for patients with breast cancer to improve prognosis and optimize overall health," *Canadian Medical Association Journal*, 2017 Feb 21, 189(7), https://doi.org/10.1503/cmaj.160464.

8. Hoffer, L John et al., "High-Dose Intravenous Vitamin C Combined with Cytotoxic Chemotherapy in Patients with Advanced Cancer: A Phase I-II Clinical Trial," *PLoS ONE*, 2015, 10(4): e0120228, doi: 10.1371/journal.pone.0120228.

9. Wang, Bingliang et al., "Artesunate Sensitizes Ovarian Cancer Cells to Cisplatin by Downregulating RAD51," *Cancer Biology & Therapy*, 2015, 16(10): 1548–1556, doi: 10.1080/15384047.2015.1071738.

10. Yunli Tong et al., "Artemisinin and Its Derivatives Can Significantly Inhibit Lung Tumorigenesis and Tumor Metastasis through Wnt/β-Catenin Signaling," *Oncotarget*, 2016, 7(21): 31413–31428, doi: 10.18632/oncotarget.8920.

11. QH Yao et al., "ω-3 polyunsaturated fatty acids inhibit the proliferation of the lung adenocarcinoma cell line A549 in vitro," *Molecular medicine reports*, 2014 Feb, 9(2):401–406, doi: 10.3892/mmr.2013.1829.

12. M McCulloch et al., "Astragalus-based Chinese herbs and platinum-based chemotherapy for advanced non-small-cell lung cancer: meta-analysis of randomized trials," *Journal of Clinical Oncology*, 20 Jan 2006, 24(3):419–430, PMID: 16421421, DOI: 10.1200/JCO.2005.03.6392.

13. P Gnagnarella et al., "Red meat, Mediterranean diet and lung cancer risk among heavy smokers in the COSMOS screening study," *Annals of Oncology*, Oct 2013, 24(10):2606–2611, doi: 10.1093/annonc/mdt302.

14. SA Kenfield, "Mediterranean Diet and Prostate Cancer Risk and Mortality in the Health Professionals Follow-up Study," *European Urology*, 2014, 65(5):887–894, doi:10.1016/j.eururo.2013.08.009.

15. C Capurso, "The Mediterranean Diet Reduces the Risk and Mortality of the Prostate Cancer: A Narrative Review," *Frontiers in Nutrition*, 2017, 4:38, doi:10.3389/fnut.2017.00038.

16. CJ Paller, "A review of pomegranate in prostate cancer," *Prostate Cancer and Prostatic Disease*, 2017 Sep, 20(3):265-270, doi: 10.1038/pcan.2017.19.

17. SA Kenfield et al., "Physical activity and survival after prostate cancer diagnosis in the health professionals follow-up Study," *Journal of Clinical Oncology*, 2011 Feb, 29(6):726–732, doi:10.1200/JCO.2010.31.5226.

18. S Krishna et al., "A Randomised, Double Blind, Placebo-Controlled Pilot Study of Oral Artesunate Therapy for Colorectal Cancer," *EbioMedicine*, 2014 Nov 15, 2(1):82–90, doi: 10.1016/j.ebiom.2014.11.010.

19. J Schwartzbaum et al., "Associations between prediagnostic blood glucose levels, diabetes, and glioma," *Scientific Reports*, 2017 May 3, 7(1):1436, doi: 10.1038/s41598-017-01553-2.

20. HI Ursu, "Functional TSH Receptors, Malignant Melanomas and Subclinical Hypothyroidism," *European Thyroid Journal*, 2012, 1:208, https://doi.org/10.1159/000339817.

21. AS Breathnach, "Azelaic acid: potential as a general antitumoural agent," *Medical Hypotheses*, 1999 Mar, 52(3):221–6, DOI: 10.1054/mehy.1997.0647.

22. "Low-Iodine Diet," ThyCa: Thyroid Cancer Survivors' Association, accessed November 7, 2017, http://www.thyca.org/pap-fol/lowiodinediet.

23. C Carella et al., "Iodized salt improves the effectiveness of L-thyroxine therapy after surgery for nontoxic goitre: a prospective and randomized study," *Clinical Endocrinology (Oxf)*, 2002 Oct, 57(4):507–13, PMID: 12354133.

24. JD Taylor et al., "Iodine Therapy for Thyroidectomy Patients Exhibiting High Thyroid-Stimulating Hormone Values: A Randomised Study," *Annals of The Royal College of Surgeons of England*, 1993, 75(3): 168–171, PMID: 8323210, PMCID: PMC2497899.

25. E Riza et al., "The effect of Greek herbal tea consumption on thyroid cancer: a case-control study," *European Journal of Public Health*, 2015 Dec, 25(6):1001–5, doi: 10.1093/eurpub/ckv063, Epub 2015 Apr 4.

CHAPTER 10

1. Courtney Davis et al., "Availability of evidence of benefits on overall survival and quality of life of cancer drugs approved by European Medicines Agency: retrospective cohort study of drug approvals 2009–13," *BMJ*, 2017, 359:j4530, doi: https://doi.org/10.1136/bmj.j4530.

2. Ian H Plenderleith, "Treating the Treatment: Toxicity of Cancer Chemotherapy," *Canadian Family Physician*, 1990, 36: 1827–1830, PMCID: PMC2280515.

3. Z Livshits, RB Rao, and SW Smith, "An approach to chemotherapy-associated toxicity," *Emergency Medicine Clinics of North America*, 2014 Feb, 32(1):167–203, doi: 10.1016/j.emc.2013.09.002.

4. HA Azim, Jr. et al., "Long-term toxic effects of adjuvant chemotherapy in breast cancer," *Annals of Oncology*, 1 September 2011, 22(9): 1939–1947, https://doi.org/10.1093/annonc/mdq683.

5. Joel A Simon, Esther S Hudes, "Relationship of Ascorbic Acid to Blood Lead Levels," *JAMA*, 1999, 281(24):2289–2293, doi:10.1001/jama.281.24.2289.

6. EB Dawson et al., "The effect of ascorbic acid supplementation on the blood lead levels of smokers," *Journal of the American College of Nutrition*, 1999 Apr, 18(2):166–70, PMID: 10204833.

7. WR García-Niño and J Pedraza-Chaverrí, "Protective effect of curcumin against heavy metals-induced liver damage," *Food and Chemical Toxicology*, 2014 Jul, 69:182–201, doi: 10.1016/j.fct.2014.04.016, epub 2014 Apr 18.

8. S Gao et al., "Curcumin attenuates arsenic-induced hepatic injuries and oxidative stress in experimental mice through activation of Nrf2 pathway, promotion of arsenic methylation and urinary excretion," *Food and Chemical Toxicology*, 2013 Sep, 59:739–47, doi: 10.1016/j.fct.2013.07.032, epub 2013 Jul 18.

9. Y Xie et al., "Curcumin ameliorates cognitive deficits heavy ion irradiation-induced learning and memory deficits through enhancing of Nrf2 antioxidant signaling pathways," *Pharmacology, Biochemistry, and Behavior*, 2014 Nov, 126:181–6, doi: 10.1016/j.pbb.2014.08.005, epub 2014 Aug 23.

10. American Cancer Society, "Known and Probable Human Carcinogens," https://www.cancer.org/cancer/cancer-causes/general-info/known-and-probable-human-carcinogens.html.

11. S Jahr, B Schoppe, and A Reisshauer, "Effect of treatment with low-intensity and extremely low-frequency electrostatic fields (Deep Oscillation) on breast tissue and pain in patients with secondary breast lymphedema," *Journal of Rehabilitation Medicine*, 2008 Aug, 40(8):645–50, doi: 10.2340/16501977-0225.

12. Roser Belmonte et al., "Efficacy of Low-Frequency Low-Intensity Electrotherapy in the Treatment of Breast Cancer-Related Lymphoedema: A Cross-over Randomized Trial," *Clinical Rehabilitation*, 2012, 26(7): 607–618, doi: 10.1177/0269215511427414.

13. Ana Elisa Bergues Pupo, Rolando Placeres Jiménez, and Luis Enrique Bergues Cabrales, "Electrotherapy on Cancer: Experiment and Mathematical Modeling," in *Current Cancer Treatment—Novel Beyond Conventional Approaches*, Oner Ozdemir (Ed.), (2011), 585–615, ISBN: 978-953-307-397-2, http://www.intechopen.com/books/current-cancer-treatment-novel-beyondconventionalapproaches/electrotherapy-on-cancer-experiment-and-mathematical-modeling.

14. A Mooventhan and L Nivethitha, "Scientific Evidence-Based Effects of Hydrotherapy on Various Systems of the Body," *North American Journal of Medical Sciences*, 2014, 6(5): 199–209, doi: 10.4103/1947-2714.132935.

15. S Blazícková et al., "Effect of hyperthermic water bath on parameters on cellular immunity," *International Journal of Clinical Pharmacology Research*, 2000, 20(1–2):41–6, PMID: 11146901.

16. V Digiesi et al., "[Hemorheologic and blood cell changes in humans during partial immersion with a therapeutic method, in 38 C water]," *Minerva Medica*, 1986, 77(30–31):1407–11, PMID: 3736976.

17. IK Brenner et al., "Immune changes in humans during cold exposure: Effects of prior heating and exercise," *Journal of Applied Physiology*, 1999, 87(2):699–710, PMID: 10444630.

18. NA Shevchuk and S Radoja, "Possible stimulation of anti-tumor immunity using repeated cold stress: A hypothesis," *Infectious Agents and Cancer*, 2007, 2:20, doi: 10.1186/1750-9378-2-20.

19. K Sugahara and M Eguchi, "The use of warmed water treatment to induce protective immunity against the bacterial cold-water disease pathogen Flavobacterium psychrophilum in ayu (Plecoglossus altivelis)," *Fish & Shellfish Immunology*, 2012, 32(3):489–93, doi: 10.1016/j.fsi.2011.12.005.

20. Ingrid Moen and Linda EB Stuhr, "Hyperbaric oxygen therapy and cancer—a review," *Targeted Oncology*, 2012, 7(4):233–242, DOI 10.1007/s11523-012-0233-x.

21. Benjamin L Hoggan and Alun L Cameron, "Systematic review of hyperbaric oxygen therapy for the treatment of non-neurological soft tissue radiation-related injuries," *Support Care Cancer*, 2014, 22(6):1715–1726, DOI 10.1007/s00520-014-2198-z.

22. Katarzyna Stępień, Robert P Ostrowski, and Ewa Matyja, "Hyperbaric oxygen as an adjunctive therapy in treatment of malignancies, including brain tumours," *Medical Oncology*, 2016, 33(9):101, DOI 10.1007/s12032-016-0814-0.

23. Noori S Al-Waili et al., "Hyperbaric oxygen and malignancies: a potential role in radiotherapy, chemotherapy, tumor surgery and phototherapy," *Medical Science Monitor*, 2005, 11(9): RA279–RA289, PMID: 16127374.

24. Skitzki, Joseph J, Elizabeth A Repasky, and Sharon S Evans. "Hyperthermia as an Immunotherapy Strategy for Cancer," *Current opinion in investigational drugs*, (London, England: 2000) 10.6 (2009): 550–558, PMID: 19513944 PMCID: PMC2828267.

25. Frey B, Weiss EM, Rubner Y, Wunderlich R, Ott OJ, Sauer R, Fietkau R, Gaipl US, "Old and new facts about hyperthermia-induced modulations of the immune system," *International Journal of Hyperthermia*, 2012, 28(6):528–42, doi: 10.3109/02656736.2012.677933.

26. Edward F McCarthy, "The Toxins of William B. Coley and the Treatment of Bone and Soft-Tissue Sarcomas," *The Iowa Orthopaedic Journal*, 2006, 26: 154–158, PMCID: PMC1888599.

27. MJ Nathenson, AP Conley, and E Sausville, "Immunotherapy: A New (and Old) Approach to Treatment of Soft Tissue and Bone Sarcomas," *The Oncologist*, 2016-0025, doi: 10.1634/theoncologist.2016-0025.

28. S Thomas and GC Prendergast, "Cancer Vaccines: A Brief Overview," *Methods in Molecular Biology*, 2016, 1403:755–61, doi: 10.1007/978-1-4939-3387-7_43.

29. AJ Muceniece and JV Bumbieris, "Transplantation antigens and their changes in carcinogenesis and viral infection." In: Virusnyi onkoliz i iskusstvennaya geterogenizatsiya opukholei (Viral Oncolysis and Artificial Heterogenization of Tumors)," 1982, Riga, 217–234.

30. AJ Muceniece, "Analysis of sensitivity of human melanomas to enteroviruses adapted to these tumors." In: Virusy v terapii opukholei (Viruses in Antitumor Therapy)," Riga: Zinatne, 1978, 175–189.

31. E Lasalvia-Prisco," Insulin-induced enhancement of antitumoral response to methotrexate in breast cancer patients," *Cancer Chemotherapy and Pharmacology*, 2004 Mar, 53(3):220-224.

32. JS Gordon, "Mind-body medicine and cancer," *Hematology/Oncology Clinics of North America*, 2008 Aug, 22(4): 683–708, ix, doi: 10.1016/j.hoc.2008.04.010.

33. G Elkins, W Fisher, and A Johnson, "Mind-body therapies in integrative oncology," *Current Treatment Options in Oncology*, 2010 Dec, 11(3–4): 128–40, doi: 10.1007/s11864-010-0129-x.

34. Alejandro Chaoulet al., "Mind-Body Practices in Cancer Care," *Current Oncology Reports*, 2014, 16(12): 417, DOI:10.1007/s11912-014-0417-x.

35. Camila Csizmar Carvalho et al., "Effectiveness of prayer in reducing anxiety in cancer patients," *Revista da escola de enfermagem da USP*, 2014 Aug, 48(4): 684–690, https://doi.org/10.1590/S0080-623420140000400016.

36. D Spiegel, "Minding the body: psychotherapy and cancer survival," *British Journal of Health Psychology*, 2014 Sep, 19(3): 465–85, doi: 10.1111/bjhp.12061.

37. Spiegel, David, "Mind Matters in Cancer Survival." *Psycho-Oncology*, 2012, 21(6): 588–593, doi: 10.1002/pon.3067.

38. Martijn Triesscheijn, Paul Baas, Jan H. M. Schellens and Fiona A. Stewart, "Photodynamic Therapy in Oncology," *The Oncologist*, 2006, 11(9): 1034–1044, DOI:10.1634/theoncologist.11-9-1034.

39. Stanley B Brown, Elizabeth A Brown, and Ian Walker, "The present and future role of photodynamic therapy in cancer treatment," *The Lancet Oncology*, 2004, 5(8): 497–508, DOI: 10.1016/S1470-2045(04)01529-3.

40. E Allan, C Barney, S Baum et al., "Low-level laser therapy and laser debridement for management of oral mucositis in patients with head and neck cancer receiving chemotherapy and radiation," *International Journal of Radiation Oncology*, 2016 March 15; 94(4):883, DOI: http://dx.doi.org/10.1016/j.ijrobp.2015.12.066.

41. JM Bjordal et al., "A systematic review with meta-analysis of the effect of low-level laser therapy (LLLT) in cancer therapy-induced oral mucositis," *Supportive Care in Cancer*, 2011 Aug, 19(8):1069–77.

42. E Jadaud and RJ Bensadoun, "Low-Level Laser Therapy: A Standard of Supportive Care for Cancer Therapy-Induced Oral Mucositis in Head and Neck Cancer Patients?" *Laser Therapy*, 2012, 21(4): 297–303, doi: 10.5978/islsm.12-RE-01.

43. HS Antunes et al., "Long-term survival of a randomized phase III trial of head and neck cancer patients receiving concurrent chemoradiation therapy with or without low-level laser therapy (LLLT) to prevent oral mucositis," *Oral Oncology*, 2017 Aug, 71:11–15, doi: 10.1016/j.oraloncology.2017.05.018, epub 2017 Jun 3.

44. Michael Weber, Robert Weber, and Martin Junggebauer, *Medical Low-Level Lasertherapy—Foundations and Clinical Applications*, 2d.Ed. (Germany: Isla-laser research-group, 2015) 341–350.

45. M Kodama et al., "[Plasmapheresis in the patients with malignant tumor]," *Gan To Kagaku Ryoho*, 1984 Jul, 11(7): 1349–55, PMID: 6378099.

46. A Kameda et al.,"[Clinical studies on plasma exchange in advanced cancer patients with special reference to the postcentrifugal filter]," *Gan No Rinsho*, 1985 Oct, 31(13): 1661–4, PMID: 4079056.

47. T Tani, K Numa, K Hanasawa and M Kodama, "Blood purification therapy in cancer treatment," *Therapeutic Apheresis*, 1998 Aug, 2(3): 182–4, PMID: 10227767.

48. Trung C Nguyen et al., "The Role of Plasmapheresis in Critical Illness," *Critical Care Clinics*, 2012, 28(3): 453–468, doi: 10.1016/j.ccc.2012.04.009.

INDEX

ACKNOWLEDGMENTS

DR. MARK: Many thanks to the people who made this book possible at Hay House publishing, including Lisa Cheng, Patty Gift, Reid Tracy, and all the staff. Many thanks to my phenomenal wife, Dr. Angela Stengler, and all her support with this book. And last but certainly not least, my God and Savior Jesus Christ.

DR. PAUL: A great deal of gratitude goes to the Hay House Team, as well as my clinical and research collaborators. I am very thankful for the support of my family and friends through the process and most importantly my incredible wife, Lori. And a special thanks to the most impactful instructor in my career regarding life and cancer, Lilly—thanks for every lesson and what you've done to change me, as well as integrative oncology.

GLOSSARY

Adjunctive—another therapy or treatment used in addition to the primary treatment.

Adjuvant—a substance or ingredient that modifies or improves the action of the principal substance.

Alpha-N-acetylgalactosaminidase (nagalase)—an enzyme used by cancer cells to develop biochemical strength and that can be a laboratory sign of a strengthening cancer process.

AMAS (anti-malignin antibody serum) test—an older, nonspecific cancer test aimed at early detection.

Amino acids—the building blocks of protein.

Angiogenesis—the growth of new blood vessels that support the growth of tumors.

Anti-angiogenesis—inhibition of the growth of new blood vessels.

Anticoagulant—a substance (natural or pharmaceutical) that makes it harder for blood clots to form.

Antioxidant—molecule that inhibits the oxidation or damage of cells. Can be found in foods such as fruits and vegetables or nutritional supplements.

Antitumor—inhibiting or preventing the formation or growth of tumors.

Apoptosis—also known as programmed cell death. It involves a series of molecular reactions that leads to cell death. It is a method by which the body eliminates abnormal cells. This process may be blocked in cancer cells.

Barium enema—a process where the patient drinks a contrast medium and has an X-ray of the colon and rectum.

Biopsy—the collection of tissue from a suspected cancer that is examined under a microscope, often collected with a needle.

Bone marrow aspiration and biopsy—the removal of fluid (aspiration) or a small, solid piece (biopsy) from the bone marrow that provides information about blood cells formed in the bone marrow.

Bone scan—test that looks for cancer that has started in or has spread to the bones. Involves the injection of a small amount of a radioactive substance into a vein, after which the entire body is scanned with a scanner that measures radioactivity.

Cachexia—the loss of muscle mass and body weight.

Cancer—a group of more than 100 diseases in which cells divide abnormally and in an uncontrolled manner. Cancer cells can spread to other parts of the body (metastasis).

Cancer stem cells—"parent" cells within (or separate from) a tumor that are left behind either during natural immune tumor killing or after standard cancer therapies. They can renew the cancer by dividing and cause the formation of other cell types that form tumors.

Carcinogenic—an agent or substance that causes cancer.

Chamomile (*Matricaria chamomilla*)—a traditional medicinal herb often used as a tea to promote relaxation and deeper sleep.

Chemosensitivity testing—method of using tumor cells in a laboratory to test the sensitivity of those particular cells to specific cancer therapies.

Chemotherapy—method of treating cancer with the use of chemical agents (drugs).

China Study diet—a diet based on extensive studies in areas of rural China where people consumed locally grown food. The diet is low in animal protein and dairy products and rich in plant foods. Researchers concluded this type of diet decreases the risk of cancer and other chronic diseases.

Circulating tumor cells (CTCs)—cancer cells that have shed from a primary or metastatic tumor and circulate in the bloodstream. The identification and isolation of CTCs can be used with or as an alternative to traditional tissue biopsies in order to evaluate what might be taking place on a real-time basis.

Circulating Tumor DNA (ctDNA)—Genetic material that typically mutates and causes cancer (oncogenes) can be found in the bloodstream.

Colonoscopy—a procedure where a thin, flexible tube with a light and camera is inserted in the rectum and moved through the large intestine to look for colorectal cancer and precancerous polyps.

Computed tomography (CT or CAT) scan—a test where, an X-ray machine uses multiple X-rays to create a three-dimensional picture of the area being scanned.

Cruciferous—a family of vegetables known for their potent cancer prevention properties. Examples include bok choy, broccoli, Brussels sprouts, cabbage, cauliflower, collard greens, kale, mustard greens, turnips, radishes, and watercress.

Cure—according to the National Cancer Institute, the term *cure* when applied to cancer "means that there are no traces of your cancer after treatment and the cancer will never come back."

DHA—an omega-3 fatty acid (docosahexaenoic acid).

Digital rectal exam (DRE)—a test where a doctor inserts a lubricated, gloved finger into the rectum to feel for abnormalities, such as cancerous growths of the lower rectum, pelvis, lower belly, prostate in men, and uterus in women.

DNA—deoxyribonucleic acid, a complex molecular structure that contains the genetic information (code) that makes a person unique and carries out body processes.

EKG and echocardiogram—test measuring the electrical activity of the heart.

Endoscopy—a test involving the insertion of a thin tube with a light and camera to examine internal areas of body parts, such as the esophagus, stomach, colon, ear, nose, throat, heart, urinary tract, joints, and abdomen.

EPA—an omega-3 fatty acid (eicosapentaenoic acid).

Fasting—abstaining from food for a period of time. There are different types of medical fasting. Some involve the consumption of water only for a limited period. Other types involve the consumption of specific juices, usually vegetable. Intermittent fasting or time-restricted eating involves the consumption of noncaloric liquids only for specific time periods of a day.

Fecal occult blood tests—a screening test for colorectal cancer, which looks for hidden blood in the stool.

Free radicals—unstable negatively charged molecules formed during normal energy production within cells, radiation exposure, and environmental toxins. Free radicals are a normal part of the immune system response to infections and disease. They can also contribute to damaged cell DNA and increase cancer risk. Certain cancer therapies (some types of chemotherapy and radiation) increase free radical production.

Galectin-3—a protein involved in inflammation.

Gamma-aminobutyric acid (GABA)—the primary calming neurotransmitter in the central nervous system, often used as a calming supplement.

Glycemic index—a value assigned to food based on how quickly foods increase blood glucose levels. High glycemic index–rated foods are considered unhealthy for weight, diabetes, and cancer risk.

Glycemic load—the amount food will elevate a person's blood glucose level after eating. It takes into account the amount of carbohydrate in addition to its glycemic index rating to more accurately estimate the effect of food on blood sugar levels. A low glycemic load is most desirable.

Human chorionic gonadotropin (HCG)—a hormone normally produced by the human placenta and the basis of pregnancy tests. Known to rise in some tumors and to potentially be a trigger for cancer growth. Used in some cases to follow cancer progress through therapy.

HER2—human epidermal growth factor receptor 2. This protein promotes the growth of cancer cells.

Homeostasis—the tendency of the body or cell to move toward balance.

Hyperbaric oxygen therapy (HBOT)—treatment that involves breathing pure oxygen in a pressurized tube or tent.

Immune system—a complex network of cells, tissues, and organs that protect the body against infections, cancer, and harmful substances from the environment.

Inflammation—the immune system response to injury, infection, cancer, or other stimuli. Chronic inflammation is known to promote disease such as cancer.

Insulin resistance—the resistance of cells to the glucose transporting mechanism of the hormone insulin. This results in abnormally high levels of insulin, a known risk for cancer, diabetes, and cardiovascular disease.

Integrative medicine—a system of medicine that considers the full range of factors that affects a person's health, including physical, mental, emotional, environmental, spiritual, and social factors. Incorporates the best conventional and holistic healing methods depending on the needs of the patient.

Integrative oncology—the combined use of the best conventional and holistic treatment methods for the prevention and treatment of cancer.

Intra-arterial—directly into an artery.

Intraperitoneal—injection into the body cavity that contains organs such as the intestines, stomach, and liver.

Intrathecal—injection in the space between the layers of tissue that cover the brain and spinal cord.

Intravenous—substances in solution that are directly delivered into a vein to be carried by the bloodstream to the rest of the body.

In vitro—study done in a test tube or artificial environment outside a living organism.

In vivo—study done in a living organism (cell, plant, animal, or person).

Kaufmann diet—a diet that restricts grains, alcohol, peanuts, mushrooms, yeast/fungi, and focuses on protein sources (animal and plant) and vegetables. The premise is that simple carbohydrates and sugar fuel the growth of pathogenic fungi that causes and promotes cancer.

Ketogenic diet—a diet that focuses on foods very low in carbohydrates, uses moderate but regular high-fiber vegetables, is rich in natural fats, and uses low to moderate protein. This results in the production of ketones, which tumor cells are unable to use for energy production and are toxic to cancer cells.

l-theanine—an amino acid found in green tea and a nutrient best known for inducing calming, tranquilizing effects while simultaneously improving alertness.

Lab tests—blood and urine tests that can help identify substances that can be a sign of cancer. They are tools to help identify cancer but are not relied upon alone to diagnose cancer.

Magnetic resonance imaging (MRI)—a test using magnets to create a magnetic field and a computer link to create a 3-D diagnostic image of body tissues to give detailed pictures of areas in the body.

Mammography—A type of low-dose X-ray that looks for changes in breast tissue, including signs of breast cancer. 3-D mammography, also known as breast tomosynthesis, is a new type of mammogram that puts the images in a three-dimensional picture.

Mediterranean diet—a diet common to the Mediterranean that generally consists of fruits, vegetables, extra-virgin olive oil, fish, whole grains, legumes, moderate amounts of wine, and small amounts of red meat. It has been shown in large observational studies to be associated with lower cancer incidence.

Metastasis—the spread of cancer cells from the primary or initial site to other parts of the body.

Mitochondria—the organelle that produces energy (ATP) inside a cell.

MUGA scan—a multigated acquisition scan that uses a radioactive tracer and a special camera to take pictures of the heart as it pumps blood with each heartbeat. Required during some types of chemotherapy to make sure they are not causing heart damage.

Naturopathic medical doctor (NMD or ND)—licensed holistic doctor trained as a primary health-care provider. These doctors combine the best of conventional and holistic healing methods to prevent and treat disease. They are graduates of accredited naturopathic medical schools in the United States and Canada. Their training includes physical exams, laboratory testing, pharmaceutical prescriptions, minor surgery, and emergency medicine, as well as holistic therapies such as nutrition, intravenous nutrient therapy, botanical medicine, counseling, nutritional supplements, and other natural forms of healing.

NF-kB—also known as NF-kappaB. A protein complex that is involved in several cellular processes, including inflammation, immunity, cell growth and differentiation, tumor formation, and apoptosis. Pharmaceutical and natural agents are used to disrupt the inflammatory and tumor growth effects of NF-kB.

Nrf2—a protein found in cells that, when activated by a substance known as Nrf2 activator, results in the production of antioxidant enzymes and genes that prevent cellular damage. This also includes protection of cancer cells.

ONCOblot test—reveals the tissue of origin of the ENOX2 protein. The ENOX2 gene encodes a particular protein involved in abnormal cell function. The cancer-associated ENOX2 (tNOX) is found on the cell surface of human cancers. Can be used to detect cancer at very early stages.

Oncogene—a gene that, when activated, stimulates cancer growth.

Oncology—the branch of medicine that deals with cancer. A physician who specializes in cancer is known as an oncologist.

Organic foods—foods grown without pesticides, synthetic fertilizers, genetically modified organisms (GMOs), ionizing radiation, bioengineering, and sewage sludge. It also refers to animal products (dairy, meat, eggs, etc.) where the producing animal has not been given antibiotics or growth hormones.

Oxidative therapies—therapies that provide the body with extra oxygen to prevent and treat disease. Examples in integrative oncology include high-dose intravenous vitamin C, hyperbaric oxygen, and ozone therapy.

Ozone—the medical use of ozone (three oxygen atoms) as an oxidative therapy. Often used medically by infusing blood withdrawn into a sterile IV bag and then infused with medical grade ozone. The oxygen-rich blood solution is then administered back into the body.

Pap test—also known as a Pap smear, a swab of cells from a woman's cervix. Tests for precancerous and cancerous changes of the cervix.

Passionflower—a traditional medicinal herb used for its calming and relaxing properties.

Positron-emission tomography (PET)—the injection of a radioactive tracer that is picked up more by organs and tissues that have cancer and then viewed on a computer image. Allows a doctor to see if cancer is present and if it has spread, and to monitor how a tumor is responding to chemotherapy. Often combined with a CT scan.

Prebiotics—substances that feed the good bacteria in the gut.

Probiotics—good bacteria.

Prognosis—the likely outcome or course of a disease; the chance of recovery or recurrence.

Proliferation—an increase in the number of cells due to cell growth and division.

Radiation therapy—a method of treating cancer by administering energy in the form of photons (X-rays and gamma rays) or particles (neutrons, protons, and electrons).

Radiation toxicity—side effects when healthier cells are damaged during radiation treatments. More common acute side effects are nausea and fatigue; chronic side effects may include irreversible problems such as organ damage and even cancer itself.

Randomized, placebo-controlled study—a type of study where people are randomly selected to receive a clinical intervention or placebo without knowing what they are receiving. Considered the gold standard in research, although not all therapies can be studied this way.

Reactive oxygen species (ROS)—an unstable molecule that contains oxygen that can cause cell damage to DNA, RNA, and proteins, as well as cause cell death. ROS are free radicals. Some conventional (e.g., certain types of chemotherapy) and integrative oncology therapies (e.g., artesunate) generate ROS to kill cancer cells.

Remission—a physical state when the signs and symptoms of cancer are reduced. Remission can be partial or complete. In a complete remission, all signs and symptoms of cancer have disappeared.

RNA—ribonucleic acid, a complex molecular structure. Carries genetic information from DNA to make proteins.

Sigmoidoscopy—the use of a thin, flexible tube with a light and camera that is inserted into the rectum and used to visualize the lower portion of a patient's sigmoid colon and rectum.

Stool test—stool samples that measure DNA biomarkers can indicate whether there is a low or high likelihood that colorectal cancer or precancer is present.

Survivorship—the transformation of cancer from a fatal disease to one in which a majority of those diagnosed receive treatments that result in long-term disease-free survivorship.

TK-1 testing—often used to monitor cancer progress during active treatment. Thymidine kinase (TK) plays a key role in tissue metabolism in acute or pathological tissue stress. Patients with intermediate and high levels of TK activity in their tumors frequently show a rapid disease progression and generally worse outcomes.

TNF-alpha—also known as tumor necrosis factor-alpha, a primary regulator of inflammation. It is produced by white blood cells in response to infection and other sources of inflammation. Dysregulation or imbalance of TNF-alpha is implicated in the promotion and progression of cancer.

Transforming growth factor-beta (TGF-beta)—a tissue factor that can be followed to monitor inflammatory and tumor specific progress or treatment.

Tumor genomics—genetic typing tests for tumor characteristics specific to certain tumor types and used to guide therapies.

Tumor markers—substances measured in blood, urine, or body tissues that are used to monitor how a cancer treatment is working or, at higher levels, may indicate cancer.

Tumor suppressor gene—a gene that slows cell division, repairs DNA, and tells cells when to die.

Ultrasound—an imaging test that uses high-frequency sound waves to create pictures of internal organs and tissues. Does not emit ionizing radiation like an X-ray.

Warburg Effect—named after German medical doctor, physiologist, and Nobel Laureate Otto Warburg. Refers to his discovery that cancer cells have a different metabolism than normal adult cells. Cancer cells are able to adapt and fuel themselves with high amounts of glucose for cell proliferation. Warburg felt that all cancers originated from dysfunctional cellular energy production. Some modern researchers agree in large part with Warburg's theory and recommend protocols that restrict glucose supply for tumor energy production.

8OHdG (8-Oxo-2'-deoxyguanosine)—one of the major products of DNA oxidation. Concentrations of 8OHdG within a cell are a measurement of oxidative stress, which is another nonspecific marker of disease regression or progression.

ABOUT THE AUTHORS

DR. MARK STENGLER is a naturopathic medical doctor who is in private practice in Encinitas, California. He is the best-selling author of more than 30 books, including *Prescription for Natural Cures* and *The Natural Physician's Healing Therapies*. Dr. Stengler is the author of "Health Revelations," one of America's most popular health newsletters. He has an expertise in combining the best of conventional and natural medicine for his patients and readers. You can visit him online at **www.markstengler.com**.

DR. PAUL ANDERSON is a naturopathic medical doctor who practices in Seattle, Washington, and Rosarito, Mexico. His practice focuses on patients with cancer and advanced chronic illness. He is a respected physician, educator, and professional writer who focuses his efforts on clinical and continuing medical education updates. He has been involved in integrative oncology practice for over 20 years, 8 of which have encompassed human clinical research. He lives in Seattle with his wife, Lori, and spends as much time as possible with his five adult children and five grandchildren. You can visit his clinic online at **www.advancedmedicaltherapies.com** or his professional site, **www.consultdranderson.com**.

Hay House Titles of Related Interest

YOU CAN HEAL YOUR LIFE, the movie,
starring Louise Hay & Friends
(available as an online streaming video)
www.hayhouse.com/louise-movie

THE SHIFT, the movie,
starring Dr. Wayne W. Dyer
(available as an online streaming video)
www.hayhouse.com/the-shift-movie

———

THE TRUTH ABOUT CANCER:
What You Need to Know about Cancer's History, Treatment, and Prevention,
by Ty M. Bollinger

FAT FOR FUEL:
A Revolutionary Diet to Combat Cancer, Boost Brain Power, and Increase Your Energy,
by Dr. Joseph Mercola

CULTURED FOOD IN A JAR:
100+ Probiotic Recipes to Inspire and Change Your Life,
by Donna Schwenk

All of the above are available at your local bookstore,
or may be ordered by contacting Hay House (see next page).

———

We hope you enjoyed this Hay House book. If you'd like to receive our online catalog featuring additional information on Hay House books and products, or if you'd like to find out more about the Hay Foundation, please contact:

Hay House LLC, P.O. Box 5100, Carlsbad, CA 92018-5100
(760) 431-7695 or (800) 654-5126
www.hayhouse.com® • www.hayfoundation.org

_____

Published in Australia by:
Hay House Australia Publishing Pty Ltd
18/36 Ralph St., Alexandria NSW 2015
Phone: +61 (02) 9669 4299
www.hayhouse.com.au

Published in the United Kingdom by:
Hay House UK Ltd
1st Floor, Crawford Corner,
91–93 Baker Street, London W1U 6QQ
Phone: +44 (0)20 3927 7290
www.hayhouse.co.uk

Published in India by:
Hay House Publishers (India) Pvt Ltd
Muskaan Complex, Plot No. 3,
B-2, Vasant Kunj, New Delhi 110 070
Phone: +91 11 41761620
www.hayhouse.co.in

_____

Let Your Soul Grow

Experience life-changing transformation—one video
at a time—with guidance from the world's leading experts.

www.healyourlifeplus.com

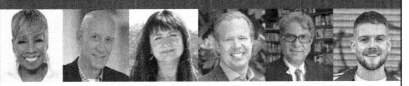